Weight Wisdom
A lighter way of thinking

Alan Jackson MSc

Weight Wisdom

First published in Great Britain in July 2023

© Alan Jackson

A catalogue record for this book is available from the British Library.

Print ISBN: 978-1-3999-6247-6

Cover image © Conckerdesign.co.uk

This book is dedicated to everyone
that has struggled with their weight,
yet, despite the unfavourable odds and
seemingly insurmountable hurdles,
they just kept on trying.

Acknowledgements

Thanks go to my long-suffering wife, who has endured this project for five long years and yet somehow, throughout, has managed to provide me with unwavering help and support; mostly accompanied with a smile.

Thanks go to my good friend Greg Hackett, who early on spotted the error of my ways and put me on the right path, guiding the project from a collection of incoherent ramblings into something that just might have some value to someone.

Gratitude goes to my amazing book reviewers, who, with their individual expertise and experience, brought enormous value to the book. Through diligent critique and robust feedback, their contributions have enhanced and clarified every chapter of the book. My thanks go to: Madelyn-Rose Hill, Kathryn Hill, Helena Jackson, Armen Lloyd, Stella Tomkins, Judith Turner-Smith, Mary Blunden, Alison Mantey, Andy Black, Lisa Ward and Jane Deacon.

Thanks also to three experts in the field of food compulsions and eating addictions, for their invaluable contributions and guidance on the section relating to food addictions. They are: Ellen Calteau, Registered Dieititan, Heidi Giaever, Nutrition Consultant, and Dr Jen Unwin, D.Psy, FBPs, C.Psychol. Chartered Clinical & Health Psychologist and Scientific Advisor to the Public Health Collaboration.

Thanks to the brilliant mathematician Sophie Jackson for help on statistics and hard sums.

Finally, thanks to my exceptional editor Michael Benge, for all his diligent work and guidance.

About this book

It is frequently the misfortune of people seeking solutions to their weight problems to find themselves under the influence of self-appointed experts. This is an unsatisfactory arrangement at best, which is why this book won't tell you what to eat or when to exercise, or how to behave in any way for that matter – as any behavioural therapist will confirm, telling people what to do diminishes the prospect of change. *Weight Wisdom* is a journey to discover the truth about yourself, by yourself, and I believe that anyone searching for a lasting resolution to their weight dissatisfaction will find their holy grail somewhere in its chapters.

During the twenty-five years I've been immersed in weight management, I've encountered many subject experts, read countless books, articles and scientific journals and authored dozens of teaching and reference manuals. I have taught and lectured for training organisations and universities across the UK, and presented at seminars both at home and overseas, supporting thousands of people to gain nutrition and weight-related qualifications and professional development. With an MSc in Weight Management, I've appeared on TV and radio and founded one of the UK's leading weight-loss organisations that has helped over 20,000 people to lose weight. I am a fellow of the UK Chartered Institute for Sport and Physical Activity (CIMSPA), having been a member for forty years.

While these experiences have allowed me a glimpse at the problem, their true value was to provide me with the opportunity and great privilege of serving people as a weight-management practitioner. These 'people moments', spanning the whole of the weight spectrum, offered me true insight, and forged my understanding of this most common of modern human conditions.

Over the years, I have seen the same constraints and barriers preventing people from overcoming their weight difficulties time after time. For most people, permanent weight loss will be their greatest life challenge, even if they have scaled the north face of the Eiger. Of course, attempting the Eiger without adequate physical and mental preparation and a good guide would be foolhardy. This book provides both the guide and the waypoints to succeed, written with the understanding that we all have unique reference points from which to start. I have learned that, with guidance and support, no matter how serious the condition, people can and do find their path to long-term weight loss.

Broadly, I have encountered two types of 'help seekers' in the world of health and wellbeing: let's call them Frank and Barbara. The doctor says: "I'm sorry to say that you appear to have contracted unusualitis; simply apply this cream three times a day". Frank, oblivious of the disorder, blithely applies the cream and hopes for the best. Barbara, however, reads everything she can on unusualitis and, armed with this knowledge, tries to figure out the best course of action for a lasting resolution (which may, of course, involve applying the cream three times a day). If you identify with Frank, and just want to be told what to do, then this book is not for you; my advice (which I seldom give) is to put it back on the shelf now.

No two people I have ever met have the same reasons for being overweight. The complex backstories that lead people into their current weight dilemmas are as unique as our DNA, and so too are the solutions. Finding that critical path is a feat that can only be accomplished by the pilot of the avatar in question – you. The one-size-fits-all approach to weight loss is now thoroughly discredited, because, if it worked, the World Obesity Federation report released in 2023 would not be predicting that more than half the world's population will become overweight or obese within the next twelve years[1]. There is only one solution, and that is to become a subject expert and a specialist in managing your own weight.

Typically, when weight becomes problematic, people are too reactive and give insufficient time or thought to developing and implementing appropriate strategies. They choose instead to lurch towards the most readily available solution, or the latest celebrity-endorsed fad, or the remedy that appears to offer the path of least resistance. But weight management is a journey of learning and development, relevant only to our individual circumstances, and each of us must carefully consider the facts in the context of our own experience and understanding of how our weight has evolved. *Weight Wisdom* will teach you how to overcome the 'yearning enigma' – that is, desperately wanting something, knowing what to do, but not being able to do it.

This book is suitable for the dieting beginner or the seasoned professional, for the social overeater or the entrenched food addict. This is because

Weight Wisdom will teach you how to think and not how to eat. *Weight Wisdom* will particularly speak to people that are worn out with dieting and are seeking a life-changing weight transformation. If you are looking for easy answers, look elsewhere, but I truly believe that somewhere in these pages are the keys that will unlock the health and weight goals for many of you. What follows is a journey of learning, reflection, self-empowerment and, ultimately, self-determination, offering life-changing outcomes. This is a search for the truth.

If you are still reading, you have probably taken the first steps of your journey on the path to weight wisdom. Now, all that you need is a notebook, a pen, and a quiet place.

Contents

Preamble

The grand dilemma confronting weight-management practitioners is a tricky one. The obesity pandemic is ultimately a result of external obesogenic[*] forces bearing down on a susceptible population, and gaining weight year after year, or struggling to lose it, is a normal response, by normal people, to an abnormal environment. At the same time, the practitioner must enable their client to realise that, ultimately, it is they who are in control of their nutritional destiny. I hope that together we can strike that balance, and I apologise in advance for when I fall short through my assumptions and assertions.

While most people don't want their food to become a religion, I don't suppose they want it to be just a functional, tradable commodity either. Sadly, however, that is what much of it has now become: mass-produced, ultra-processed cargoes, barely resembling food and with little connection to the land from which it came. We have severed the ancient and spiritual connections between the earth, our food and our bodies, in favour of wrapping ourselves in multiple sterile layers of refined calories, each representing another barrier between us and the great giver of life.

Over thirty years ago, travelling India on the 3rd class rail network, holed up in a six-birth sleeper with an unknown family of meagre resources, I learned something important about food. Due to a logistics oversight, my companion and I found ourselves without food on a thirty-six-hour train journey. Early in the evening, our unacquainted family set about unfurling their food canteen. They didn't speak English, and our Hindi was decidedly ropey, but without hesitation, once the food was set, they gestured for us to join them to eat. Embarrassed but hungry, we made token signals to indicate that we were fine, but they dismissed our feeble ruse and insisted that we join them. They shared all their food with us evenly as if we were part of their family. This meant that they all had less. We had nothing to contribute, and they absolutely would not accept payment. Those beautiful people shared more than just calories that day, they shared a lesson about the gift of food. It is a precious gift, it is life, and we must always cherish it. Take care of our food, and it will take care of us. Look after the people that look after our food, and they will reciprocate.

---

[*] Causing, or increasing the likelihood of, obesity in a person or animal – Dictionary.com

According to the World Health Organization (WHO), in 2016 there were around two billion overweight adults in the world, representing 40% of the global population. Of these, 650 million were classified as living with obesity. These figures have tripled over forty years, and now most of the world's population live in countries where overweight and obesity kills more people than food shortages or malnutrition. A scientific study published in 2008 predicted that, by 2048, all Americans would be overweight or living with obesity[2].

In the US, in 2017 almost three-quarters of adults were overweight, with 43% of these living with obesity[3]. In the UK today, collectively around two-thirds of adults are overweight or living with obesity, with more men than women crossing the BMI threshold of ≥25kg/m2 (about 69% vs 54% respectively). Interestingly, younger men are far less likely to be overweight than younger women, but older men are far more likely to be overweight than women of a similar age. Of the fifty-three countries in the WHO Europe region, the UK ranks fourth, behind only Turkey, Malta and Israel as the most overweight[4].

Over the years, I have witnessed the ever-changing villain of nutrition. First, it was fats that were considered bad for us, and specifically saturated fats. Then it was carbohydrates, and specifically sugars, and now it appears it is proteins, specifically animal proteins. While I am being a little flippant here, my point is far from mocking the collective wisdom of the day, but more to point out that the science of human nutrition is still evolving, and the pursuit of a blueprint for optimum human nutrition is far from concluded.

When we look back in 100 years, I think we will find that each of these iterations in the search for the ultimate diet for human health was correct in the context of what was known at the time. Personally, I still believe that eating processed fats and sugars is a risky habit, and I'm currently considering the prospect of animal proteins as being deleterious to human health, too, but I have yet to reach a position on this as I don't believe there is sufficient compelling evidence to support such a radical idea. But that isn't to say that this won't change in time.

At this point, I presume that you are reading this book because you are struggling with your weight. I hope you will take comfort in the fact that it is not your lack of willpower or asserted gluttony or sloth that has gotten you to where you are now. The vast numbers of people affected – encompassing all ethnicities, socio-economic groups, geographical parameters and cultural, religious, or political persuasions – rule out a delinquent lifestyle as the root cause of the obesity pandemic.

Millennia ago, governments realised that cheap and plentiful food was the bedrock for a stable political landscape, and this is as true today as it has ever been. To threaten the supply of inexpensive food is to threaten the establishment. Subsequently, obesity is a consequence of ubiquitous, affordable, calorie-dense and convenient food, woven into the geo-genetic and social lottery of life. It is these factors that will largely determine your risk of becoming overweight or obese.

I frequently hear discussions about where the responsibility for the obesity pandemic lies; is it personal responsibility or does it sit with our governments? Do we need to be telling people to eat less and move more, or should we be tackling the obesogenic environment (OE)? The answer is that we should be doing both. It is important to support people to eat less (or, more precisely, eat more healthily) and to move more, and yet at the same time, all of society – including politicians, educators, policy makers, food producers and suppliers, and environmental designers – should be tackling the OE. It is not one or the other, it is both. To make the travelling public safer, sensible governments legislate for and ensure the increasing safety standards of both highways and vehicles. Why should we not also expect them to do the same for the food we eat?

With respect to the individual or the establishment, it helps me to think about the obesity pandemic on two levels. Firstly, I consider matters at a population level – my high street, my town, my city, and so on, each with its environmental, political, economic and commercial landscapes that create and perpetuate weight gain. These are the embedded structural systems and processes that work gradually and pervasively to dominate their populations, despite the best efforts of those communities living amid the onslaught, such as food supply chains and multinational corporate power structures. The resulting obesogenic pressures exerted on these unsuspecting populations are entrenched and intractable; they will be very difficult to change in a hurry. Testimony to this is the litany of well-meaning attempts by governments of all persuasions over thirty years to try to curb and reverse the ever-expanding waistlines of their electorate. Not one of them has scratched the bloated surface, and we are collectively still getting heavier.

Then, of course, I consider the second and more apposite matter (for you and me), which is weight at an individual level. The person who is with me in practice, the foot soldier, battling against a tsunami of weight-promoting products and practices that shape our lives and bodies. Each overweight person has their own story to tell, their narratives are totally unique. Similarly, each person's path to a healthier weight is as inimitable as their journey into overweight was in the first place.

When in practice, before I start a consultation, I take a moment to remind myself that this person has probably tried to lose weight 100 or 1,000 times before. In most cases, they will be experts in every diet known to mankind and will have tried all sorts of weird and wonderful eating and exercise regimes to control their weight. They will have had temporary success making them feel amazing; their aspirations and life plans could not have looked brighter. Ultimately, however, the diet ended, the weight returned (with interest) and all their efforts came to nought.

They suffered the humiliation and pain of having put their heart and soul into something only for it to fail. Why would they put themselves through that again and again? But wait! They're still here; they are sat with me right now. Despite the hurt and disappointment of the past, they are still trying; they still believe that one day they will achieve their goal. I am full of admiration for them; they exude strength, determination and fortitude. I'm reminded that these people are not quitters, they have grit, and I know that, if together we can find their path, then they will surely walk it.

My hope and beliefs are that this book will help you to find your path, but the path you are seeking is hidden, for now. To find it, you must search in a different place, and you must look from a new vantage point. Central to change is being able to see things in a different way. Because, when you can see things differently, you can start to think about them differently. Crucially, only when you can think differently can you start to behave differently. In a nutshell, we must see things differently to think differently so that we can act differently.

You may be new to weight management, but the chances are you're probably not. You may well be thinking how or why will it be different this time? I suggest that this time it will be different because, en route, you will change your outlook on key aspects of your life and the world around you. You will recognise both the internal and external disrupters of weight and the balance needed for health and happiness. You will learn how to overcome engrained unhelpful behaviours, habits and thoughts that have thwarted you in the past, and you will adopt these new ways of thinking to ensure a future that is free of weight turmoil. You will learn things about yourself that you never imagined. This is the journey of *Weight Wisdom*.

A typical weight-loss journey

As I'm sure you are aware, most people can lose weight. The problem is that weight lost normally returns, and this is very demoralising for the dieter. Most diets start with a wave of optimism and determination – this time it will be different! Primary and secondary goals drive the changes needed for weight loss and these commonly include a desire to improve appearance, self-confidence, be more active and improve overall health. Meal plans and exercise projects are scheduled, and a general air of excitement and positivity gets things off to a good start. With early weight loss comes optimism, enhanced confidence, and a brighter outlook; all is well with the world.

However, weight loss takes considerable time and effort, resolve, strength, abstinence, and several other virtues in generous helpings if it is to be guaranteed. Typically, diets run into one of two problems during or at the end of the diet. As events progress, life gets in the way of our best intentions and, sooner or later, weight loss diminishes, the target weight becomes a distant hope, and any faith of remaining in control evaporates. At this point, there is a realisation that neither the weight-loss goals nor the dreams of becoming a slimmer person will be realised. Lapses become more frequent and turn into relapse, which finally succumbs to total collapse[†]. Weight gain at this point is inevitable. The other primary drawback with diets is that, if the dieter successfully reaches their target weight, motivation to maintain the 'temporary' changes required by the diet wanes and it isn't long until a full-scale return to previous eating habits and sedentary living occurs, followed by a return of the weight.

This is a crushing time for anyone. For the dieter, there can be no other conclusion than that their frequent attempts to control their weight are not worth the considerable effort required (let alone the brutal effect it has on their mental health) and, as a result, they abandon any plans for future weight loss.

[†]   A **lapse** (or 'slip') is a brief return to old habits after a person has made a commitment to change. A **relapse** is a longer but still temporary (medium term) return to old behaviours and a **collapse** is a full-scale return to previous lifestyle and the causal behaviours, with no apparent intention to change.

Many diets set out a weight-loss phase followed by a 'mythical' maintenance phase. To me, this is rather like asking someone to take a perilous walk across a treacherous, icy, high-altitude ravine. Once safely across to the other side, the instructor says, "Oh, you can't stand here on terra firma, you need to get back out there in the middle and stay there!" There is no maintenance phase, there is either the lifestyle you are living now, or the lifestyle that you intend to live. Both are on firm ground.

It appears, though, that most people blame other individuals or themselves for weight gain. In an article published in the international journal *Appetite* in 2013 entitled 'Who is to blame for the rise in obesity?'[5], the authors asked 800 US citizens who they thought were most contributing to the rise in obesity (assuming it was a representative sample, 70% of them would have been overweight). Respondents were asked to pick from: food manufacturers, grocery stores, restaurants, government policies, farmers, individuals, and parents. Eighty percent said individuals themselves were primarily to blame, with parents the next-most culpable group, blamed by over half of respondents.

A further problem is that many people reading this will have had their weight 'medicalised' by a lifetime of traversing the healthcare system, consulting doctors, nurses, dieticians, pharmacists and endocrinologists. Following these interactions, it may be difficult to consider your weight in the context of the social, environmental and behavioural factors that may well provide the answers. Keeping an open mind is essential for getting the best out of this book.

This book is structured in a way that enables you to take the lead in finding the path that is right for you (as would happen in normal face-to-face behaviour-change practice). You may be nineteen years old, or seventy-nine years young, either way you must work through the Five Insights in a way that is relevant to you, as they are the foundations upon which your rehabilitation will be constructed. And may I brazenly suggest that this involves much more than a few brief notes in your book. How carefully you think about the questions raised by the Five Insights, and the integrity and depth of your answers, will greatly influence your future voyage.

Weight-loss myths

At this point, it's worth revisiting and examining any advice you may have previously been given, or perhaps any that you are still getting. Be sure it is evidenced, or, at the very least, that it makes good sense to you. By way of example, I recall lots of 'experts' telling people not to weigh themselves more than once each week (I think, over concerns that people might spiral into obsessive compulsive weight neurosis), but I always found this notion odd, and I avoid advocating any weighing regime, simply leaving it to the preference of the individual. Recently, research has shown that more frequent weight monitoring assists weight loss, leading to greater adoption of weight-control behaviours. Apparently, people don't drive themselves crackers doing it either![6]

A further myth is that losing weight gradually is better than losing it rapidly. For years, weight-loss professionals (including myself) have followed the prevailing recommendations and advised gradual over rapid reductions, because we wrongly, it appears, accepted the hypothesis that the longer the duration that people spend losing weight, the more likely it is that their new lifestyle will 'stick'. To test this, Australian researchers randomised 204 overweight people to either a twelve-week rapid weight-loss programme on a very low-calorie diet (450-800 kcal/day) or a thirty-six-week gradual weight-loss programme, reducing intake by about 500 kcal/day (which was for years the standard advice). They found that, while the overall calorie deficit for both groups was the same (over twelve weeks or thirty-six), 80% of the quick losers achieved the target weight loss of 12.5% compared to only half of the slow losers. After three years, there was no noticeable difference between the group's weight regain[7]. Therefore, contrary to Aesop's fable, in a straight race, the quicker beast wins. Importantly, I must mention that I am not advocating very low-calorie diets and don't recommend them for weight loss.

Despite how many times you have heard it, "Don't skip breakfast, it's the most important meal of the day, particularly if you are watching your weight", Wicherski et al looked at all the available evidence to date and promptly poured water on that particular firework when they showed that skipping breakfast does not correlate with being heavier[8]. While this will not be the best breakfast bulletin Kellogg's have ever had, it will be music to the ears of people that practise time-restricted eating to support their weight loss (more on this later).

9

You've also got to keep an eye out for the flaky science. Having read thousands of scientific journal articles, I'm frequently surprised by published articles that have somehow escaped the scrutiny of peer review (sometimes, in journals that should know better). One example was a 2020 study published in the 'Bulletin of the Association of Medicine of Puerto Rico' looking into sociodemographic factors affecting weight loss in adolescents. The researchers determined that female adolescents were more likely to lose weight if they felt unhappy about their appearance whereas males were less likely to lose weight if they were unhappy with their appearance[9]. Could you take that to the bank? I don't think so. You can't always rely on what you read in a scientific journal. Make your own mind up, scrutinise all information from 'the experts', including anything you read in this book. If it makes sense and it seems to work, that's not a bad starting point. If not, be very wary.

In writing this book, I have tried to balance the things I have learned in practice against the more nebulous machinations of the evidence base. My aim in melding these two uneasy bedfellows is not only to seek the truth, but to make sense of it all. Each section represents an important contribution towards the objective of solving for the reader the great enigma that is unwanted weight. The book strives to bring enlightenment and empowerment, with the aim that you become a self-weight-management expert. I believe that this is the only sure way to discover your path to success.

I have always believed that what accompanies learning and development is great power, in this case the power to change your life. You will learn about the biology of weight gain from before the moment of conception, and the forces that act upon our weight as we grow and develop. You will come to understand the intricate interplay of appetite control and energy management, and how hormones work to support or undermine our hopes. *Weight Wisdom* offers every relevant fact, scenario, situation and opportunity that I have encountered in twenty-five years of weight-management practice and study. Each contribution is integral in building the cache of tools and knowledge that will lay the foundations for your successful journey.

The early part of the book provides information to build your essential knowledge base and adopts a heuristic and enquiring approach. Therefore, don't look for solutions at the end of each section and do not expect me to give you the answers as we go along. Remain patient, take notes, and carefully consider the relevance of each issue in the context of your own situation. Take sufficient time to reflect on the aspects that have the most relevance and resonate with you and your life. Think about them over days or weeks, if necessary. Share your thoughts with family and friends, and discuss ideas or hurdles, listening to and considering the views of those that you trust the most. This is fundamental in transforming information into knowledge and knowledge into wisdom.

The latter stages of the book will focus on changing the way you think. But this will only be successful if you are in receipt of and have processed all the relevant information to enable your brain to make valid judgements. If your hard drive is not in command of all the facts, how can you expect the CPU to make accurate decisions and calculations.

A sense of balance

I often read that, when setting out on a weight-reduction journey, people should avoid unrealistic goals. My question is this: what is an unrealistic weight-loss goal? For example, for someone weighing fifty stone and electing for gastric bypass surgery, losing half of their body weight – while challenging for certain – would seem like a sensible target. Losing 10% would appear largely pointless considering the risks involved. On the other hand, someone with a BMI of 28 might consider that they would be happier if they were half a stone lighter, and some would say that this is a more realistic target. This target, however, could in fact be as unrealistic as the first example, because even if achieved, people rarely make their weight loss permanent, so it should be assumed that the weight will return. In this case, then, either all weight-loss goals are unrealistic, or none are. I prefer to think that none are.

Saying I want to lose a stone in weight is all well and good; it states what you would like to achieve, which isn't bad as a starting point. An accompanying question might well be: how do I lose a stone in weight? There are lots of different approaches and some are likely to work better for you than they do for me, and therefore perhaps some trial and error may be required. However, the most appropriate question would be: how do I become motivated to make the changes needed to lose a stone in weight? This is because, if we are sufficiently motivated, we will always find the right way to achieve what we set out to do, and the key to long-term weight loss is finding the right approach for you.

Another important consideration is to stay realistic. If you think that losing weight will not involve restrictions on your life, you have been reading too many fad diet books. Life is balance, which involves placing restrictions on the excesses that are damaging us. It is important to accept that there will be disadvantages and sacrifices associated with losing weight, with the most obvious being that you will not be able to eat some of the foods you are used to eating. Ironically, if your journey goes to plan, in the future you will consider these to be advantages.

Overweight people know all about populist weight-loss strategies and, with respect to dieting and slimming, many could probably write a book. But, of course, diets don't work, and I'm guessing readers of *Weight Wisdom* have long figured that out. I know that people I have worked with are aware of the daily behaviours and choices they make that foil their weight-management efforts. Each could describe an effective lifestyle plan that would permanently resolve their weight, if only they had the power to adopt it and maintain it. And this is why knowing what to do only loosely correlates with behaviour change. *Weight Wisdom* has two primary purposes: the first is to convince you that change is the only path to long-term weight management, and the second is to show you how to convert your (currently concealed) lifestyle plan into reality and realise the weight loss that you desire and deserve.

While it is entirely a matter for individual preference, I don't necessarily think that setting out with a weight-loss target in mind is the most effective way to go about things. I would suggest that the best targets to set yourself would be behavioural, nutritional and psychological. When you can make these targets stick, then your weight-loss 'target' will sort itself out, and you'll find the balance point that is right for you in terms of weight and lifestyle. The first important rule is to focus on change goals, not weight-loss goals.

I believe that the great thinkers and philosophers of the world mostly reached the same conclusions when it came to the big question: what is the meaning of life? They broadly settled on happiness and contentment being at its core. I would suggest that balance is at the heart of this. Balance is paramount: without it, we are lost, all of us, and the Earth, and the universe. If you are overweight or in debt, or unhappy, or discontent or unwell, or don't feel loved or valued, or whatever, I would suggest that, somewhere along the line, the balance in your life has been disrupted. The only possible remedy is the restoration of equilibrium. Throughout this book, I hope to convince you that it is not weight loss or thinness or 'the body beautiful' that will bring about health and happiness, but balance (which may include one or all of the above). I believe that the purpose of this book is to help you find balance, which in turn will move you closer to lasting happiness and contentment, and a beautiful and respectful relationship with your faithful avatar.

The lifestyle continuum

I'd like you to consider your lifestyle on a one to ten Likert scale, where one is the dregs, characterised by Wayne and Waynetta, the fictional slobs from the hysterical 'Harry Enfield and Chums' show. With respect to health and balance, Wayne and Waynetta's lives are an absolute train wreck. Ten on the scale represents the 'Health Saints', the most health-conscious souls of both mind and body that you could conjure up. These saints maintain a strict palaeolithic diet of organic fruit and vegetables, a few nuts and seeds, and drink only pure, fresh mountain water. They've eradicated stress from their lives and walk daily in the tranquillity of ancient woodlands culminating in the calmness and silence of an hour of solitary Zen Yoga.

Then there's the rest of us, somewhere in between the slobs and the saints. As the months and years go by, we vacillate between these normal operating parameters on our own lifestyle continuum. Where we are at any one time depends upon how we have reacted to all the external forces that are pressing down upon our lives at that time. This is normal. Most of the time we are striving to escape Wayne and Waynetta, but, perhaps at the same time, not wanting to get too close to the saints either. When our lives are in control and events around us are stable, we naturally gravitate in an upwards direction on the continuum. All is well, we are happy, we are healthy, we are eating well, and we are moving freely.

Then a significant something comes along to disrupt our plans (life has a habit of interfering with our best-laid plans – Covid-19, for instance). Illness in yourself or your family, the rigours and demands of work, economic hardship or just the plain old stresses and strains of life. Disruption occurs, commotion ensues, and our positive behaviours and choices falter, convenience and comfort become the order of the day and we slide back down the continuum, closer to Wayne and Waynetta.

Fortunately, it is innate in humans to try to do the best that we can. Following adversity, when things settle down and normality returns, we pick ourselves up, dust ourselves down and start again. Typically, we re-engage with our healthful activities and gradually we escape the sphere of influence exerted by the slobs. As our lifestyles improve, we feel happier and more in control, our mind and body are contented; we sense the balance returning to our lives. That is, until the next inevitable disruption. This is the reality of the lifestyle continuum, upon which we are all long-haul passengers.

Once you recognise the lifestyle continuum as reality, it relieves the stress and guilt associated with 'falling off the wagon' and diminishes the imperative of always doing the right thing. This understanding enables you to think one day at a time, and you can relax in the knowledge that you can simply try to do better today than you did yesterday. If that doesn't work, you can try again the next day. What's more, if you buy into the concept of the continuum, then you have a plan that anticipates and expects lapses and provides a realistic framework to turn things around when things go awry. In time, if you embrace the continuum, I believe that you will observe an ascending ratcheting effect, where the backward slides aren't so precipitous, and the recoveries are swifter and more sustained. The key is not necessarily to question where you currently are on the continuum, but what is your direction of travel, and what are your intentions?

Don't lose the path. As on any journey, you will from time to time stray, but don't dwell upon these transgressions, the key is that you search until you find the path once again. It may be that you join the path further back than where you were previously, but that is OK – the point is that you are back on the path once again. This is the imperative.

In a moment, you are going to close your eyes and think of a period in your life when you were in a good place and feeling great about yourself and all that was around you. Don't make the mistake of confusing the intoxicating vibrancy and resilience of youth with the harmony and contentedness of a balanced, mature life that is available to us at any age. Don't open your eyes until this vision is clear and you can recollect when and where it was.

During this time, you are most likely happy with your behaviours and choices, you appreciate moving freely and are energetic and active. Time pressures seem manageable and stress, for now, is kept at arm's length. You recognise your good fortune and enjoy your rewarding life. It might be that you are eating foods that you enjoy, and you don't feel like you are denying yourself the things that are important to you. You feel fulfilled and might think of these times as carefree. You are probably at your happiest and most likely your healthiest as the two are inextricably linked. The result is high self-esteem, mental wellbeing, and a positive body image. Consider where this point would be on the lifestyle continuum, what number would you place on it? I suggest that this is most likely to be a good indicator of your preferred balance point. In fact, it is your actual balance point! Write down in your notebook: MY BALANCE POINT IN LIFE IS ...

Now it's time to determine where you currently are on the lifestyle continuum; what is the reality of your situation right now? To do this, you will need some reference points regarding all the measures of 'lifestyle', such as diet, sleep, stress, physical activity, social interactions and other interests, use of stimulants (caffeine, nicotine, alcohol or drugs) and anything else that is relevant that you can think of. Determining a perceived lifestyle value will probably also involve considering behaviours and choices that you think you ought to be making, but aren't. In your notebook, write down a number from one to ten and then make some notes on why you have reached this figure. Write down in your notebook: MY CURRENT LIFESTYLE POINT IS ....

It's not fair!

I've heard it many times from my clients: "It feels so unfair that some people can eat what they want, but I can't have a biscuit when everyone else can". Well, here's news for you: life's not fair! I have a friend whose fourteen-year-old son has a very severe nut allergy, and he can never have biscuits or chocolates, or sweets or ice cream, or pastries or cakes or puddings or breakfast cereals or grain breads or takeaways or eat at regular restaurants, and he must always check every food label as if his life depended upon it – because it does. Sometimes, life isn't fair, so you need to decide how fair your situation is. Thinking that it is unfair that you can't have 'junk food' because instead you choose health and happiness over diabetes and emotional turmoil is dysfunctional thinking.

You may also be surprised to learn that most healthy-weight people don't just eat what they want when they want, despite what they may tell you or what you might think. Healthy-weight people realise that they must adhere to certain eating parameters if they are to stay lean and healthy, and while they don't necessarily have the same struggles as someone that is overweight, they still need to be vigilant because life makes you fat. Furthermore, you might not have considered that, for people that don't have weight problems, exercise is also hard and tiring and time-consuming, and often needs a good dollop of motivation to get it done.

I often wonder if the difference between people with or without weight problems is simply that healthy-weight people have learned (most probably from their parents) to train their brains to be more harmonious in terms of their cognitions and their wants. If your thoughts and beliefs (which control your behaviour) are at odds with your wants, you will never have what you desire. Achieving our goals is simply a matter of learning how to think in a way that connects our wants with our actions. *Weight Wisdom* will teach you how to do this, but, for now, just try to think about how your thoughts and beliefs influence your actions.

Another thing to think about for now, is whether you have allowed yourself to fall into the trap of developmental procrastination. When it comes to the things that we want to do, people say: "I'm looking forward to doing all these things when I have lost some weight. I can't join the dance group now, I'm too heavy, I'll do it when I've lost a bit of weight. I'll get my bicycle out of the shed when I'm two stones lighter. I'll join the chess club when I feel a bit better about myself." But it doesn't work like that. Doing these things now will help with your weight because they make us feel stronger and more positive about ourselves. These things give us tangible reasons to keep working at the changes in our lives that make things more meaningful and rewarding. They bring friendship and camaraderie and the social support that is required if we are to make positive changes in our lives. Taking the steps that enable you to do the things that you want to do in life brings self-credibility.

Self-credibility

You know that you are not happy with how things are, and you desperately want to change – you have ideas about change, and you are just waiting for the right moment to make your move. You need some space and time in your life to overcome a few obstacles before you can start – now is not the right time and there are lots of good reasons for this. Also, the status quo of the moment is serving its purpose – it's familiar, comforting and reassuring, and nothing seems that immediately threatening. What's more, you are worried that if you try to change, and you are not ready or prepared, then you may fail, and you're afraid of what this would mean, which makes it difficult to take the first step. If this sounds familiar, you are not alone. I feel like this regularly.

But by seeking help, or pursuing self-help, or buying this book, you have taken the first step. You have accepted that there is irregularity or disturbance in your life, and you must believe that there is a realistic prospect of a satisfactory outcome or you would not have taken the first step, which you have. Jointly, your actions, supported by your beliefs, confirm your readiness to embark upon this journey. Remind yourself daily that, simply by the power of your thought, you have reached the conclusions that have enabled you to act and engage in self-help, this is the first logical act of therapy. By taking this step, you are already moving away from the irrational beliefs that have held you back in the past, and you are now travelling in the direction of a more positive, productive and rational life. You are now gravitating along the 'lifestyle continuum', and this gives you self-credibility.

Credo is the root of the word credibility, and means 'I believe' in Latin. For years, I worked in general management and the theme of professional credibility was a constant bubbling undercurrent. When competing ideas or strategies clash and corporate tension escalates, so too does the notion of professional credibility. What usually follows is a palpable 'credibility display' by each party, determined to press home their own professional credentials in a bid to win support for their proposals. As petty as it seems, credibility displays are central to commerce, because being able to believe in someone is ultimately what drives business. Having left that surreal world, I've thought a lot more about the concept of credibility and how it applies to the self.

The issues of credibility and relatability are also important considerations for people attending support groups. A crucial element that creates the all-important group chemistry lies in the bond between the facilitator and the group members. This is why ex-users make the best drug rehab leads, and why weight-management practitioners with higher BMIs tend to get better results from their clients[10]. I learned early on that most overweight people were not going to take dietary advice from a lanky stick insect like me, which is one of the reasons I stopped giving it! (I think this is also one of the main reasons that I still suffer terribly from imposter syndrome). My friend who is a dietitian of many years also told me that patients don't like dietitians if they are too fat or too thin – as she says, "You just can't win!"

Developing self-credibility is probably the most important foundation for your growth and development. It is the framework upon which you will build all the skills and techniques required to achieve your weight-loss goals. The more that you think about it, the more likely it is that you will reach the unavoidable conclusion that, without self-credibility, you can't believe in or trust yourself, in which case, you really are in a spot of bother. Take a couple of moments to think about this.

We all regularly deceive others to benefit our own cause ("Sorry I can't make Friday; I'm taking my gran to the cinema"). But why would we deceive ourselves? The general theory is that self-deception evolved to make it easier and more convincing to deceive others – if you first deceive yourself, you don't have to lie to anyone else. Self-deceit is a common feature of human nature but we don't do it only to aid deception of others, but also to distort self-truths or suppress painful realities and memories, thus avoiding uncomfortable feelings associated with things we don't want to face up to. A thief that doesn't get the opportunity to steal considers himself to be an honest man.

Central to this theme is the question: how can you achieve self-credibility and learn to trust yourself if there is no core honesty? If, every time we get something wrong or make a mistake, we rationalise it away or lay the blame elsewhere and allow it to settle as a distorted memory, where is the growth? If we make excuses for ourselves and put the blame elsewhere and justify our actions with untruths, where is the learning? Each time we turn our faces from the truth, we loosen our grip on reality a little further and fall further into the abyss that is an irrational world of make-believe.

Research has shown that we all lie to ourselves, and this is known as cognitive dissonance. First proposed by Leon Festinger in his 1957 book *A Theory of Cognitive Dissonance*, Festinger proposed that we desire our attitudes and beliefs to always be in harmony, but that they can become conflicted or dissonant because of our behaviours. When this happens, we lie to ourselves to avoid the mental torment that such conflict brings. An example of this might be someone that steals from their employer and then convinces themselves that this is to justify the low wages that they are paid. Maintaining a firm handle on self-reality provides a basis upon which to make decisions and control the direction of our lives. By making ourselves aware of our self-deceptions, we can regain self-credibility, followed by control, and finally find the true direction in our lives.

A good starting point to build or restore self-credibility is to acknowledge that you do lie to yourself, and accept that it has probably become habitual.

In this case, you are going to need a plan to develop the healthier habit of self-honesty, with the goal of making this a core life principle. Self-honesty will often involve facing up to your fears and accepting your limitations, which can be challenging. Only when we truly know that our words, decisions and actions are tethered to reality can we start to trust ourselves and reclaim self-credibility.

Take a moment to think of some examples of how you might have deceived yourself in the past, or perhaps instances of ongoing deception that you use, possibly as a coping strategy. Write them down in your notebook. Here are a couple of self-lies that I sometimes fall into the trap of using, that erode my self-credibility and core self-trust:

"I can't go to the gym today; my knee is sore from the long dog walk yesterday."

"I don't have time to make a healthy lunch today because I have to keep writing this book and get it finished, so I'll just have something quick and convenient."

"I didn't get time to help my son with his homework tonight as I was too busy with research."

Here, in contrast, are the truthful words that will rebuild and sustain my self-credibility:

"I didn't go to the gym today; I couldn't find the motivation and I was comfortable at my desk."

"I just ate junk for lunch today because I couldn't be bothered putting in the effort to make anything better."

"I didn't help my son out with his homework today because I prioritised my work over his."

Such reality checks might not always lead us to the gym or to eat more healthily or whatever, but they will make us feel better because we are being honest with ourselves. This in turn will help us to make the right decisions, so there is more chance of us doing the right thing simply by being honest with ourselves. This is important to keep us on track – we all want to be better people.

We all know that the short-term consequences of making poor lifestyle decisions are marginal, but over the long term, if we maintain the self-deceit that is perpetrating these bad decisions, then we are aware that things won't turn out well. The penalties for successive bad life choices are going to include physical and psychological distress, the consequences of which, in time, could become calamitous. Everyone makes mistakes, but lying to ourselves to justify them only makes matters worse.

Furthermore, frequent, conscious poor choices will ultimately diminish our faith in our own judgement. We all need to be cognisant of our decisions and be vigilant against taking too many easy or selfish options and passing them off with lies and excuses. Being honest with ourselves and truthfully rationalising our decisions (and owning them) helps to stop the self-duplicity and grounds us back in reality. Being true to ourselves enables us to take responsibility for our decisions and to trust in our judgement. This gives us self-credibility, the characteristics of which are:

Respect – Respect, love and care for the person that you are, and for your avatar.

Expertise – Be competent in your field. Be a self-expert in weight management

Self-truth – Self-deceit and disloyalty will undermine all self-credibility. If you make a mistake, immediately acknowledge it and correct it if possible.

Practice Authenticity – Don't try to be someone else, realise who you are, and grow and develop that person.

Emotional intelligence – Feelings and emotions guide us. Be aware of emotional strengths, weaknesses and vulnerabilities to help avoid impulsive actions.

Credibility – Take ownership of your actions and be responsible for them. Don't make excuses for bad decisions or choices.

True Integrity – Alignment between thoughts and actions. Do the right thing for the right reasons – especially when no one else knows.

Things to practice when developing self-credibility

■ Practice listening to yourself – what am I saying to myself?

■ Practice fact-checking yourself – is that what I really believe?

■ Practice reasoning with yourself – is that really what I want?

It is also important to remember that past performance is no guarantee of future results, and a successful life relies upon us trying hard each day to achieve the things in life that we feel are important. At the same time, an essential aspect of achieving and maintaining self-credibility is building a bridge from the past to the present, which we can then project into the future. This is because time links all things together, and you can't just cut off the past or ignore the future. Our past does not define us, but it helps to remind us, and acts to guide us for the future. Take some time to consider the journey that you are on and use your experiences of the past to give you strength and direction for the future.

Purpose

We all need purpose in life. Without purpose, life has no apparent meaning or direction. A life without purpose is surely just a confusing cycle of pain and pleasure, leaving us bobbing around in the yin and yang of existence. Without purpose, you can try to make sense of the chaos all around, but the meaning is lost. In the absence of purpose, we are simply coping and surviving, lurching between triumph and disaster. But life is meaning, and purpose validates our existence and helps to answer the age-old question of why we have been gifted this the most precious commodity of all – being.

Now, while it has been said of me that, if I were a swimming pool, I would have two shallow ends, I don't agree. For instance, I regularly muse over the meaning of life, which normally involves me thinking about who or what I am, and trying to fathom what my purpose is in life. When I delve into what I am, it helps me to consider myself as a symbiotic organism, with two parts – the mind and the body. My body (including my brain) is the physical form that allows me to exist. My mind is the product of this physical form, and it is the master, where my body is the servant. Throughout my life, I'm ashamed to say that my mind has meted out some dire treatment to my body, abused it, and taken it for granted. My mind has relied on my body to always come through, to be there irrespective of how it treats it. My body has taken the knocks every time and has always been there when I've needed it. I've punished it, truly, but it never complains, it does its best and always obeys the command of its master.

I know what the body needs, and I know what nourishes it and protects it, but the master doesn't always care about that, sometimes the master wants gratification and pleasure, and the avatar must suffer the consequences. When it gives up, I am gone, 'we' are gone, but I don't see my body as an equal partner. I don't value it as I should, or I wouldn't abuse it in the way I do. If I am to achieve all that I want in life, I need to develop an equitable relationship between my mind and the beast of burden that is my body.

My body has always looked after me, cared for me and protected me. My body has always been my guardian. My body truly loves my mind, and this is evident in everything that it has ever done for me, and everything it continues to do, in spite of my ungrateful disregard for its welfare and often abhorrent treatment of it. My body provides me with unmitigated devotion, but I, the mind, do not always reciprocate.

As a younger person, my behaviour was delinquent. By the age of sixteen, mostly as a result of my reckless actions, I had spent three weeks in hospital with serious burns, managed to spear myself through my calf muscle, and almost died from pneumonia brought on by self-neglect. Shortly after leaving school, I spent another long shift in hospital with septicaemia and endocarditis (a potentially fatal infection of the inner lining of the heart) because of treading on a broken bottle and ignoring the wound. In my mid-twenties, I ruptured a ligament in my knee playing football (absolute disaster) and almost fractured my skull cliff diving while on holiday in Yugoslavia (got away with twenty stitches). Aged thirty, I travelled the world for a year, during which I contracted a bad dose of malaria, spent another three weeks in hospital in New Delhi suffering from typhoid (very, very nasty!) and brought home a few parasitic worms in my intestines and liver (bilharzia), which needed several visits to the unit for tropical diseases at Kings Cross to exterminate the blighters.

I remember watching TV one evening sometime later and seeing one of the BUPA ads you may recall – 'You're amazing' (you can still see them on YouTube). These ads catalogued a series of astonishing facts and images about the body and portrayed this magnificent organism in all its glory. At that moment, I had an epiphany: "I'm no longer going to be the abuser in this relationship. I commit that, from this day, the servile relationship ends, and this becomes a true symbiotic partnership with common respect and reciprocated caring and love for this most precious thing, this wonder of creation, this body that loves me and cares for me and protects me. I would never treat anyone else in this way, why am I treating this faithful and loving friend in the way that I do?"

Shortly after, I changed career and moved from general management back into the wellness sector where I had previously worked in phase four cardiac rehabilitation and exercise referral programmes. I considered the growing obesity pandemic and re-retrained, specialising in weight management. I started to take my health more seriously and learned everything I could about human nutrition and non-communicable lifestyle disease. I applied what I learned to myself, and tried wherever possible to make better choices. I was starting to earn credibility with myself, which I still strive each day to maintain as best I can.

I am glad to say that, since this awakening, I haven't had any major medical skirmishes and I have been more responsible in taking care of my avatar in the same way that it takes care of me. I truly believe this way of thinking has helped me to make wiser lifestyle choices in the face of all the temptations that are thrust upon me, and all of us, daily. It was the start in giving me self-credibility and purpose. If I can't have respect for my own body, how on Earth can I have credibility when it comes to helping others to think about their bodies in a similar way? Maintaining self-credibility continues to keep me grounded and validates my work with others, which is, I think, what gives me purpose.

I believe that the most important (or sole) purpose of humankind is to make life better for others. But this must include taking care of ourselves (perhaps the most purposeful thing that we can do). For how can we help others if we are gone?

Feeding nurture

There is no doubt, your weight today is the result, to a large degree, of what and how much you ate as a child. From the moment of conception, your nutritional environment will have played a significant role in plotting your lifetime weight trajectory. The earlier the influence, the more profound the effect. I will ask you to consider this in detail when you undertake the five Insights of *Weight Wisdom*, because without a clear understanding of your journey into your weight, you will be unable to find the path to your new life. More about this in Insight 2.

All infants (humans and other animals) rely on their parents to teach them what to eat. This is fundamental to survival and is, in my opinion, one of the most crucial responsibilities a parent assumes when they bring a child into the world. Every mammal undergoes a nutritional apprenticeship, and the head teacher is typically the mother. In highly socialised animals such as elephants, siblings and other family members are also important teachers. In the case of our closest relatives (primates), this education can last for twelve years. During this time, children and other young animals spend much of their days observing and learning from their parents which foods are nutritious and which are to be avoided.

One aspect of this that you may not have considered is the permanence of such lessons. Something learned about food or feeding in childhood is held sacred, and unless challenged, will most likely become a lifelong 'belief' about how to behave around that food or that feeding behaviour. Nature has a way of 'imprinting' valuable knowledge to safeguard it for future generations. I experienced the power of this when I was about six or seven, but I did not realise its significance until some thirty years later when it occurred to me why it had such prominence back then.

My friend Gerald, or Jez, as he was known to us, was a real character, as tough as old boots. He had five older brothers with eight people living in a tiny two-up two-down next to Bank Hall colliery in Burnley where his father and some of his older brothers were working, 'down pit'. When I first heard the poem Timothy Winters by the poet Charles Causley, I instantly thought of Jez (and still do). The first verse goes like this:

Timothy Winters comes to school
With eyes as wide as a football pool,
Ears like bombs and teeth like splinters:
A blitz of a boy is Timothy Winters.

I recall asking my mum if Jez could come round to our house one day for tea (dinner) after school. Knowing of his family, Mum was resistant at first, but eventually caved in under my persistence. And so, sure enough, after a school footy match Jez came along. On walking into the house, Jez spotted the table was set for five people. He stopped in his tracks and gave me a look of real surprise:

Jez:	"Are we having a party?"
Me:	"What?"
Jez:	"Why then the table and chairs and tablecloth etc?"
Me:	"Because we are going to have our tea!"
Jez:	"Oh…"

We didn't speak about it after that, but that conversation stayed with me. Why on Earth did he say that? I would muse over it for weeks after. I knew that Jez had a big family and I supposed they didn't have the room in their house for a table big enough for eight. Perhaps they all sat in a circle on the floor to eat their meals? What on Earth did they do when it came to tea time? I just couldn't fathom it out.

Of course, what I realised many years later was that we had both been socialised differently regarding eating as a family; to do anything different would be utterly absurd. I imagined their family to be huddled in a circle on the floor, and Jez thought we had a tea party every evening. The message, I hope, is clear. If you think that what you believe about food and feeding is correct, if you learned it in childhood, you need to check that it is valid. What is more, even if it was appropriate back then, you need to determine whether it is still the case.

> Throughout the book, lookout for sections of text that are greyed out. These provide more detailed technical information that will be at the preference of the reader.

The obesity pandemic

In an article in *The Lancet* ('Where Next for Obesity?'), Harry Rutter wrote:

> *"There is a seductive simplicity to the conceptualisation of obesity as a straightforward problem of energy balance calories in versus calories out. But the physiological, behavioural, and environmental influences on this relationship are asymmetrical. Therefore, although the basic arithmetic holds true, in practice it is much easier for people, and populations, to gain weight than to lose it."*

I would prefer not to bore everyone with lots of statistics, however I think it'll be helpful to summarise the scale of the pandemic and examine its influence in countries as diverse as the USA and Kuwait. There have been many unfortunate milestones passed, and yet the situation just keeps getting worse. It was in the year 2000 when the World Health Organization (WHO) first declared obesity as a 'global epidemic'. Later, in 2004, they announced that for the first time ever there were more overfed than underfed people on the planet. Then, in 2014, the European courts set a precedent by ruling that severe obesity qualifies for protection under disability protection legislation. In 2022, 42% of the global population had central obesity, the annual cost of which is estimated to be four trillion dollars, or 3% of global GDP[1].

As significant as the prevalence is the degree to which people are gaining weight. In developed countries, the fastest-rising category of weight gain is severe or morbid obesity. In the twenty-five-year period between 1978 and 2003 in the US and UK, while obesity levels doubled, the number of people with severe obesity tripled and this worrying trend is set to accelerate[11]. The costs associated with this pandemic are astronomical: in a 2020 survey in Italy (a country with lower rates of overweight and obesity than the UK), the costs attributable to excess weight amounted to over €13 billion per annum[12]. According to the Centres for Disease Control (CDC), the cost in healthcare alone in the US is $173 billion each year. Globally, the cost is set to become $17 trillion by 2030[13].

Today, next to the climate emergency, excess body fat is arguably the greatest avoidable threat to the health of mankind, yet it is expected that its continued expansion will lead to the first decline in the life expectancy of humans. Virtually all people living with obesity will develop symptoms of chronic disease by the age of forty, and the majority will require medical intervention before they are sixty. Maladies related to an expanded waist, in particular type 2 diabetes, liver disease, heart and vascular disease, have overtaken smoking as the primary cause of preventable death in adults in the UK, the US and most other developed countries. Surely, the time has come for something to change?

Professor Katarina Borer of the University of Michigan knows her stuff, and, in very few words, summarised the drivers of the pandemic in the USA[14]. She says it's a combination of genetics; a lack of motivation to be physically active; labour-saving appliances; a built environment designed around the car; food dependence and cravings; increased stomach size and hunger from overeating and overly large portions; cheap junk food; slowed metabolism and enhanced fat storage; and government dietary advice that increases insulin resistance. She suggests the best defence is an understanding of the causes of obesity and appropriate strategies to change our behaviours accordingly[‡].

Recently, Theis and White from the University of Cambridge asked the question: "Is obesity policy in England fit for purpose?" They examined fourteen government strategies published between 1992 and 2020, containing 689 wide-ranging policies, and found that, generally, these proposals do not lead to implementation. That is, governments rarely commission evaluations of previous government strategies or learn from policy failures. Instead, they adopt their own 'shiny new' ideas which are invariably less interventionist and which favour strategies that make high demands on individual behaviour changes, rather than tackling the external influences that are actually responsible. This is why obesity strategies in the UK (and elsewhere) have singularly failed to achieve anything over thirty years of trying, and what is worse is that the researchers concluded these failures have led to little policy learning[15].

In 2010, Zoe Harcombe released her book *The Obesity Epidemic: What caused it, how can we stop it?*[16]. The book is a critique of current dietary advice and centres around the belief that it is carbohydrates and processed food rather than fat in our diets that is causing obesity. While I don't agree with everything in the book (fats aren't culpable), we agree on more than we disagree. Harcombe was spot on in her advice to governments about what needs to be done to curtail obesity, which can be broadly summarised as:

---

‡   Katrina, thanks for summarising the reasons for and purpose of this book!

- A dramatic reduction or elimination of refined carbohydrates and ultra-processed foods (more real food, less processed food).

- Establishing one government body to manage obesity, thus providing coherent and evidenced messages on diet and exercise.

- Removing the conflict of interests where 'Big Food' infiltrates the debate and calls the shots.

Thirteen years on from this advice, not a single step forward on any of these sensible suggestions has been taken. In March 2023, the UK government's own adviser on obesity, Henry Dimbleby, quit his post amid criticisms that the party's approach to tackling obesity "makes no sense". On reading the details, it appears to be just another example of the government getting all the right data and advice, but then failing to take the tough decisions. They shelved plans to restrict junk-food advertising and tax high-fat, high-sugar products, in favour of the now discredited and worn-out line of: "Working with industry to help people make healthier choices". If you are waiting for governments to sort out the food landscape, you are in for a long wait.

Obesity in China

Until very recently, China was traditionally one of the leanest populations on Earth, but this has now changed dramatically. In 1975, the proportion of adults living with obesity was fewer than half of 1%. By 2022, the Chinese Nutrition Society reported that this had risen to 16.4%. In under fifty years, the number had multiplied 35 times, currently standing at almost 200 million adults.

A 2021 study reported that, by 2030, two-thirds of adults and one-third of children in China could be overweight or obese if no effective interventions could be implemented[17]. With more than 700 million overweight people, China now has far more unhealthy weight citizens than any other country, with the more dangerous visceral obesity (fat around one's organs) being a significant confounding factor. The health consequences of this are colossal, and China is already dealing with a tidal wave of diabetes.

The reasons behind this obesity eruption in China are no different to that experienced elsewhere in the developed world, but just happen to have occurred more swiftly, due to China's move from relative poverty to a global superpower in just fifty years. It has been facilitated by rapid economic growth, modernisation, urbanisation, food processing and the globalisation of food markets, a phenomenon known as the Global Nutrition Transition (GNT). The substantial changes in dietary patterns include eating more animal-source foods, more refined grains, and significantly more highly processed, high-sugar and high-fat foods. All of this has coincided with significant declines in physical activity levels, resulting from people moving from rural to urban areas, where office and factory jobs take the place of field work[18]. It is interesting to note that China is not able to blame the policy limitations imposed by the revolving door of governments in the West for their inability to curb obesity, which illustrates the power of the GNT, which is able, it seems, to override democracies and autocracies alike.

Obesity and climate change

Let's consider the global obesity calamity, which shares environmental and social similarities with the gravest of all human threats, the climate emergency. Both obesity and climate change are significant threats to mankind, each with its own unique formula for misery and mortality on a vast scale. Both are a result of bad administration of our resources by the majority of wealthy people on the planet, to the detriment of the poorest.

We have the knowledge, science and means to rectify both catastrophes should we choose to, yet we collectively choose not to. Both obesity and climate change and their causes are worsening despite growing alarm, financial cost, lives lost and planetary destruction. The loss of biodiversity caused by modern food-production techniques, destructive commercial fishing, and the demand for meat, is an unmitigated disaster for our planet and all that inhabit it (especially those individuals and species that are no longer inhabitants as a result). According to the Food and Agriculture Organization of the United Nations, an estimated 75% of the world's food is produced from just twelve plant and five animal species!

The size of the average person on the planet continues to increase, as does the total number of people. Data published in the journal *Obesity* in 2020, estimated that the greater biomass of human obesity creates extra emissions of up to 700 megatons per year of CO_2 equivalent. This is about 1.6% of worldwide climate-destabilising emissions[19]. In 2012, science writer Tim De Chant, using data from the Global Footprint Network, suggested that, if everyone on Earth lived like the average American, we would need four planets to sustain us, and if everyone lived as they do in the United Arab Emirates, we would need five.

Human behaviour is complex; what appears to one to be an absurd position, seems perfectly acceptable to another. Your own view of these two unfolding scenarios will probably determine how you respond. Some will be alive to each threat and take both personal and societal responsibility and act accordingly, while others deny there is a problem at all, and blithely continue as they always have, choosing instead to rubbish or cancel those that appreciate the magnitude of each parlous situation.

Water

Mexico is one of the most obese countries in the world, where three-quarters of adults are overweight with half of them living with obesity. The country also suffers from water scarcity. Therefore, it was fitting that a team of innovative Mexican scientists investigated how these two problems relate, and how, by reducing one problem, they might ameliorate the other. They noted that food production represents 90% of a person's water footprint, and the unhealthier the diet, the more water is needed to produce such foods. Their results showed that the average Mexican diet requires an astonishing 6,056 litres of water per person, per day, which is 55% higher than the water footprint of international healthy diets[20]. Consumption of beef, milk, fruits, chicken and fatty cereals represented 56% of total water footprint, and the more calorific the diet, and the higher the BMI of the person, the more water is required to produce the products. The diets of people who are overweight required 729 litres per day of extra water. The researchers concluded that following a healthy diet would benefit the individual and help to mitigate the problem of water scarcity[21].

This book is about weight and not about climate change, but I can't help thinking that the underpinning human characteristic central to both catastrophes is the innate human flaw to consume until all is gone.

Human evolution

Our evolutionary lineage follows a route that branched from the apes around seven or eight million years ago (chimpanzees being our closest living relatives). Over the next several million years, a number of ape-like creatures appeared, living concurrently for various periods until the first hominins (primitive pre-cursers to Homo sapiens) appeared around 2.5 million years ago with the emergence of Homo habilis and Homo nalidi. Thereafter, several primitive hominins competed, and Homo erectus (appearing two million years ago) became the predecessor to Homo heidelbergenisis (600,000 years ago), Neanderthal (400,000 years) and Homo sapiens (meaning 'wise human') around 300,000 years ago. It is known that Homo sapiens lived alongside Neanderthals for some time and traces of Neanderthal DNA can be found in people today. It's strange to think that Neanderthals were still around as recently as 40,000 years ago.

Finally, a further change spawned larger brains than the earlier sapiens and, around 160,000 years ago, the modern human arrived – Homo sapien sapien (wise, wise human). These same humans, around 70,000BC, were developing 'modern' behaviours and cognitive traits including abstract thinking and planning, alongside symbolic behaviour such as music and dance. Hunting and blade technology were also evident in this period, as were cultural foundations, social norms, language and extended cooperation. All the above, including our direct ancestors the chimps, are likely to have been omnivorous (chimps regularly hunt for meat).

Throughout our evolution, since long before we were modern humans, famine has been a major threat to human survival. This omnipresent menace has resulted in a species well-equipped to deal with frugal environments, but totally ill-equipped to deal with a continuous abundance of food. A fundamental pillar of survival is to eat nutritious things and reject flavours and smells that signify danger. The evolution of food-reward mechanisms in the brain, alongside exquisite olfactory (smell) and gustation (taste) structures, exemplify a control system that acts as supreme guardian over the survival of humankind. Rather than being background functional circuitry, these primal networks are central actors in energy management and food selection and rejection. They are intertwined with our learned approaches to eating, and together with food availability, combine to determine our overall diet.

It is believed that our predecessor, Homo erectus started cooking 1.8 million years ago. Compared to earlier hominins, Homo erectus had very small teeth, a small body, and a much larger brain, probably enabled by the technological revolution that was cooking food. As well as killing off nasty pathogens in meat and making many inedible plant foods edible, cooking allows the extraction of more usable nutrients from the same amount of food, thus providing more calories per bite. This means less time hunting, scavenging and gathering, and more time developing social skills and technical developments to improve survival chances. Cooking food was therefore a major leap forward in the development of humankind.

Only as recently as 12,000 years ago did humans 'invent' farming. One bright Palaeolithic spark decided it would be a good idea that, at the end of the growing season, the group should gather up as many wild grass seeds as they could and store them in a dry place so that they could eat them during the barren months. Furthermore, they could choose the biggest seed heads and plant them for the next year's crop, thus increasing the size of the edible seeds each year (our modern-day grains are derived from these early wild grasses). "That's a great idea!" said another, "But I can go one further. Why don't we go out and catch some grazing animals like goats, which we can pen in and feed and fatten them up, and then we can kill them and eat them when we need to – they'd be like a walking larder! If we're feeling really bold, we could lure the young, most docile wild Ox into captivity, and they will provide us with lots of meat. We could drink their milk, too." These were the ancestors of our modern cattle.

Before the advent of this second technical revolution (fire and cooking being the first), survival required, among other things, continual vigorous physical activity, nomadic lifestyles with the frequent building of shelters, constant gathering, scavenging, hunting and tracking the migratory paths of wild herbivores. Higher-energy foods such as nuts and seeds were an ephemeral annual boon, depending on the season, but the staple foods were low-energy sources such as tubers, shoots, vegetation and fruits, with an approximate energy density of 400 calories per kilo (kcal/kg); our ancestors had to eat a lot of food for little energy reward. Therefore, for 288,000 of the 300,000 years that Homo sapiens have been around, it was the nomadic, scavenging, gathering existence that shaped our genes to survive in a harsh and frugal environment. This was, and is, what we can assume as a 'normal' environment for humans.

Throughout our evolution, we have fought against famine. In Africa, considered the cradle of humanity, failure of annual rainfall is estimated to occur, on average, every seven years. Climatic disturbances causing drought or flood leads to widespread failures of plant growth and the resulting famines can be devastating. Ultimately, in the absence of intervention, when vegetation fails on a wide scale, animal life perishes, and human starvation is inevitable. Against this background of ever-present food shortages, humans have evolved biological processes to defend against starvation. They are primal and powerful, and selected to accumulate additional energy stores at any opportunity. They are also complex and unified with the behaviours of management of feeding and acquiring food; two complementary skills that ensure our survival. The frequent hunger experienced by our ancestors has hardwired us with a primary insurance policy: eat whenever there are calories to be had.

Contrast this with our recent history (the past fifty years), where people are habitually sedentary and regularly consume extremely energy-dense food: chocolate (5,500 kcal/kg) French fries (2,500 kcal/kg) and crisps (5,300 kcal/kg). The last fifty years represent 0.017% of our species' time on the planet, or, if our 300,000 years was a twenty-four-hour clock, then, at 15 seconds to midnight, our world changed dramatically, and our genes have had no time to adapt. While over the years starvation has killed many millions, the irony is that today, in the absence of food shortages across much of the world, hundreds of millions of people are amassing extreme levels of excess energy, which is proving in many cases to be just as fatal.

Collectively, this helps in part to explain why there has been so little progress in resolving the current obesity pandemic using medication. Current prescription drugs have very low efficacy, and those that did work moderately well, were swiftly withdrawn due to their serious detrimental side effects. A new drug called semaglutide (sold as the brand Ozempic or Wegovy) is available in the US and UK. It can be bought over the counter at around £200 for a one-month supply and may be available through the NHS for people who have at least 1 weight-related comorbidity and a BMI above 35kg/m². The drug is based upon the body's natural gut hormone glucagon like peptide 1 (GLP1) and is designed to suppress appetite and increase satiety. Let's wait and see how this latest magic potion works out. 25 years of practice has taught me that people do not reverse their obesity through drug therapy. If you speak to people that successfully lose weight for the long term, they will tell you that they change the way that they eat, think and behave. I believe The Verve hit the nail on the head when they sang: The drugs don't work (they just make you worse)!

Dieting, which swiftly reduces body fat, signals famine, triggers a slowing of metabolism, conservation of fat stores and a voracious hunger, where food-seeking completely occupies the mind – sound familiar? Today's problem, of course, is that the exquisite systems that regulate our appetite were developed at a time when food was in its natural form and was far from abundant. 'Natural' means that food contains all the organically occurring fibre, water, vitamins, minerals and phytochemicals (micro-nutrients) without the supplementary sugars, fats and profusion of contemporary artificial additives that modern processed foods contain.

In contrast, we now have open access to highly modified, ultra-processed foods (UPFs), the GNT has resulted in the mass production of high-calorie, low-nutrient, long-life, cheap foods that taste good. A hallmark of these 'dysfunctional foods' is that they are high in macro-nutrients (fat, carbohydrate and protein) but low in the essential micro-nutrients (vitamins, minerals, fibre and phytochemicals), making them energy dense and nutrient poor. Chocolate, confectionery, puddings, high-fat, high-sugar, high-salt foods, takeaways, biscuits, cakes, crisps, sugary drinks and so on, are all UPFs; the question is, are they food? I don't think so, which is why I tend not to refer to them as food, but instead as edible products that are calorific, refined, appetising and processed. For the sake of brevity, I'll use the mnemonic CRAP.

Obesity can and does exist in a paradoxical state of excess calorie intake and simultaneous malnutrition – too many macro-nutrients and too few micro-nutrients. Deficiencies or imbalances of essential micro-nutrients will significantly affect daily performance, intellectual and emotional state, and the physical state of the body. As a consequence of eating too much CRAP, many adults and children in the modern world are overfed and undernourished – the shocking double whammy of malnutrition.

The overweight evidence base

There are only a few contexts in which the word 'losing' is deemed positive. Weight management is one of them.

Over the years, I have learned that people hold greatly differing views about their size, weight and body image. I particularly recollect working in the West Midlands alongside a group of delightful midwives who were primarily from the Afro-Caribbean community. The subject matter for our gathering, of course, was weight gain before, during and after pregnancy. One of the themes that cropped up (as it did regularly when working with health professionals) was "How can I ask someone else to lose weight when I'm overweight myself?" A lively discussion ensued during which one lady in the room said something along the lines of, "I'm too heavy at the moment; I'd like to be lovely and slim like her", pointing to one of the now blushing ladies in the group, who I would estimate to have a BMI of around 35. At this moment, I realised how subjective weight is and the absolute imperative of recognising all goals as legitimate, irrespective of whether they fit anyone else's ideal.

It is worth noting that the generally established estimates or measures of fatness are there for convenience; a way to provide a baseline that can be used to compare and evaluate change. Of course, metrics like BMI, skinfold and waist circumference have clinical and epidemiological validity, and as such help to guide clinicians in their assessments. But, for an individual, the most important measure is that which they feel most comfortable with. Is it weight, clothes size, appearance, body shape, or is it related to functionality, fitness and mobility? Whichever works best, this is what you should use.

Measuring weight

One reason for this is that people are not very good at assessing their weight using the established categories of BMI, and when asked if they are underweight, a healthy weight, overweight, or obese, they are wrong about half the time, with underestimates being more common than overestimates. Of those that do overestimate, most are women[22]. In case you wanted to use some of the established measures, I have detailed some of the more commonplace ones here.

Body Mass Index (BMI)

BMI is calculated by dividing weight in kilos by the square of the height in metres. It is the standard measure used by most clinicians for classifying under/overweight. It is by no means perfect, but, on balance, I'd say it's more helpful than not. You can just go online and punch the numbers in, but it is a simple calculation that works like this: if you weigh 95kg and your height is 1.75 then you will have a BMI of 31. Below is an example:

$$BMI \quad \frac{Kg}{M^2} \quad = \quad \frac{95}{1.75 \times 1.75} \quad = \quad \frac{95}{3.06} \quad = \quad 31$$

BMI Ranges	
Underweight	<18.5
Normal Range	18.6 - 24.9
Overweight	25 - 29.9
Obese Class 1	30 - 34.9
Obese Class 2	35 - 39.9
Obese Class 3	>40
Super Morbid Obesity	>50

Waist circumference

For those seeking to reduce their risk of health complications, a useful measure would be waist circumference (WC). WC is a good proxy measure of the amount of fat accumulating around and infiltrating vital organs (known as visceral fat), which, as you can guess, is not particularly helpful. Visceral fat is closely linked to a disruption in blood lipids and the loss of insulin sensitivity, and therefore waist measurement is a better guide than BMI in assessing diabetes and cardiac risk.

Waist circumference is normally taken by measuring midway between the pelvic crest and the lowest rib (this can be tricky to locate consistently and, as it is normally around the navel it may be best to just aim there). The chart to the right shows the waist circumference and relative risk of coronary heart disease (CHD).

Men	>94cm	Increased risk of CHD
Men	>102cm	Severely increased risk of CHD
Women	>80cm	Increased risk of CHD
Women	>88cm	Severely increased risk of CHD
Asian men	>90cm	Severely increased risk of CHD
Asian women	>80cm	Severely increased risk of CHD

One group at higher risk from an expanded waist is Asian people, because Asian people have a genetic tendency towards a less favourable fat-to-muscle ratio at a comparable body weight to other ethnicities. Because muscle is highly cardio-protective, having more fat and less muscle leaves you at more risk of metabolic disease. Furthermore, the location of body fat determines the impact on health, and Asian people carry more visceral fat (around the organs) which can infiltrate the organs. Finally, Asian people have fewer adipocytes (fat cells) for the same relative fat mass, meaning fewer safe storage spaces for fats and potentially more 'lipid spillage' (fat leaking from the fat cells and into the blood). Taken together, this accounts for the increased risk of metabolic disease compared to non-Asian people with a comparable BMI.

While I was recently looking into the clinical legitimacy of these guidelines, what cropped up was a scientific publication written by the Faculty of Education, Health and Wellbeing at Wolverhampton University, in conjunction with Coventry Uni[23]. They were arguing that waist-circumference guidelines were unfair, stating that NICE's latest advice, to keep the size of your waist to less than half of your height, "...unfairly penalised shorter people and lulled taller people into a false sense of security". So, for all you six-footers out there, watch out, your three-foot waist is coming to get you!

Percentage body fat

In 1995, the World Health Organization defined obesity based on having a percent body fat more than 25% for men and 35% for women. I'm not being gratuitous when I mention that the maximum body fat likely to be measured on a walrus is 35%.

Ideal body weight (IBW)

Ideal body weight is based upon information related to morbidity (disease) and mortality (death) and can be used as a guide, but should not be seen as a weight target. Frankly, I don't think they have much value at all, but I include them for information. There are two valid methods for calculating ideal body weight (IBW):

Devine formula

1. This method is widely used, but, unless you enjoy maths, it can be a bit fiddly. Like with BMI, though, you'll be able to find a calculator for this online.

   Men = 50kg + 2.3kg per 2cm over 1.5m Women = 45kg + 2.3kg per 2cm over 1.5m

   (There is a + or – allowance of 10% for big or small frames)

   Therefore, if you are female and 1.65m, your IBW would be 45kg + (7.5 x 2.3 = 17.3) **IBW = 62.3kg** (+/- 10% for frame size)

2. A simpler formula for both men and women is 22kg multiplied by the square of height in metres. **IBW = 22kg x m2**. Therefore, if you are 1.75m tall your IBW would be 1.75 x 1.75 = 3.06 x 22 = **67.4kg**.

Somatotype (body type)

We are born with a build type that is primarily inherited from our parents. This is known as your 'somatotype' and, broadly speaking, there are three types, as shown to the right. Each has different characteristics with respect to gaining weight. It is endomorphs that typically struggle with weight gain.

Endomorph	Small bones, short limbs, wide hips, generally round, gain weight more easily.
Mesomorph	Heavy bones, broad hands, broad chest, triangular shape.
Ectomorph	Long bones, slim, little body fat, low potential for muscle growth.

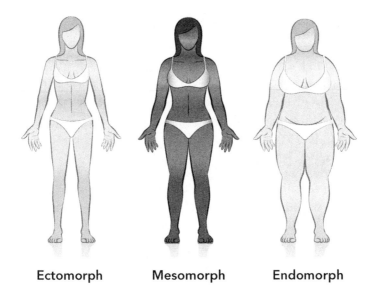

Ectomorph   Mesomorph   Endomorph

Weight composition

When considering your weight, it may also be helpful to think about the five general components that make up the majority of body weight (if we exclude fluids such as water, blood and plasma).

1. Organs: brains, liver, gut, heart etc. Vital to life and tightly controlled in terms of size and proportion.

2. Bones. good bone mass is a sign of health, particularly for women who can suffer from fractures if peak bone mass is not reached and maintained in later years. Resistance and load-bearing activities and a healthy diet throughout life are highly beneficial.

3. Muscles. Not only essential for mobility, but critical in maintaining insulin sensitivity and protection from metabolic disorders. A target of maintaining a good musculature throughout life would be wise.

4. Subcutaneous fat. Held directly under the skin (think pear shape, large bottom and thighs). Not considered harmful, and pear shapes are linked to lower metabolic risk.

5. Visceral fat (apple shape) gathers inside the abdomen and infiltrates the organs (ectopic fat) particularly the liver, pancreas and arteries.

Lifetime weight trajectory

One hurdle standing tall in the face of change is the difficulty that people have in projecting their weight into the future. They consider their weight as it is right now and assume that this is where it stops. While unhappy with their current weight, many people don't pause to think about the consequences of keeping on treading the same path. To counter this myopic view of the future, I use the lifetime weight projector, somewhat of a blunt instrument, but more often than not it will have the desired effect.

At the initial consultation, I would ask clients to recount their journey into weight. I would normally do this by using a crude graph to plot their recollections of weight over the passage of time. Using one of my client's data as an example (let's call him Yusef), here's how the predictor works. I ask Yusef to think carefully about how his weight has progressed over the years and to think of any time points when he can remember his weight. Yusef was good at this, as he was a weight trainer up until the age of about twenty-five, and so kept a close eye on his weight. Back then, he laughs, the aim was to get his weight up, but now it's the opposite!

We plot his recollections on the graph (the thin line running from bottom left) up until his current age of forty-four years, which is where the solid black and dashed lines start. These conversations usually go something like this: "So, Yusef, you came to see me because you're worried about your weight (Yusef was only short in stature, and at 96kg for someone just 1.53m tall, his BMI is 41) and you say that this is the heaviest that you have ever been, and now you have developed type 2 diabetes. We can see that your weight has been steadily rising since you were sixteen and stands at 96kg today."

Next, I would draw a horizontal line across to age 65 (dashed line). I'd then ask Yusef to look at the graph and tell me that, if nothing changed, would this represent reality? In other words, is it a decent prediction of his weight over the next twenty-five years? As you can guess, put like this, most people figure out that it is most unlikely. At this, I hand the pen to Yusef and say, "OK, judging by what's happened up until now, please have a go at predicting where you think you will be at age 65". Yusef takes the pen and, with a bit of a grimace, cautiously draws a line (solid black line): "Something like this?" We make the estimate around 117kg, which is well over three stones (42lbs) heavier than he is now. At this weight, I'm sorry to have to tell Yusef that his BMI would be 50, putting him in the very severely obese category, and for a sixty-five-year-old, not only would this be dangerous, but in terms of what he can expect for his quality of life at that point, a future without change does not look bright.

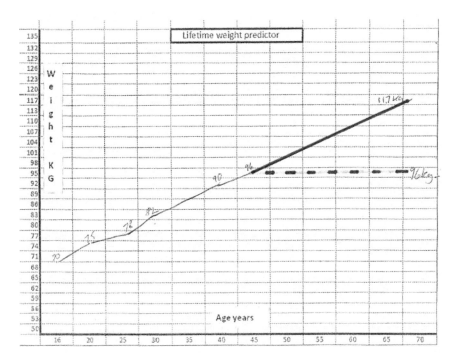

On taking Yusef's body fat percentage via bio-impedance, we discover he has a fat percentage of 39%, and while far from optimum for a 44-year-old man who is fit and strong, it's not the end of the world – he has the youth and strength to manage this level of surplus inert mass. I don't want to put the boot in, but I feel the need to explain to Yusef that, unfortunately, the graph does not present the whole picture. As we pass the mid-point of our lives (around thirty-five – forty years), we start to lose lean mass such as skeletal muscle and bone. But fat mass continues to accrue, meaning that by age sixty-five, if Yusef was to become 117kg, his body composition (fat-to-lean ratio) would skew dramatically more in favour of fat than it currently is. I estimate that if he does go on to become 117kg at age sixty-five, his body fat percentage could well be over 55%. His prognosis were this to happen would be very poor.

Of course, the purpose of this exercise is to encourage Yusef to think about the long-term lifestyle changes that will ensure that he does not become that person entering his later years with all the difficulties that will bring. The lifetime weight predictor, as rough as it is, acts as a reality check, a glimpse of what might come if Yusef is unable to find another path. One aim, at the very least, is to get people to draw a line in the sand: from now on, no more weight gain. Of course, if you can successfully put in place changes to halt weight gain, then it is only a small stretch, a few more incremental alterations to daily routines, to put weight into decline. So, this is our plan to safeguard Yusef's happiness and significantly improve his diabetes, and, perhaps more than each of these, enable Yusef to experience the profound comfort and reassurance brought about by successfully piloting the ship.

If you are under 50 (not much point after that) it may be worth having a go at the lifetime weight predictor. You can download this and many other free weight-related resources from www.weightwisdom.co.uk

To illustrate the extent to which humans can gather body fat, the late Jon Brower Minnoch of the USA (the heaviest ever recorded human being) reached a colossal 100 stones (635kg). An average-sized person carries around 150,000 kilocalories (kcals) in fat reserves; however, I'd estimate at this weight, Jon's onboard lipid cache was over four million kcals. That's enough fuel for an average-sized person to run almost two thousand marathons, equivalent to around fifty thousand miles, or twice around the circumference of the Earth! The human body can store a lot of energy and uses it very sparingly.

Metabolic rate

With respect to weight management, pondering the vagaries of metabolism is probably as useful as gazing at your navel. However, it is important to understand how it works, if nothing else to counter the many myths surrounding it. In simple terms, the metabolic rate is the speed at which our bodies burn the fuel that we eat, to produce the energy that we need for everyday life.

Metabolic rate is controlled by many varied factors and is a complex system of signals and feedback loops. Age, gender, weight, fitness levels, physical activities, food consumption and genetics all play their part. Cells and tissues have different metabolic rates depending upon their function. Consider the huge requirement of energy needed by the organs, which form only 6% of total body weight yet use almost 60% of energy. Generally, lean mass burns approximately 20kcal/kg/day, while fat mass at a more sedentary

4kcal/kg/d. Therefore, provided there are no metabolic disorders such as hypothyroidism, resting metabolic rate (as it is known) is largely set by the fat-to-lean ratio and the individual amounts of both lean and fat tissue present in any person.

Your metabolic rate will mainly determine how many calories you'll burn over a twenty-four-hour period, but there are two other contributors. When collated, this is referred to as the total energy expended (TEE). The contribution of each of these three energy requirements to TEE is entirely individual, based upon the factors mentioned above, but some approximate values have been provided for an average-sized person.

1. **BMR – Basal Metabolic Rate**

   At rest, the body requires energy for the heart to beat, circulation to pump and respiration to continue, as well as for body heat, digestion and other bodily functions. This is your BMR, sometimes referred to as Resting Metabolic Rate (technically slightly different, but, practically, means the same) and it accounts for around 60% of daily energy requirements.

2. **Activity Levels**

   The activity levels of an averagely active person will contribute around 30% of TEE each day. This figure can increase to 60% for very active people and can be as low as 5% of total energy output for sedentary people.

3. **Dietary Induced Thermogenesis – DIT**

   All food has an energy requirement needed to break it down and digest the various components before it can provide us with energy. Also known as the thermic effect of food, it can account for up to 10% of our daily energy expenditure.

Therefore, it is not true to say that people are fat or thin because they have a high or low metabolism.

Weight regain following weight loss

It is accepted that, in most cases, voluntary weight loss is a temporary state and the cycle of relapse for those trying to lose weight is a continual and demoralising torment. There are several reasons for this, but one significant factor is how much daily energy we need, which can change quite drastically. As we have seen, we all have different energy needs based upon variables such as age, gender, body composition, and, for those with a high fat-to-lean ratio, their energy requirements are proportionately lower.

Consider two people weighing 85kg: one has a body fat percentage of 20% and the other 35%. The first person would therefore have around 68kg of lean mass and the second would have around 55kg of lean mass. Imagine they both have the same activity levels and are eating the same amount of food (seems reasonable, as they both weigh the same). The low body fat person could require 400kcals more each day simply because of the metabolic requirements of fuelling the extra 13kg of lean mass. If they both ate the diet required for the leaner person, then, the second person would have an excess of 400kcals each day and would gain even more weight. Therefore, calorific requirements can't be based solely on weight.

Having said that, one might assume that if a person previously weighing 100kg with high body fat slimmed down to the same body composition and same weight as our 85kg lean person above (that had never been overweight), they should now require about the same number of calories per day, because they weigh the same and have the same body composition. However, weight loss interferes with anticipated energy requirements based upon weight and body composition. What occurs following weight loss is a dramatic reduction in energy requirements, disproportionate to the amount of weight lost, and can mean needs are 28% lower (at least temporarily – see below) compared to someone of a matching weight (that has not lost weight).

In an acclaimed study conducted in 1984[24], researchers looked at two groups (people with obesity [OB] and those without [NO]). Each were examined for energy requirements in a closely controlled experiment that lasted many months. The OB group were put on a precise liquid formula, restricted diet where average weight loss was 60kg and their energy requirements were accurately measured before and after weight loss. The average weight of the NO group was 63kg (no weight loss required). The resulting energy requirements for both groups reported as calories per kg of weight (metabolic rate), and total daily calorie requirement are shown in the table below, and are not what one would expect:

Group	Av weight	Kcal/kg/day	Total Kcal/day
OB start weight	160kg	24	3,651
OB after weight loss	100kg	19	2,171
Never obese	63kg	36	2,280

The OB group's energy requirements declined dramatically as weight was lost, to the point that they had energy requirements for their body mass well below the NO group (19 kcal/kg v 36 kcal/kg), so that, remarkably, even though the OB group were still heavier by around 40kg, their total daily energy requirements were lower than the NO group (OB 2,171kcal/day v NO 2,280kcal/day). In other words, the weight loss had made them far more energy efficient, requiring substantially less energy per kg of body weight, even though their fat-to-lean ratio was now more favourable (24/kcal/kg/day v 19/kcal/day).

The researchers conducting this study suggested that this was 'metabolic resistance' to long-term weight loss, which may be nature's way of returning the body to its natural weight after a period of famine. Their work suggests that, following weight loss, a further 25% reduction in food consumption is still needed. Similar findings have been seen in other studies in which weight regain is greatly enhanced following a period of food restriction. These results throw the previous wisdom of metabolic rate being tied to body composition and amount of lean mass up in the air, because this does not consider the metabolic brakes applied following weight loss. To add insult to injury, following weight loss, not only do energy requirements decline, but changes in circulating hormones involved in appetite such as leptin and ghrelin shift in favour of increased hunger. The body likes to maintain a constant mass, which is why reaching adulthood as a healthy weight is so important.

However, there is good news. Another study found that metabolism only slowed during the reducing phase of weight loss, and concluded: "Our findings do not provide evidence in support of adaptive metabolic changes as an explanation for the tendency of weight-reduced persons to regain weight"[25]. In other words, in time, metabolism will stabilise at 'normal' levels at the new weight.

As for hormonal changes after weight loss, studies conflict on how long they last. Some say up to one year and others that it is a transient state that normalises when energy balance is resumed. The majority of changes in fasting gut hormones seem to occur in early weight loss and then stabilise, with starting BMI having little influence on the degree of hormone change[26]. Yet another study[27] added to this by reporting a significant lessening in cravings for high-energy foods over time following weight loss.

Of course, 'weight rebound' mechanisms would surely be beneficial in our evolutionary past, when most humans faced cyclical famine, but in the modern world with its abundance of food, this evolved biology is the blight of every 'bon vivant'. In conclusion, though, it appears that weight reduction *does* alter metabolic rate and the hunger hormones in favour of weight regain, but that this is only temporary until the body can re-adjust to the new weight. The key is to allow the body (and behaviour) time to adjust to the new weight.

Finally, it is suggested that persistent attempts at weight loss may make matters worse in the long run. A rat experiment put a group through two cycles of dieting and refeeding. After dieting, the animals showed significant increases in weight gain. This became more significant after the second cycle, where weight loss occurred at half the rate of the first cycle and regain at three times the rate. At the end of the experiment, cycled animals had a four-fold increase in food efficiency (and therefore weight gain) compared to obese animals of the same weight who had not cycled[28].

Therefore, yoyo dieting makes weight loss and weight maintenance much harder, and the sense of failure and the magnitude of dejection is proportional to the total investment placed in each failed diet. To compound matters, following these futile cycles, the dieter's body composition has unfavourably shifted towards less lean mass and more fat mass, adding to the demoralisation brought on by yoyo dieting.

Diets don't work

I see so clearly now the futility of popular approaches to weight loss. Get-thin-fast remedies are ubiquitous and it's big business, estimated to be worth $150 billion annually in the US and Europe alone. Millions of people are on weight loss diets at any one time. These people are old, young, rich, poor, fat, thin, educated and illiterate, and from every country and culture. The merry-go-round of fad diets, endorsed by celebrities and grinning waifs wielding florets of broccoli claim, "You will never be hungry on this diet!" But they lie to you. Diets inevitably lead to voracious hunger; but if you believe the spin, you won't be expecting it. You will blame yourself for caving in. "No one else feels hungry on this diet, it's typical of greedy guts me; I'm such a failure when it comes to dieting!"

Diets don't work because they are temporary, fostering a bunker mentality – I must just keep my head down and plough on, swimming against the tide until I reach my target weight. But as any crustacean will tell you, if you swim against the tide, eventually you get exhausted and get swept away. Long-term studies show that, for successful dieters, most weight is regained within one or two years, with at least one-third regaining more fat than they lost. Thus, diets deliver the opposite of their intended purpose.

Perhaps the most malign form of dieting is the once-popular crash diet featuring dramatic calorie reduction. For the average person, maximum 'fat' loss is about 1-2kg in a week, and it won't be a stroll in the park. Theoretically, 1kg of fat loss is equivalent to about 7,700kcals (as body fat also contains water), so to lose 1kg of fat you will need 1,100 fewer kcals than your requirement every day for a week. That's a huge deficit! Normally, to get into the realms of 2kg a week weight loss, bariatric surgery is required. Whether the 1,100 calorie deficit each day works in principle, is a contested matter.

I regularly recall that, after stepping off the scales, one of my clients would bemoan: "What! Just 250g of weight loss! Oh no, what's that in pounds?" At which, I'd have my lard bags at the ready (no self-respecting weight-management practitioner should be without lard bags). I'd grab the 250g (half a pound) bag of lard and say something like: "Absolutely brilliant effort this week Doris – over half a pound! In this bag is almost two thousand calories, so I know how well you've done this week. I know that you've eaten 300kcals fewer than you need every day of the week, which is amazing. Take a look at it (fat is quite voluminous so a quarter kilo looks like a lot), it's pure energy in a bag, and what's more, that was on your butt last week!" Most of the time, I got away with that one!

So, even under severe calorie restriction, fat loss will remain relatively slow because when food is dramatically restricted, the body assumes famine and starts conserving fat stores. The fuel of choice becomes glycogen, stored in the muscles (80%) and liver (20%). Glycogen is one-part glucose and three-parts water, so you are burning sugar and releasing water. Great, you may think… well actually no, glycogen is the muscles' primary fuel source and so you'll feel sluggish and fatigued.

An average-sized person has around 2kg of glycogen on board, so that's 500g of sugar and 1.5 litres (1.5kg) of water. The frequent toilet trips during the first few days of a crash diet are a release of the water (and weight) locked up in the glycogen. This 2kg weight loss in the first few days often leads to the belief that everything is going well, reinforcing the theory that drastically cutting food intake is the way to lose weight. However, when losing weight, the only desirable reduction is fat, and you haven't lost any yet!

As 'famine' continues, the body takes drastic steps and starts to break down muscle, converting it to sugar (gluco-neo-genesis [sugar-new-creation]). Since active muscles are the most efficient fat-burning tissues in the body, shrinking them is a bad idea for dieters. Also, as lean mass is depleted, basal metabolic rate (BMR) will be reduced proportionally. Severe calorific restrictions of this type can suppress the metabolism by as much as 28%. As metabolism slows, so does the dieters' ability to operate at normal levels; exercise becomes difficult and general lethargy sets in. The body has successfully adjusted to the new low levels of available energy and can now survive on less food than it could previously – evolutionary adaptations have served their purpose!

After two or three days on a crash diet, you probably won't have burned much fat at all. Only as the diet progresses, will your body have no alternative but to turn to its fat stores to make up the daily energy deficit. When this happens, there will be a battle in the body as the fat cells resist shrinkage by releasing their primary defensive cell signalling proteins known as adipokines. These signal to the brain: eat, eat, eat! And forget the lettuce, we want pies, chips, cake and chocolate!

When the diet inevitably comes to an end (which is why they don't work as a vehicle for permanent weight loss) and previous eating patterns resume, calorie requirements are now significantly lower than before the diet because you have reduced your BMR, creating a large energy surplus on the hitherto 'normal diet'. Additionally, dieting is frequently followed by rebound binge eating. An uncontrollable urge to overeat as the body attempts to quickly get back to the weight to which it had previously become accustomed – driven by shrunken fat cells and those pesky adipokines.

At this stage, it is worth mentioning that very low-calorie diets (VLCDs), which provide intakes as low as 600Kcal each day, do have their place in health care. VLCDs are medically managed, high-biological value commercial products normally taken as liquids. Typical daily minimum macronutrient compositions would be protein 75g, carbohydrate 30g and a minimum of 13g essential fats, as well as current established daily values for vitamins and minerals. VLCDs are now being used with great effect to reverse the effects of type 2 diabetes in many cases. They are also effective at reducing the size of the liver before bariatric surgery; an important safety consideration. Under these circumstances (and possibly other medical situations), VLCDs, are important medical instruments, properly supervised by a health professional who is qualified to do so. However, for someone with no underlying medical condition wishing to lose weight for the long term, I would not recommend them.

I'd say now is a good time for me to mention an important principle that I always ask my clients to keep in mind. I'll recount this by way of an encounter with Steve, aged about forty-five (a lovely fellow, a carpet fitter).

Me: "Hi, Steve, nice to see you. How've you got on this week?"

Steve: "Great, I've had a really positive week. I got up at 5.30am every morning and did a 40-minute run!"

Me: "What the Dickens did you do that for?"

Steve: "To help me lose weight. I thought you'd be pleased!"

Me: "Steve, I really do admire your enthusiasm and determination, but I need to ask you an important question and you need to think about the answer. Is it realistic that to control your weight you'll get up every morning at 5.30 for the rest of your life and run for 40 minutes?"

Steve: "Probably not, but I might do some running."

Me: "Which is why I would have been thrilled if you'd said, I'm taking up running, I've been out twice this week."

The key to permanent weight loss is through change. Before you make any change aimed at weight loss, ask yourself the question that I asked Steve: "Is it realistic that I will maintain this change for the rest of my life in order to help control my weight?" If the answer is probably no, think of something else.

Quacks in the business

One of the challenges of being a weight-management practitioner is that you can get a lot of quacks in this field; the trick is to hope it doesn't rub off on you! I've done my best to call out and challenge the quacks, as in some small way it probably helps to legitimise what is a genuine and sincere profession; needed more today than ever before. I hope that many more people will consider becoming qualified weight-management practitioners.

If you are unfortunate enough to stumble across a quackers marketing site, it won't be too long before you are reading something along the lines of: "Doctors just want you to be sick so that they can further their profession, and big pharma just want to make millions from selling you drugs that you don't need." What the quacks don't say, but should, is: "Instead of that, buy my supplements or invest in my 'wellness guru' programme."

Health gurus – enter the wellness-sphere

Q: What do you call alternative medicine that has been proven to work?

A: Medicine

I really love health gurus; don't they just make life worth living! I had so much fun researching this section that I almost took to drinking dried lizard soup and undergoing rebirthing therapy. Lifestyle or health gurus position themselves at odds with medical experts, their charismatic mystique blended with pseudo-science alludes to secret or sacred information that cannot be accessed through modern medicine: "We know the things that they, the establishment, don't want you to know". Their treatments, which go from the slightly potty but mostly innocuous, to the totally crazy and downright dangerous, are out there, and you might be surprised how widespread they are. In March 2018, it was reported that a fifty-five-year-old Spanish woman died after undergoing what I'm told is all the rage at the moment – bee sting therapy. While some swear by it, I say don't get stung by this craze!

Wellness entrepreneurs marketing themselves as 'therapists', who just happen to be fanatical about banging a huge gong near your affected parts or placing lit candles in your ear, will relieve you of a handsome sum for the privilege, but other than that, no harm done (unless the candle falls out onto the oily towel). But you need to be wary of some of the more dangerous practices and stay shy of them like you would avoid having your skull drilled (trepanning). Which just happens to be promoted on several websites for "do it yourself" skull drilling surgery.

Peter Halvorson, who runs the International Trepanation Advocacy Group (AKA the lunatics' convention) and who drilled a hole in his own head in 1972, claims that the 9mm-wide hole increased his metabolism and got rid of his depression. Incredulously, people believe this madness, and several years ago, a *British Medical Journal* article reported the case of a Gloucestershire woman who drilled a 20mm diameter hole in her own thick skull. Miraculously, she survived, but I'm told she turned down the marketing opportunity offered to her by Black and Decker.

You might however be taken by a bit of snake massage therapy using constricting serpents to soothe those now rapidly tensioning muscles. Or keep an eye out for the Ear Seed Kit (for sexual wellness) sold on Goop – they are an absolute steal at just $45. Advocates of cryotherapy swear that stepping into a chamber chilled to minus 120 degrees Fahrenheit shocks your system, sending out a jolt of hormones that will have you running 100m faster than Usain Bolt. The only shock you are likely to get though is when they hand you the bill.

Herbal therapies for weight loss are never far from the classified ads in the tabloid press, presumably aimed at those people that have plenty of cash about their person but appear to have misplaced their senses. A few of the current gems doing the rounds include clean berberine; glucomannan and chromium; ashwagandha; chitosan; and chromium picolinate (I've no idea either!). Now, I have to say that I am a big fan of herbs, but normally this is when they are infused into a hearty casserole. In my opinion, relying on herbal treatments to lose weight is the financial equivalent of hoping to pay off real liabilities using imaginary assets, a truly ruinous situation.

Also trending currently is urine therapy, and it appears there is almost no ailment that a decent swig of your own liquid waste won't cure. Of course, the advocates of this repulsive practice are all nutters, amply demonstrated by Christopher Key, of the anti-vax website 'Vaccine Police', who swears that drinking your own urine is more efficacious than the Covid-19 vaccines – why let the truth get in the way of a good story?

Will Blunderfield, wannabe pop star, now known as the Wild Naked Man, is also a big fan of taking the piss, and has added his own quaint variation. If you are male, then you can get enhanced benefits by capturing some semen and mixing it in before you slurp this yummy elixir down the hatch. As well as quaffing his own body fluids, Will offers other great therapies, and frankly you'd be mad not to cough up the $999 for one of his semen-retention courses, or enrol for some sexual kung fu! Or, for just $360 each month, you could join the online nutrition programme 'Ultimate Lifestyle Transformation', which will provide you with some shakes and an assortment of catchy-sounding nutritional supplementary tat.

Will is a genuine health philanthropist, a real friend of humanity, but sadly he lives in fear of the predatory capitalist structure, which, as I'm sure you will appreciate: "Cuts us off from our juiciness and full power". However, despite his devotion to Bikram yoga, I think the avaricious cat was out of the holistic bag when he recently said: "When you feel juicy in your own skin, that's when the record deals come, that's when the money comes!"

Nonetheless, I think I'm going to give this urine therapy lark a go, but I'll just make a couple of minor modifications. I'll probably switch the urine for a kiwi and banana smoothie and the spermatozoa for a cod-liver oil capsule. The main thing, though, is that I'm sticking with the core principle of having a nutritious and tasty start to the day. I've always thought that tweaking someone else's pioneering health innovation to suit yourself is the way to go.

Detoxing

A real favourite of mine is the detox. Why would you bother with a healthy diet, plenty of tap water, and a spot of brisk walking, when you could enter the sacred temple of the commercial detox. Yes, that's you lot I'm talking to, the unclean eaters, shame on you! You ought to be mulling over a four-day raw juice cleanse, or a commercial tea-tox for breakfast lunch and dinner. Better still, I suggest you follow the example of Freelee the Banana Girl, who reportedly eats fifteen bananas, forty pieces of fruit and a couple of kilograms of potatoes every day, which she claims has cured her weight issues, depression, irritable bowel syndrome, chronic fatigue, poor digestion and acne (obviously, not her madness though). Well, I'd say she really is bananas, as this amount of potassium is enough to give a horse tachycardia, and if her number twos are normal, then it's nothing short of a medical miracle.

While I'm at it, let's have a look at some of the most bonkers weight-loss products out there now. A good place to start is the fat-burner keto gummies that are currently flooding the internet. Apparently, they will stimulate a metabolic shift from carb dependence, improve endurance, weight management, cardiovascular and digestive health, enhance mental clarity and focus, and detox and clean you. While some products offer a measly 2000mg of active ingredient (presumably ketones), the eye-catching 25 million mg looks like great value (particularly if you are plotting your own departure). Not bad for what is essentially apple vinegar and pectin, and, at £36 per jar, it's a real snip!

The stomach 'Lipo' fat burn machine destroys those nasty adipocytes without inflicting any damage or harm on your body whatsoever. What can I say, other than dash out and get one before they are all gone! If you've completely lost your marbles, you could try the succinctly named 'Portable lymphatic drainage slimming botas pressure compression preso-therapy machine'. Or how about the 'Fat freezing system easy fat loss with cold body sculpting wrap belt'? Both available at the annual masochists and self-harm Expo.

I love all these great products, and to cash in on the action I'm set to market my very own guaranteed weight-loss gizmo. This brilliant idea was spawned in the Royal Oak one Saturday night following a substantive dose of ethanol. It involves an oral contraption that sits between the teeth rather like a mechanical brace. This clever gadget can measure calories consumed and each month you simply set your preferred 30-day daily calorie consumption limit on your smartphone, and when your daily limit is reached, SLAM! You can up your calorie allowance for weekend binges and reduce for frugal Mondays. Please send your application for shares in this winning idea to my publisher (strictly no time wasters!).

Understanding weight gain

The myths and misinformation surrounding weight, nutrition, dieting and all things related are legendary. My favourite so far: "My neighbour says if I eat too little I'll put on weight". To set you on the right course, I'd like to take an in-depth look at the causes of weight gain and dispel some of the daft notions that are out there.

The cause of an expanding waistline appears obvious; calorie intake exceeds energy expenditure, leading to energy surplus. However, this incontrovertible law of human biology belies the intricacies involved. In fact, the causes of excess weight are complex and multi-factorial: psychological, physiological, neurological, endocrinological, behavioural, environmental, nutritional, genetic, social, and, less frequently, pathological or drug related. The interplay between these contributors is extremely complex and is further convoluted by the fact that people respond differently to calorie consumption, environmental variables, and, of course, behavioural attitudes to change. Therefore, recognising the unique treatment needs of everyone seems sensible, as the one-size-fits-all approach has long been discredited, and failing to acknowledge these variations is perhaps one of the reasons that treatments are so frequently ineffective.

Even the differences between men and women regarding weight loss needs to be acknowledged. For instance, men who attempt weight loss are more likely than women to increase exercise and eat less fat, while women are more likely to join weight-loss programmes, take prescription diet pills, and follow special diets. Women tend to eat more calorie-dense foods even though they report the desire to eat healthier more than men[30], and men are also more likely to lose and maintain weight loss than women following a programme[31]. There is a suggestion that many women suffer diet burnout and have become accustomed to the merry-go-round of weight loss and weight regain in the classically described yoyo diet cycle, whereas, for men, weight loss is perhaps more of a new experience.

While on the little-discussed theme of men and weight loss, it is apparent that many men appear reluctant to engage with dietary interventions for weight loss. Often men will attribute their weight to external factors such as the food industry or spouses who are 'in control' of food and cooking. Sometimes entrenched eating practices and engrained habits can make change difficult for men, bringing significant risk of becoming 'set in our ways', which is a banker for physical and psychological deterioration. Moreover, overweight men, like women, feel despondent and experience the shame and embarrassment brought on when they internalise weight stigma. This leads to low self-worth and a downward spiral of low self-confidence, and an erosion of the essential constituent required to bring about change – self-efficacy.

The good news is that, in my experience, when men do engage in weight management, their outcomes are very good, and while men can often be cited as the barrier to dietary change in a family, if they are engaged in the educational aspect of nutrition, they can often become a driving force for change in the household. One potential reason for this is that weight-loss services are primarily run by women (and perhaps for women), which is ironic, considering more men are overweight than women. I would urge commissioners of weight-management services to also consider commissioning services that cater for men-only groups.

I say this because results obtained from the FitFans weight-management service for men, designed from the bottom up and rolled out to thousands of men by my great friend (and by far the most competent and innovative weight-management practitioner I have encountered) Rob Ward, taught us that, if you design and implement a service specifically for men based upon physical activity with straightforward healthy-eating messages, and wrap it up with a sporting theme, then, while you won't catch every male, you will catch the majority, and the ones you will engage are likely to be the target audience you are seeking. The FitFans programme is the best example of a men's weight-loss service I have ever come across. Rob, you are a weight-management legend and a men's health hero.

Is it calories in, or calories out?

Over the years, there has been a lot of debate about which is the most influential contributor to weight gain; is it poor diet, or physical inactivity (calories in or calories out)? This discussion is now concluded, and the consensus from the scientific community is that, while the couch potato lifestyle is problematic, the primary reason for the obesity epidemic is diet. I agree one hundred percent (but I happen to also believe that trying to solve weight problems using diet alone is a fundamentally flawed strategy, the reasons for which I cover in the section on physical activity). For now, suffice it to say that if you are having difficulty with your weight, the main cause is almost certain to be your diet.

Despite the individual complexity of weight gain, there are some common drivers of the obesity pandemic, primarily the increasing consumption of highly processed, energy-dense, nutrient-poor CRAP products. The resulting calorie overload is compounded by a marked reduction in physical activity, reflecting profound changes in society and in behavioural patterns of communities over recent decades. This is the obesogenic environment, and, for the individual, it sets up a self-sustaining circuit, where obesity and unhealthy lifestyles are interwoven with increased demand and consumption of CRAP foods alongside the accompanying lethargy created by such a lifestyle. It is this obesogenic cocktail that creates the downward spiral into the inescapable incarceration of established obesity in which many people feel trapped.

Our way of life has changed dramatically in recent years. We drive more, move less, consume more food made by others than by ourselves, we have most things delivered to our door and our phones are never far from our fists. This convenience helps us to cope with the demands of our stressed, hurried, information-overloaded and competitive lives. Edible CRAP products are available, palatable and affordable, and marketed to encourage us to eat more. As urbanisation is the order of the day, diets high in fresh, fibrous, water-based plant foods, become more expensive and give way to cheaper options with longer shelf lives, containing more fats and sugars (macro-nutrients) and fewer vitamins, minerals and phytochemicals (antioxidant micro-nutrients from plants). A predictable outcome of the Global Nutrition Transition.

Most daily physical activity has been lost from our lives in pursuit of convenience and time efficiency. Remote controls, escalators, washing machines, dishwashers, power tools and gadgets of every conceivable form, take the effort out of almost everything that we do. I often speculated with my students that, if I could invent a 'duvet cover fitting machine', I could sail off into the sunset. As a consequence of these changes, we are now supposedly half as active as our parents were, and our children are less active than we were at their age. According to one study, Britons are now around 600kcals per day less active than we were only forty years ago, which is the equivalent of running a marathon every four days!

Set point theory

Set point theory[32] states that each of us has a genetically pre-programmed set weight point that our bodies would prefer to maintain (under normal environmental circumstances). It can and does alter, but all things being even, our body will try to maintain a genetically programmed preference. For simplicity, let's consider that our total body weight represents either fat mass or lean mass. Our lean mass (muscles, organs, bones etc.) is rigorously defended, and any deviations brought about, such as a reduction through famine or an increase through heavy weight training, will spring back to 'set' levels and the 'normal' environment is resumed. This is because the size and number of organ, intestine, bone and muscle cells etc. are strictly controlled as determined from the moment of conception.

Fat mass, however, is far less stringently controlled, and like any fuel reserve, needs to be able to fill or empty. For this reason, fat cells are happy to grow; they can expand 100 times from the size they were created, and as you've no doubt experienced, they will grow quickly under the right circumstances, leading body weight to drift away from the 'preferred' value. Any weight lost quickly 'rebounds' after temporary fasting, though, annoyingly, weight gained is less inclined to 'spring' back following feasting. Some people suggest that, if weight gain is maintained long term, it becomes established, perhaps even re-setting the 'set point' at a higher value. If this theory of weight progression is correct, it underpins the reality for many people, which is the upwards-only ratcheting of 'set' weight through the life course.

Proof of this came in 2000, when a study overfed rats a high-fat, high-sugar diet to the point of obesity, and then put them on a diet returning them back to their previous healthy weight. What happened then was a relatively rapid return to the obese state once the rats were allowed free access to almost any diet (healthy or unhealthy). The researchers unearthed changes in neuroendocrine function before, during and after restriction, suggesting that the brain may be the determinant of the higher body weight set point[33]. Therefore, the activation of this coordinated response (to favour upward-only return to the highest previous weight) supports the view that as weight increases, so too does the body's 'set point', and efforts to reduce weight below this new point are now, as before, vigorously resisted.

Body fat and distribution

Fat is stored in specialist cells called adipocytes, bound together and collectively known as adipose tissue (or, more precisely these days, the adipose organ). Adipocytes safely hold fat (lipid) and release it when there is an energy requirement. The preferred storage site is just below the skin, known as subcutaneous or peripheral storage. This enables significant amounts of fat to be stored over a large surface area, thus avoiding one big bump (think camel), which would create mobility and agility issues, making tight plumbing jobs trickier. As well as being a vast energy reserve, subcutaneous fat is an important and effective insulator from the cold, which is why thinner people feel the cold more readily. It's also why people with more body fat find exercising in warmer temperatures more difficult, as the heat from their muscles can't readily escape, and internal temperature quickly soars.

Subcutaneous fat cells are a safe vault for lipids, which, if allowed to linger in the blood, can cause havoc. But under continuous calorie overload, fat cells in the periphery become full, and so the body has no alternative but to direct fat away from the 'safe' confines of the subcutaneous storage sites, and instead send it to the ever so slightly different fat cells located in the abdomen. This produces camel-esque features, but around the girth. This kind of waist expansion is referred to as visceral fat (viscera meaning gut organs) and it signals fat infiltration of the vital organs and vascular system (known as ectopic fats), where it may affect the structure and function of each organ prompting illnesses such as cardiovascular disease, fatty liver, fatty pancreas and T2D.

The good news is that visceral and ectopic fat deposits respond to weight loss more readily than peripheral fat stores, presumably because the body does not want fat in these places, and therefore gets rid of it first (if you worked in a warehouse, you would refer to this principle as LIFO – last in first out). Furthermore, this is why small amounts of weight loss offer exponential health benefits, because the weight initially comes from the most dangerous places first. But the only way the body can do this is when you burn more calories than you consume for a prolonged period. As such, a reduction in waist circumference is an excellent health aspiration for any weight-loss programme, as any decrease greatly reduces metabolic disease risk.

Body shapes vary markedly, and men and women tend to have different patterns of weight, with men being described as apples and women pears. The primary difference in these gender-related patterns is determined by the sex hormones oestrogen and testosterone, as oestrogen tends to favour peripheral shunt, moving fats to the extremities, whereas testosterone seems to favour central adiposity. Forty years ago (before the advent of widescale obesity), if smoking was taken out of the equation, visceral weight appeared to be the main difference explaining the disproportionate numbers of men succumbing to cardiovascular disease.

Puberty and menopause are key times for changes in body fat accumulation and distribution, mediated in women by oestrogen production. Puberty signals the change from the lean, pre-pubescent figure, to a more rounded and curvaceous shape, through an increase in fat storage around the hips, buttocks and breasts. Oestrogen causes an increase in the fat-storing enzyme lipoprotein lipase, instructing fat cells to take up more fat in circulation and to store it in specific subcutaneous sites. This movement of fat to the extremities ('peripheral shunt') has some advantages in protecting women from the harmful build-up of intra-abdominal fat. Of course, it keeps the waist slimmer during the fertile years, but, at menopause, when oestrogen falls away, so too does the effect of peripheral shunt. At this, many women would complain to me that, since the menopause, they had noticed they had developed a 'tummy' for the first time.

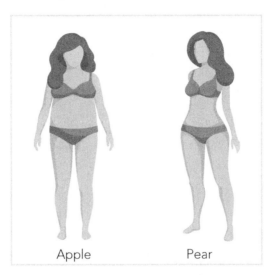

Apple   Pear

Genetics also play an important role in body-fat distribution, with families following discernible similarities in body shape. There are also clear differences in how people interpret body shapes, with some individuals and cultures embracing a corpulent body while others reject it. This reminds me of a frequent request I'd get from clients requiring 'spot fat reduction' (targeting one area of body fat while leaving others intact). "How do I get rid of this big butt, belly or bingo wings?" they would ask. Well, I'm afraid the truth is that you can't spot reduce; when you lose weight, where the fat loss comes from is in the hands of the mythical God Obesius.

Why liposuction doesn't work

Fat cells can trigger their own death (apoptosis) which is reserved for conditions such as a life-threatening famine. In such situations, when energy restriction threatens life, the (empty) fat cells are sacrificed, allowing other tissues to use the small amount of energy that the adipose cell may have been using. The secondary benefit is that the body can scavage the constituent components of the cell to reuse, collectively offering a slightly increased chance of survival. At this life-and-death stage, it is all about fine margins, and in such a precarious situation, you really are drinking in the last chance saloon.

No one knows how many millions of people have faced this terrible fate since time immemorial, some will have perished, and some will have survived. For the lucky ones that did make it and endured, albeit with many fewer fat cells, the body has another trick up its sleeve. It knows that when (if) the good times come again, it can repopulate its fat cells from an abundant supply of undifferentiated fibroblasts that reside around the body. These pre-curser cells change to form new adipocytes and reconstruct the energy reservoir needed for life. One interesting aspect of this is that, remarkably, when the fat cells return, they repopulate to the exact previous number, and nobody has any idea how the body does this – how does it remember?

Perhaps you can recall Birhan Woldu, the Ethiopian girl saved from starvation by the 1985 Live Aid project. As a child, Birhan was found by a Canadian camera crew at a feeding station in northern Ethiopia moments from death by starvation. She was saved. Twenty-three years later, at Live8, she appeared on stage with Bob Geldof as a healthy-weight adult. Her body had clearly repopulated those fat cells that had surely self-destructed in that terrible famine. Therefore, if you hoover out your fat cells, they will just come back if you keep on eating, which is why liposuction was abandoned as a weight loss therapy.

Homeostasis

When environmental changes occur or when our bodies need to adapt to shifting conditions, our biological systems must quickly and efficiently respond, swinging across a range of parameters to cater for prevailing needs. It is equally important that when conditions return to normal, the system can then restore itself to a steady state, thus re-establishing the symmetry required for optimum performance. This is homeostasis, the self-regulatory systems, where dynamic equilibrium ensures uniform conditions prevail, which in turn safeguards our resources and maintains balance and coherence.

Homeostasis operates to maintain balance over many systems including hydration, oxygenation, pH, body temperature, ion and saline concentrations, blood sugar and blood pressure. When we are too hot, we sweat, and heat is carried away from the body in the evaporating water. When we are too cold, we shiver, and since 75% of muscle energy is released as heat, this acts to warm us up. These are dynamic processes and continue to work night and day to ensure our bodies maintain optimum operating conditions without us having to think about them most of the time. But disruptions in homeostatic balance appear to be a feature of weight gain.

As a weight-loss practitioner, it soon became apparent to me that the more overweight a person became, the more difficult sustained weight loss was for them. For many (thin) people this may sound counterintuitive, imagining that weight must be easier to lose if you have more of it. However, the reality is that as weight takes a grip, a combination of physiological, biological, and psychological adaptations occur, leading to disruptions to homeostasis. Consequently, when energy input through food increases, rather than return the body to a previous, steady weight, the weight-induced changes bestowed on the individual appear to have the opposite effect and encourage further weight gain.

This is known as the 'asymmetry of appetite', and while we automatically eat more following weight loss, there appears to be no reverse side of the coin – we don't spontaneously eat less when energy needs are low, explaining why it is so easy to put weight on and so difficult to take it off. We must eat to survive, and hunger is very powerful, but satiety cues are weak and easily overridden by external factors such as the sight or taste of food. A practical example is the contrast between the difficulties of skipping a meal, compared to the ease of succumbing to a dessert or cheese board even when satiated.

If anyone required proof of the difficulty of losing weight once a certain threshold has been crossed, a 2015 study published in the *American Journal of Public Health*, looked at the probability of people living with obesity returning to a normal weight over the next nine years[34]. Their results make for bleak reading for would-be dieters. Not only were the chances for people living with obesity very low, but as people became heavier, their prospects of acquiring a healthy weight diminished exponentially.

Prospect of returning to a healthy weight		
	Men	Women
BMI >30	1 in 210	1 in 124
BMI >40	1 in 1,290	1 in 677

Some of the earliest work on this theme came from the eminent Boyd Swinburn, who, in 2004, published his paper 'The runaway weight gain train: too many accelerators, not enough brakes'[35]. His paper describes how, once started, weight gain is difficult to stop. He noted that the accelerators of weight gain are powerful, but the brakes are weak, postulating that the strongest brakes are psychological such as the social penalties of excess weight, the discomfort and reduced quality of life, and the disease threat associated with obesity. The physiological brakes are the increased basal metabolic rate of a bigger person and the increased leptin concentrations in circulation because of larger and more numerous fat cells.

Swinburn says: "While all these brakes seem to be substantive, they are clearly not strong enough to halt the increasing momentum of the weight gain train". He describes the "downhill obesogenic slope" compounded by key accelerators which you will recognise as the vicious cycles mentioned throughout this book. He notes that this is one train ride that children will definitely not want to take.

Humans possess highly evolved and exquisitely tuned appetite mechanisms that can cater for all manner of calorie variability. If we eat the foods we are supposed to eat, our bodies will have no problem regulating weight, just as it has no problem regulating our body temperature in summer or in winter. However, when you start consuming things that are ten times more energy dense than you were designed to eat, the system becomes overwhelmed. Not only is this the case for humans, but obesity affects other domesticated animals that we feed with foods they were never meant to eat – weasels don't become obese, even amid a plague of mice.

Hunger hormones and energy management

Understanding the biology of hunger and how it governs our dietary habits will help you to manage appetite and hunger-related challenges, an inevitable requirement of weight management. When considering appetite, the most important contributor is the drive to eat. This is independent of dietary habits, food preferences and food reward, which are heavily influenced by culture and the environment. The drive to eat arises from the biological requirement to keep vital organs functioning and other energy requirements. Physical activity also contributes to the drive to eat, but the immediate need is more weakly felt, which is rational from an evolutionary perspective. In fact, in the short term, physical activity (particularly vigorous activity) switches off hunger, presumably to keep you hunting and gathering until successful.

Let's start by considering the four primary appetite and energy balance hormones: leptin (signals satiety); ghrelin (drives hunger); insulin (stores nutrients); glucagon (releases nutrients). Hormones are chemical messengers that are released from organs and glands around the body and tell different cells what to do, at what rate, and how long to do it for. Hormones tend to work in concert, which is to say, one is responsible for instructing a cell to act in one direction, while an opposing hormone notifies the cell to do the opposite as and when required. This is the principle of homeostasis. It is when hormones become imbalanced that problems arise.

Leptin

Leptin, from the Greek *leptos* meaning thin, was discovered in 1994 and is a hormone released exclusively from fat cells. Leptin's main role is to control feeding by acting on the hypothalamic receptors in the brain to induce satiety. In case you have any doubt as to the power of leptin to suppress appetite, I have previously read about a leptin-deficient child whose parents restricted his food intake in a desperate attempt to control his weight. What was reported is that the child ate the family goldfish!

Concentrations of leptin in the blood are directly proportional to fat mass, effectively informing the brain of the total volume of energy reserves within the body at any given time; for how else would the brain know? Therefore, leptin is the body's background appetite suppressant, constant and relative to our current levels of fat mass. As fat mass increases, then so too does the level of leptin in circulation which should dampen appetite, returning

65

body fat levels to equilibrium. If fat mass becomes low, so too do leptin concentrations and as leptin diminishes, appetite dramatically increases. A classic negative feedback homeostatic system.

Overweight people have more body fat, therefore they have more circulating leptin. A logical enquiry therefore would be, as they have more appetite suppressant, how come they are overweight? The answer is probably leptin resistance, postulated as a central feature of obesity and caused by too much leptin exposure, unsurprisingly known as 'leptin-induced leptin resistance'. Leptin targets cells within the hypothalamus in the brain, and possible malfunction of the hormone receptors on these cells are the cause of the resistance. Once the leptin feedback system malfunctions, fat cells can no longer signal to the brain to stop eating – leptin is knocking, but the cerebral response is: "Talk to the belly, the brain isn't listening!" Therefore, the experimental therapy of giving overweight people more leptin (to great expectations) was doomed before it began.

It appears that years of excess weight (and thus excess leptin) overwhelms and blunts the leptin receptors in the hypothalamus. This, it is argued, is no different to years of excess insulin secretion, which does the same to receptors on target cells designed to enable glucose to enter, the cause of T2B. Therefore, perhaps leptin resistance is no different to insulin resistance in its cause. Very recently, evidence is emerging that this is the case and studies in animals and humans show that diets high in fat, carbohydrates, fructose and sucrose are drivers of leptin resistance[36]. Weight gain therefore leads to leptin resistance and leptin resistance inevitably leads to further weight gain, due to constantly elevated hunger, another demoralising vicious cycle.

If you've been overweight for some time now, you'd be excused for thinking that climbing the Eiger is starting to look more achievable than long-term weight loss! The previous section may have led you to a question that I have been asked dozens of times by my clients: "If, because of my weight, I've become leptin resistant, then if I lose the weight, will I become leptin sensitive?" After twenty-five years, much research and the anecdotal evidence of hundreds of clients, my answer remains the same: "Well, it works for insulin resistance and my guess is it will work for leptin resistance, too."

In 2020, researchers put forward a theory about how people can become re-sensitised to leptin by reducing circulating leptin, which, they say, triggers a high degree of leptin sensitisation and improves leptin action[37]. The procedure for this involves sustained weight loss: lose weight, lower leptin (increase hunger temporarily), improve leptin sensitivity, normalise appetite, lower chances of weight regain – a heartening virtuous circle. Maybe my twenty-five-year hunch was right all along! There are other things that you can do to favourably shift your hunger hormone balance. Studies show that fish oil and reducing diet-induced inflammation (less CRAP) may also help reverse leptin resistance. Better sleep is also known to be beneficial.

Ghrelin

The opposing hormone to leptin is ghrelin. Produced mainly in the gut, ghrelin is a potent stimulus to feeding and crosses the blood-brain barrier, targeting the hypothalamus, where it signals to the brain that you are hungry. Ghrelin levels increase during fasting (peaking after twenty-four hours) when appetite will be at its greatest. Ghrelin levels take thirty minutes after eating to dissipate, which is why you need to allow time after your meal to feel fully satiated.

The illustration below shows the peaks and troughs in circulating ghrelin relative to mealtimes. Notice how ghrelin (the black line) builds gradually between meals and then drops dramatically following feeding. As ghrelin starts to peak, this signals to the brain that you are hungry. After feeding ghrelin plummets and leptin (the grey line) once again becomes the dominant hormone signalling to the brain that you are full . The grey line represents your leptin sensitivity; above the line represents hunger, below, satiety. The lower the grey line (leptin sensitivity) the more you will eat.

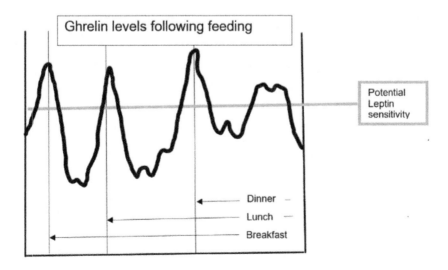

Insulin

Insulin is intrinsically linked to feeding and metabolism. It is released following the consumption of food and is particularly attuned to sugar or carbohydrate intake. Insulin has long been associated with weight gain as it is known to promote the storage of fats and sugars. Insulin is secreted from the pancreas and, once in circulation, instructs muscle and fat cells to take up nutrients, also directing the liver to stop releasing sugars into the blood (because there is a surplus from food).

Glucagon

Glucagon is the opposing hormone to insulin, reversing its effects. It is secreted from the pancreas when blood-sugar levels fall too low, and acts to raise blood glucose levels by stimulating the liver to release glucose, thus maintaining equilibrium.

Hormone summary

Collectively, these hormones and the corresponding appetite networks in the brain represent an exquisite energy-management system that has regulated human weight for millennia. An 80kg active male who is weight stable, will burn around one million calories in a year. Without even thinking about it, he will eat one million calories; it is an impeccable system of wonder. It functions perfectly in all mammals, too (hibernating animals such as bears can become very fat, but this is necessary to get them through half a year without food).

At this point, I'd desperately like to be able to write something clever and totally captivating about these hormones, the sort of thing that you are likely to read from trending articles about 'hormone balancing' or the highly implausible 'bio-identical HRT'. Instead, I can only tell you that if you want these four hormones to work the way they were intended, to manage energy balance and regulate your weight, then you need to stop overwhelming your system with calories!

Dietary determinants of weight gain

"One cause, which made it necessary to study the art of restoring lost health, was the great difference to be observed between the diet of the healthy and that of the sick."

Hippocrates, 400 BC

Too many fats, too many carbs, too much protein?

The controversy over the macronutrient balance of our diets has rumbled on for years. What is the optimum balance of fats, carbohydrate and protein? Is there a human optimum, or is it individual to each of us? Do some people better 'tolerate' more carbohydrate than others, for instance? Is it that our genes have evolved around our traditional diet and any deviation from this causes problems? Is it that the current dietary advice is wrong? Do people listen to dietary advice in any case?

What is the current advice?

Here it is for the UK, launched as the 'Balance of Good Health' in 1994, it was updated in 2007 and renamed the 'Eatwell plate'. In 2006, it underwent another (cosmetic) update and is now called the 'Eatwell Guide' (EG).

The idea is that, rather than lots of wordy information about what to eat and what to avoid, people can look at a simple visual depiction of what is considered a balanced diet. I like this idea. Many people are not fans of the EG, with its most vociferous critics stating their opposition to the amount of starchy carbohydrates depicted. I agree that it is not perfect, nothing ever is, but my view is that if people adopted the EG wholesale, we would have considerably less chronic disease, less obesity and less environmental carnage.

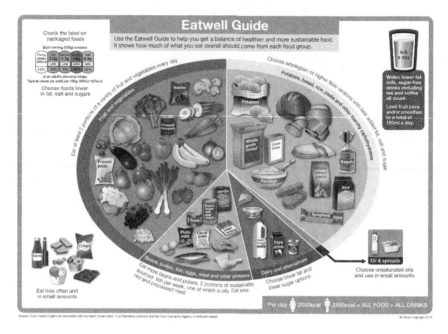

The problem, of course, is that people aren't adopting it. If you don't believe me, go to your local supermarket (not M&S or Waitrose, but Asda, Morrisons, Lidl or Aldi) and spend a couple of hours looking at people's shopping trolleys as they checkout. Pay particular attention to those with children.

The US has gone for a more basic version of dietary advice, that looks like a complete waste of time to me. In any case, dietary advice in the US has been hijacked by 'Big Food', designed in my view to keep multinational companies earning vast profits rather than helping people to stay well, which is why they are suffering the greatest obesity epidemic of all.

Calories consumed

In terms of overall calories consumed, according to data published by the UN Food and Agriculture Organization (www.fao.org), all major regions of the Earth have increased food consumption in the period 1961 to 2018.

Most individuals on the planet are now eating more than people were sixty years ago (some are eating considerably more). And this is our problem. **It is only when humans eat too many calories and too few micro-nutrients that our bodies can't adapt**. I am firmly of the view that the macronutrient debate is somewhat of a distraction. Eat real food, but not too much, and you will be a healthy weight and in the best shape to avoid chronic disease.

Regional calorie increases

Region	1961	2018	% calorie increase
Africa	1,993	2,604	+ 31%
Asia	1,783	2,833	+ 59%
High-income countries	2,862	3,432	+ 20%
North America	2,685	3,471	+ 29%
South America	2,327	3,084	+ 33%
China*	2,230	3,206	+ 44%

*data starts 1934

However, for those who say that government dietary advice is all wrong, I say you are missing the point. Telling people what to eat has never worked (for me or for governments). If the government want people to eat proper food, they must simply change the playing field so that healthy foods are cheap and the CRAP and UPFs are expensive (not the other way round, as it is currently). Anyone and everyone knows this.

Should we all go back to the palaeolithic diet?

Over tens of thousands of years of human migration from Africa, our diets have become extremely diverse, from those eating the high carbohydrate diets of central Africa, to the protein and fat combinations of those in the coldest regions on Earth. For instance, residents of central and east African countries such as Rwanda and Burundi, diets of around 80% carbohydrate (plantains, cassava, peas and maize) are common, with meat eaten in small quantities. Just thirty years ago, cardiovascular disease (still by far the biggest killer in developed countries) was very low in such countries. However, these people are also subject to the Global Nutrition Transition (GNT) and increased urbanisation and their diets and lifestyles are succumbing to the disease-promoting combinations of the developed world: more ultra-processed food, more calories, more smoking, less activity, and therefore more disease.

Icelandic people and those living in the coldest parts of the world eat the highest proportion of protein and fat. For example, a traditional Inuit would get approximately half their calories from fat, around a third from protein, with only a fifth coming from carbohydrates. The carbohydrates they do consume come mainly from the glycogen locked up in the muscles of the animals that they eat (it's tricky to grow corn at minus 40°C on an ice-bed). The Inuit people have been famed for their low cardiovascular disease risk, and indeed this has often been the basis for promoting a diet low in carbohydrate. Sadly, even the Inuit people are now succumbing to risk factors as more UPFs, smoking and obesity blight their lives[38].

Proponents of the palaeolithic diet (paleo, caveman, pre-modern etc.) suggest that we ought to eat only what was available before the development of farming and agriculture. There are several problems with this, primarily that there was probably no single definable paleo diet, as what you ate back then would depend on where you were living and what was available to you (as the above examples illustrate). To suggest a macronutrient composition of the caveman would be as absurd as proposing the protein content of the diet of a Martian. What's more, on a strict paleo diet, you couldn't be seen to be chomping on broccoli, cauliflower, sprouts, cabbage or kale, as they were all relatively recently cultivated by humans from one original species of plant (*Brassica Oleracea*). So, the paleo diet is very restrictive and probably eliminates many very beneficial foods. It is also wrong that the paleo diet is treated as the pinnacle of human feeding, as it is just one segment in our long, meandering and continuing evolutionary and dietary history. I accept that we are probably currently at the nadir, but as most people can't even adopt a reasonably balanced diet, what are the prospects of maintaining the paleo diet?

What all of this says to me is that homo sapiens are amazingly flexible and can adapt to enormously varied diets. This is due to several factors, including our ability to cook food, our diverse range of teeth, and our ability to digest a wide variety of nutrients. In addition to our physical flexibility, we also have a great deal of cultural adaptability. We are able to adopt new foods and learn new ways of eating, and share dietary information and ideas with others, allowing us to adapt to new environments and to new food sources. While it takes many generations to adapt to dramatic dietary changes (when we started drinking the milk of animals, for example, it took a while for the gene coding for lactase to remain switched on after infancy and thus allow us to digest it), given time, people do adapt to accommodate their available options. It is this flexibility that is a great strength of our species. Perhaps the time will come when we do define the optimum diet for humans, and we will all be in a position to be able to adopt it, but I'm not convinced about this either.

Proper food

As a youngster, I had the best dietary start anyone could wish for. We didn't have a lot of money, my dad worked as a hospital porter and my mum worked in factories during the day and in a fish and chip shop a few evenings a week. When it came to food, my mum was a visionary, way before her time, making sure that, with the limited resources at her disposal, we all ate proper food. Back in the 70s when I was growing up, food was still a functional commodity, you ate three times a day, and as food back then was mainly unprocessed, that was sufficient for all your needs. For all the time I was at home, I watched as my father ate a paltry breakfast, take a sandwich prepared by mum to work, then came home and had tea (us northerners refer to dinner as tea and lunch as dinner). I never once saw him have a snack other than a handful of nuts at Christmas time.

I remember so many occasions when I would ask my friends on the way home from school what they would be having for tea. They'd respond with delights such as sausage egg and chips, or omelette and chips or potato pie chips and beans (always chips – everyone had a deep fat fryer!). If only we could have sausage egg and chips, just once, I thought, I would drool at the prospect. Once home, "Mum, do you think we could have sausage egg and chips sometime?" "Stop your bleating and eat the lentil stew!"

Mum and Dad had an allotment, and they worked it hard to grow all manner of things. We think food is dear now, but in terms of proportion of available income, back then it was much more expensive, so growing your own was an important aspect of improving your quality of life. Mum would always have her nose in a book or magazine looking out for healthy recipes or foods that were supposed to be good for us, and that would be it – next thing we knew, it would appear on the table. "What's that?" we'd enquire cautiously. "It's black-eyed peas, with stewed onion and tomatoes, and it's good for you so eat it." "Bloody hell, just once, please, sausage egg and chips!"

And as if to get in on the nutritional torment, my dad would occasionally knock up one of his own delicacies. I particularly remember the occasion when he called us down from our room: "Lads, come and look what I've got". We flew downstairs to find my dad with something very large and heavy in his arms, bundled up in newspaper. "Come and see, come on, get closer." Then with our noses up to the newspaper, he quickly removed the paper to reveal an enormous pig's head, complete with eyes, hairy nose and huge teeth. "Whoooooaah, what the!?" We were off, but Dad was right behind us, chasing us up the stairs with the pig's head biting at our backsides.

Then he would set to work with his vast cooking pot. In went the head, water, herbs, carrots and liver... I think! This cauldron of cranial swine juice seemed to be boiling on the stove for an eternity. Eventually, Dad ceremoniously removed the now pristine skull and set about decanting the remainder into various pots and pans, some for eating as stew now, and some that he would press down into a solid paté in the yard using bricks to weigh the vessels down and press the liquid out. Once set, he would then cut off a chunk and eat it with some rock-hard oat biscuity-type things that tasted like something from the bottom of a bird's cage. This he proudly referred to as 'Stew 'n' Hard!' Hard to stomach, I'd say! It all went though, every last scrap. The dog got the skull bone and the ferrets got part of the snout. I didn't dare ask what happened to the eyeballs just in case they stayed in the meal (I suspect they did).

So, I grew up on proper food and I'm eternally grateful for the food wisdom of my mum, in particular, who, at a time when processed foods were pervasively sneaking into the daily diets of most Britons, stuck to her principles of feeding us kids properly. Thanks, Mum.

What are the healthiest of healthy foods (The Good)

An observational study published in the *British Medical Journal* looked at diet and mortality in around 11,000 vegetarians and other health-conscious people. The aim was to measure death and disease rates against the population norm, and variations within the 'healthy group' with a particular emphasis on healthy foods. They chose a range of foods to act as independent variables (wholemeal bread, bran cereals, nuts or dried fruit, fresh fruit, and raw salad), with the dependent variables being death (from all causes), ischaemic heart disease, stroke and cancer. The group was followed for 17 years. Unsurprisingly, this healthy cohort had a mortality about half that of the general population, and the daily consumption of fresh fruit provided a further 21% protection from death and disease within the 'healthy' group[39].

Vegans v vegetarians v omnivores

In a comparison of the diet quality of 1,475 participants who were either vegan, vegetarian, semi-vegetarian, pesco (fish) vegetarian and omnivores, researchers rated the health value of the diet using two established instruments (The Healthy Eating Index[40] and The Mediterranean Diet Score[41]). They determined that a vegan diet had the highest score, and an omnivorous the lowest. The 'more prudent diets' (vegetarians, semi-vegetarians, and pesco-vegetarians) were better in terms of nutrient quality than the omnivores. But it wasn't all roses for the vegans, as the researchers found that calcium intake was lowest for vegans and below national dietary recommendations (in the USA, where the study was conducted)[42]. It seems, therefore, that the diets listed as 'prudent' are nutritionally optimum for humans.

Mediterranean diet

The Mediterranean diet (MD) has long been associated with health and longevity and is the primary dietary advice to protect against vascular disease. It is rich in plants such as cereals, fruits, vegetables, legumes, tree nuts, seeds and olives, and primarily uses vegetable oils (unsaturated fats). It is a low-energy density and high dietary-fibre diet, with high to moderate intakes of fish, moderate eggs, poultry and dairy products, and low red meat.

Ultra-processed foods (The Bad)

This genre deserves brevity – the more ultra-processed foods (UPFs) you eat, the more overweight you will be, the more disease you will encounter, and the sooner you will die[43]. I considered leaving it at that but I thought, while true, perhaps it is not the most helpful message given in isolation. I therefore thought I'd provide a little more on what UPFs are, the risks involved and the ways that you can avoid them, just in case shuffling off this mortal coil prematurely is not in your grand plan. To illustrate the extent of the problem, more than half of daily energy intake is coming from processed and ultra-processed foods in most Western countries[44].

In a Spanish study[45], scientists followed 55,000 people and grouped them based upon UPF consumption (fewer than two UPFs/day or more than four per day). They found that the higher UPF eaters were 62% more likely to have died after ten years. In a similar French study[46] following 105,000 people, the low group got an average 7.5% of their energy from UPFs compared to 31% for the highest. After just five years, the high group had a 28% increased risk of cardiovascular disease compared to the low group. Both studies controlled for saturated fat, salt and sugar intake, thus it was not these elements found in ultra-processed foods that were responsible for their toxicity. A third study[43] observed over 100,000 people and concluded that a 10% increase in ultra-processed foods in the diet was associated with a 10% increase in the risk of cancer.

The concept of UPFs was first proposed by Brazilian nutrition researcher Carlos Monteiro in his paper published in 2009 in the journal *Public Health Nutrition*[47]. Since then, NOVA, a food classification organisation, has categorised foods according to the extent of their processing. The premise of their work is that it is not simply the nutrients contained in a food that matters, but what has happened to that food along the way. Their classifications follow the general principles laid out below:

Unprocessed foods are fresh and in their natural state. They are washed and presented with their vitamins, fibre and phytochemicals intact. **Minimally processed foods** are slightly altered, which may involve trimming of inedible parts, drying, roasting, freezing, pulping etc., primarily for convenience and storage purposes. Unprocessed or minimally processed foods would include all fresh foods such as fruit and vegetables, pulses, fresh meat and fish and eggs.

Processed foods are changed from their natural state usually by adding salt, oil, sugar, and other additives. They include canned foods and those in syrup, breads, cheese, pies and pastries. Most processed foods have two or three added ingredients.

Ultra-processed foods have more than five added ingredients (and often many more) and contain industrial substances and chemicals such as preservatives, colouring, sweeteners, emulsifiers, stabilisers and flavourings. UPFs are normally made primarily from extracts using fats, starches, added sugars and hydrogenated fats. Examples of these foods are processed and cured meats such as sausages, hot dogs and tinned meat, convenience foods, ice cream, soft drinks, most fast food, salty snacks, baked goods, frozen ready meals, cakes, sugary breakfast cereals, packet soups, puddings and crisps, and many more foods that come in packets and have a long shelf life.

If you are unsure, check out the label, and if there are a lot of ingredients in there that you don't recognise, think UPF!

Sugar (The Ugly)

The main body of work on sugar in this book is in the section about food addictions, because of the effect that sugar has on the brain. However, it would be careless of me to have a section entitled 'Dietary determinants of weight gain' without including a few words about sugar.

The most likely theory for our liking of sugar stems from the fact that it is a great source of energy, and if we gorge on it, then excess sugar can be converted into fat in the liver or in fat cells and stored for the long term. Millions of years ago, the apes that got the biggest brains were those that ate the most sugar, which is obvious considering sugar is the primary fuel of the brain. The smarter they got, the more they evolved to like sweeter or riper fruit because it had more sugar, thus bigger brains, and better survival prospects through being smarter and storing more calories.

A 2015 article in the *Journal of Public Health Nutrition* reported a positive association between sugar intake and BMI (the more sugar you eat, the heavier you are, and vice versa). However, this association was only apparent when the researchers analysed urine samples to establish exact sugar intake. When they referred to the seven-day food diaries, the sugar/weight correlation completely disappeared[48] – surprise, surprise!

If you are interested in further reading about sugar and its detrimental effects on the body, then the best source I can direct you to is a splendid book called *Fat Chance: The bitter truth about sugar*, written by the American Paediatric Endocrinologist Robert Lustig[49]. In this entertaining and enlightening tome, you'll learn all that is required to change your path with respect to the sweet stuff. As Lustig says, "Your fat is not your fate, provided you don't surrender".

I would say that *Fat Chance* is a must-read for all those interested in how our food has got into the state it has, and how this is impacting our lives, the planet, and our health. The politics and economic aspects of food production and distribution are fascinating. In terms of impact, this book is up there with *Fast Food Nation* by Eric Schlosser[50], which twenty years after its publication, is perhaps more relevant today than it was back then – the mark of a real visionary. I'd read this, too, if I were you.

While I thoroughly recommend reading *Fat Chance*, I do take issue with Lustig's insistence that weight is nothing to do with personal responsibility, with all the culpability sitting with governments and corporations. People do make food choices, and while some people's choices are limited because of their circumstances, we still have choice (for ourselves or for our children). Despite their difficult circumstances, some people still manage to make good food and lifestyle choices. To totally disassociate our ability to choose from health outcomes seems bizarre to me. Lustig also says that "Weight loss is next to impossible". Now, while I know that long-term weight loss is not easy, my experiences tell me that the right approach at the right time makes weight loss probable.

Sugar-sweetened beverages (SSBs)

Sugary drinks have always been out there in a league of their own in terms of their effect on weight, but it is not one hundred percent established how this effect occurs. There are two most likely reasons. One is the compelling evidence for the weak satiety effect of calories that accompany drinks. This means there is little or no compensation made for the energy taken in via drinks – you could drink 1,000 kcals in sugary drinks and it would not impact your next meal. The other mechanism involves the role of hedonic effects of sugars on the regulation and cognitive control of food reward. The principal idea behind this theory is that consuming concentrated forms of sugar in this way teaches the brain to want more. Either theory is likely to be correct, and probably both have an independent effect on promoting weight gain.

In terms of the relationship between SSBs and weight, from 1997, soft drink consumption increased globally from 9.5 gallons per person per year to 11.4 gallons thirteen years later, and this was a significant contributor to the increase in obesity and diabetes worldwide[51]. One 330ml can of cola contains around 35g of free sugar and the current UK recommendations for daily consumption of free sugars for adults is 30g/day. Children aged seven to ten should have no more than 24g per day and those aged four to six should have no more than 19g per day[52]. If you consider these numbers, then the sugar factor alone explains much of the disease burden of the modern world.

One public health initiative that seems to be gaining momentum is the sugar tax. Evidence to date shows that when applied to SSBs, such a tax does reduce consumption and also leads to the reformulation of drinks to lower sugar content, which has a positive impact on obesity levels – one of the only strategies to show an effect on population obesity[53]. In Spain, researchers looked at the popularity of such policies and found that two-thirds of people supported a sugar tax, but that this support was lower in people that ate the most sugar, as well as with groups that hold anti-establishment ideologies[54]. More scientists are now pressing their governments to adopt taxation as an evidenced method to improve the health of their citizens. Bravo!

In developed countries, the volume of SSB consumption is inversely linked to affluence, and according to data from the US National Health and Nutrition Examination Survey, people on the lowest incomes consumed almost twice as many calories from SSBs than those on the highest incomes. Hunt Allcott, Associate Professor of Economics at New York University and his colleagues took an in-depth look into the health economics of taxing SSBs and published their findings in the *Journal of Economic Perspectives*, entitled "Should We Tax Sugar-Sweetened Beverages?"[55]. Unsurprisingly, they concluded that we should, and they offered seven concrete suggestions for policymakers:

1. Focus on counteracting the causes of disease rather than minimising consumption.
2. Target policies to reduce consumption among those most affected.
3. Tax grams of sugar, not ounces of liquid.
4. Tax diet drinks and fruit juice if and only if they also cause health harms.
5. When judging regressive taxation, consider long-term benefits not just who's being taxed.
6. Implement taxes nationally.
7. The benefits of sugar-sweetened beverage taxes probably exceed their costs.

No such thing as unhealthy foods

Early in my wellness career, I remember hearing the food industry mantra 'There are no such things as unhealthy foods, just unhealthy diets'. At the same time, food producers would be banging on about all the benefits of their healthy ranges. Surely, if there are no unhealthy foods, then there can be no healthy foods – just food. But, of course, there are unhealthy foods. While my hypothesis – that ten Mars bars a day will kill you quicker than ten Marlboro a day – probably wouldn't get through ethics to test it, my money is still on the Mars bars. Whichever of these is the most lethal must for now remain a moot point, but there is no doubt: either of these regimes will have you pushing up the daisies before your time, and I'd say that makes them unhealthy. I accept that one Mars bar won't kill you, but neither will one cigarette, so I suppose the new corporate defence line from the tobacco industry should be 'There is no such thing as unhealthy cigarettes, just unhealthy smoking regimes!'

Energy density

Calorie consumption has increased significantly in developed countries worldwide since the 1970s and is now accepted as the main contributing factor in the obesity epidemic in both adults and children. The evidence that increased calorie consumption is the cause of the obesity epidemic is further supported by rises in food supply and distribution, which have escalated in parallel with obesity[56]. Calorific, refined, appetising and processed (CRAP) edible products are perhaps the most significant contributor, and they promote weight gain in a number of ways. These 'hedonistic' products overwhelm appetite through their high energy and low mass, therefore avoiding the feeling of fullness until vast numbers of calories are consumed – quite the opposite of a more traditional low-energy diet containing considerable water and fibre.

The energy density (ED) of our food (calories per bite) has been steadily increasing for decades. It is measured by the number of calories per 100g, and as food labels must list this information, checking on ED is now simple. Look at the chart to the right to see examples of high-energy foods and compare them to the overall ED of a healthy diet. Some of the most energy-dense foods that are available are regulars in most people's diets. Now referred to as Energy Dense Nutrient Poor food and drinks (EDNP), they are considered a primary candidate for the starring role in the obesity pandemic.

Basically, EDNP is another definition for Ultra-Processed Foods (UPFs) and includes the usual suspects of cakes, sweets, crisps, cola, chocolate biscuits etc. A Danish study headed by the food scientist Biltoft-Jensen gave this considerable thought and suggested that for the benefit of a healthy waistline, consumption of EDNP should be restricted to around 5% of the energy requirement of the diet[57]. Therefore, roughly 100kcals per day from EDNP or UPFs, which would be the equivalent of two-thirds of a regular 330ml can of cola, under two custard creams or 1.8 fingers of KitKat. That's how energy dense these things are. Check out a few labels in your cupboard and start to get your head round ED.

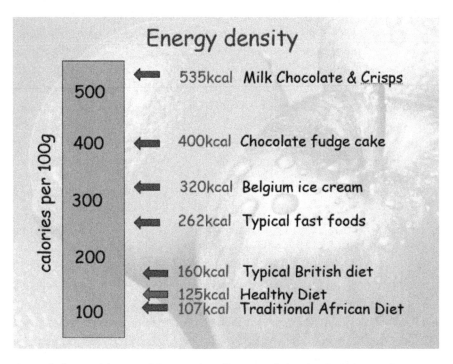

One of the problems with popular dietary advice is that it can focus on nutrients rather than food. Therefore, it is understandable that people get confused by the continually conflicting messages about single nutrients, such as the imperative of reducing saturated fat this week and free sugars the week after. But this approach overlooks the fact that these nutrients invariably coexist in CRAP, resulting in a diet high in both saturated fats and free sugars, and this is likely to have a synergistically damaging effect on health. For this reason, dietary guidelines which focus on foods rather than their constituents could help avoid inadvertent increases in one nutrient of concern at the expense of another.

One group of researchers were interested in this idea and so they looked at the main dietary causes of disease and narrowed it down to a small and easily understandable set of dietary guidelines. They found that the main dietary pattern associated with disease and early death was characterised by high intakes of confectionery, butter and free sugars, and low intakes of fresh fruit and vegetables and whole grains[58]. This is probably not news to many people, but it does emphasise the importance of thinking about the things we eat, as well as the individual elements of which they are composed.

Researchers in Canada wanted to pinpoint the contributors to weight gain in an obesogenic diet and calculated factors for foods that may be obesogenic or protective and gave them weightings. They found three obesogenic categories: fast food (+ 0.32), carbonated drinks (+ 0.30), and salty snacks (+ 0.19). Six broad categories were protective: fruits (-0.40), vegetables (-0.32), whole grains (-0.26), dark-green vegetables (-0.22), legumes and soy (-0.18) and pasta and rice (-0.17)[59]. These weightings speak for themselves and should act as a guide to anyone trying to re-engineer their diet to improve their health and weight.

Two studies funded by the Bill and Melinda Gates Foundation and published in 'The Lancet' in 2019[60] and 2020[61] found that poor diets were now a bigger killer than smoking, cutting one in five lives short every year from the eleven million people in the 195 countries that were examined. The study extrapolated information from the 'Global Burden of Disease Study' of 2017, finding that poor-quality diets are damaging hearts and causing cancer. The key findings show that dangerous diets are those that have too much salt, too few whole grains and too little fruit. Other contributors were a lack of nuts, seeds, vegetables, omega 3 and fibre. Salt is a major problem, as most premature deaths in the study came from cardiovascular disease and hypertension leading to heart attack and stroke. The studies estimate that 14% of UK deaths are related to diet.

The follow-up study found the largest increases in global health risks related to high BMI, poor glycaemic control, and elevated blood pressure – the latter two no doubt a result of the former. A leading risk factor was also identified as child and maternal malnutrition. What a shocking situation: too many people on Earth eating too much while too many children are sick because they don't have enough food.

Warning labels

Graphic warning labels on cigarette packets that display shocking images of the diseases associated with smoking have worked. Taken together, a total of thirty-five studies demonstrated that such images increase awareness of health risks and achieved the desired outcomes of changing beliefs about smoking and increasing quit rates[62]. Using this technique to highlight the dangers of consuming SSBs, UPFs and CRAP would, in my opinion, work in much the same way. Experimental studies have demonstrated that even simple 'worded' sugar warning labels on snack items leads to reduced consumption and encourages producers to reformulate their products in a healthier way[63], which helps people to lose weight. Now that obesity has overtaken smoking as the number one killer in developed countries, I see no rational argument for not using graphic warnings on CRAP products.

There are countless examples of people being poisoned by contaminated drinking water. Britain's worst mass poisoning event involved the accidental contamination of the drinking water supply to the town of Camelford, Cornwall, in 1988, where twenty tonnes of aluminium sulphate entered the water supply. The result was the production of several tonnes of sulphuric acid, which led to the leaching of lead and copper from the pipe networks and the formation of other noxious chemicals, causing serious health issues for the residents drinking the water.

When the things we ingest toxify us (causing sickness or death), if you didn't see it coming, it's fair to claim you've been poisoned. If you get sick and die prematurely because of what you are being provided as food, then is that not the same as what happened to the residents of Camelford? As shown in the aforementioned studies, we are being toxified by CRAP in our food chain, but can you really say that you didn't know? Is it justifiable to continue claiming we are unaware of what's going on or is it easier to turn the other cheek? The difference is that water contamination events are unintentional accidents and the residents of Camelford could not see it coming. But what is happening with our food is in plain sight, and it is no accident.

Perhaps more people need to be aware of the effects of CRAP and UPFs, and this is where the graphic labelling would help. So, once again, while there is no one magic bullet for the obesity pandemic, there are a multitude of solutions out there, but governments are just too weak to implement them. It's sad to realise that, in terms of the obesity epidemic, there is no such thing as government help, there is only self-help.

The Fat Switch

Richard Johnson, an American physician, claims that we may be getting fat because we are activating our survival switch all the time. In his book *The Fat Switch*[64], he shows how this is used in the wild as a survival mechanism to regulate the energy reserves of animals in the face of wildly varying food availability. For instance, migratory birds and hibernating animals in autumn suddenly start eating two to three times more food in preparation for winter. The reason for this gorging, Johnson postulates, is that at the end of summer, when fruits are very ripe (with lots of fructose), bears and birds will eat thousands of berries and fruits at a time. He showed that this fructose binge leads to leptin resistance (leptin is the satiety hormone) fuelling an ever-increasing appetite, triggering an autumn binge in preparation for the long winter ahead or the extensive migrations that birds face. The fructose leads, therefore, to a voracious appetite and the subsequent gorging leads to obesity. For a bear in autumn, it's the perfect storm.

Johnson found that fruit-eating animals preparing for winter were not only storing fat in their adipocytes and becoming obese, but also storing fat in their liver (and developing fatty liver), and in their blood (and getting hyperlipidaemia), and becoming insulin resistant. In fact, they were developing metabolic syndrome. It's known that when you become resistant to insulin you become a better storer of fat, making more energy available for the brain, perfect for survival during hibernation. The logical conclusion is that metabolic syndrome is a disease of humans because we don't do the lengthy fasting of hibernating animals, or fly 5,000 miles overseas, or live through the frugal, long winter months with little food. Instead, we adopt the default of feast, rest, feast and repeat. In animals, leptin resistance, obesity, insulin resistance and fatty liver are simply adaptive traits to assist them with the bust and boom scenario of seasonal food availability. The question Johnson asks is: "What turns on the fat switch?"

In his animal experimentation, he says that it took about a month of fructose loading in the lab to make his experimental animals leptin resistant, at which point they lost control of their appetite and started eating much more, becoming very overweight and insulin resistant. Johnson argues that one of the reasons for the 'switch' being thrown is that, compared to glucose, fructose acts differently at a cellular level, leading to uric acid production, which tricks the body into thinking that it is starving – even though there is an abundance of food. A further problem according to Dr Johnson is that, when the switch is activated for a long time (such as in a typical Westerner's diet), it reduces our levels of mitochondria, which explains the progressive fatigue and lethargy that many overweight people report. This in turn makes it harder to lose weight – another perfect storm! Johnson asks: "Are we essentially getting fat because we are activating the survival switch all the time?"

I think that Dr Johnson's account is a compelling and novel explanation for the parallel explosion of human obesity and sugar (50% glucose, 50%

fructose) consumption of the past sixty years. His work complements previous explanations about evolutionary survival, and how feeding occupies large parts of the brain's computing capacity which controls powerful emotional and instinctive drivers for a guaranteed supply of food. Currently, though, these systems are simply overwhelmed and rendered insensible to continuously high leptin levels during ongoing feasts that are no longer interrupted by frequent famines.

Food waste

When I was growing up in Northern England in the 1960s, it was the cultural norm not to waste food, and the mantra of 'Asia's starving millions' was constantly ringing in our ears. I'd say it worked, and my generation seems to understand the importance of not wasting food; a virtue as applicable today as it has ever been. Currently, according to the UN Environment Programme, approximately one-third of all global food produced for human consumption is wasted, the cost of which is around one trillion dollars each year ($1,000,000,000,000).

Every year, consumers in rich countries waste almost as much food as the entire net food production of sub-Saharan Africa (230 million tonnes). Food loss and waste reveals further squandering of other precious resources, such as water, land and energy, and needlessly produces additional greenhouse gas emissions exacerbating the climate emergency. If just one-quarter of the food currently lost or wasted globally could be saved, it would be enough to feed 870 million hungry people in the world[65].

It is apparent to me that most people living in the developed world today don't consider food waste particularly relevant to them. Even in my micro-bubble, I am mortified by the regularity with which I see good food go to waste. We appear to have ditched any notion of the folly of food waste in favour of the idea that you should throw food away rather than eating it; presumably because it is so cheap, or perhaps to protect yourself from becoming overweight. Well, hello, food is no longer cheap, and as for avoiding weight gain, wasting food will have zero bearing on that, despite what some of the squiffy science will tell you. I advise caution over some of the messages that escape the number-crunching confines of statistical software.

According to one study that relied upon participants answering a food questionnaire (already looking very suspect), plate-clearing adults had a higher than average BMI[66]. But correlation is not causation, and without accounting for portion size, in my opinion their results were meaningless. I'd say the message of avoiding plate clearing to avert weight gain is complete hocus-pocus. Just another, "OK, listen up everyone, look what us clever folk have worked out, this is what you ought to do to control your weight – waste more food!"

Food should be cherished and treated with the utmost respect; wise societies have done this for millennia. Making too much and serving too much is obviously not going to help if you are concerned about your weight, and as we all have a responsibility to waste less food, try to put in place measures to cook the right amount or have handy freezer tubs at the ready to store meals for later in the week. Wasting food is decadent irrespective of your weight, and telling people not to clear their plate to stay slim is just plain silly. At a time of food shortages, where some people cannot afford to adequately nourish themselves, food waste is indefensibly profligate and wholly unethical. Funnily enough, if you are concerned about food waste, you waste less, and it does not in any way relate to your BMI[67]. We need to adopt the notion of food appreciation and conservation, and perhaps change the theme of 'Asia's starving millions', to 'the West's bursting billions!'

Should food be cheaper or more expensive?

As Abraham Maslow taught us in his work on the hierarchy of needs, to endure and flourish, people must first satisfy the basic requirements of survival before they can enjoy the indulgences of other life experiences. This is why the need to eat is at the base of his ascending triangle of needs. Excepting the novel and ludicrous food inflation of the post-Covid-19 years, food in the UK has never been so affordable. Of course, it is not the actual price of food that is relevant, the key is what proportion of your income does the cost of your food devour.

In the 1950s in the UK, most families spent around one-third of their income on food. By 1975 this had decreased to around 24% and has continued dropping ever since. In 2020, people in the lowest-income households in the UK spent just over 17% of their household expenditure on food and (non-alcoholic) drink, and those in the top-income bracket just over 10%[68]. This continued decline in the 'cost' of food in the West represents one of the greatest recent advances in quality of life for millions, allowing more of the population to spend more of their income on pursuing more of the fun and enlightening interests on the ascending stages of Maslow's triangle. This is progress.

I've often thought that food in this country needs to be more expensive. My reasoning behind this is that I imagine it will enable growers to continue to produce good food, while at the same time allowing them to make a decent living out of what is a pretty grinding vocation. Halting and reversing the current race to the bottom in terms of food prices could prevent growers of quality food from going to the wall, while avoiding the need for dwellers of this fertile land to eat ever more food imported from overseas.

Investing more in existing farms could prevent further devastation of the ecology through current farming sprawl and empower farmers to concentrate on getting larger yields from a finite biobank. However, considering the parlous state of the current economy and the cost-of-living crisis, this principle of dearer food won't win me many supporters. I maintain, however, that the imperative of adequately investing in our food growers is one of the most vital considerations facing all people of all countries. The economic and environmental arguments for maintaining a healthy domestic food industry are indisputable.

I've realised, however, that my preference for more expensive food only considers half of the equation. There is a widely held belief that healthy eating is expensive (although I'm not entirely convinced by this). I agree that fresh, healthy foods are in many cases more expensive than mass-produced, non-perishable CRAP foods, but many healthy fresh foods are also very cheap. The pertinent discussion in this case is that healthy food needs to be more affordable (many already are) and toxic foods need to be considerably more expensive.

I hear commentators say that taxing CRAP food is a regressive tax on the poorest in society but that is a false narrative (does it apply to taxing cigarettes and alcohol?). If certain foods lead to your demise while others do the opposite, responsible governments would conjure financial instruments to fix what is currently an economic incentive to eat ourselves into an early grave. In ten minutes, I could probably scribble the basics on the back of a Krispy Kreme doughnut packet.

When considering the expense of food, this needs to include the cost of time. By way of example, I could go to most typical high street CRAP food outlets and buy 1,000 calories (large fried chicken and chips with a large fizzy drink) for around £5. Or I could get a couple of frozen pizzas, put them in the oven (pay for the heating) and get even more calories for my cash. That's 50p for every 100kcals, or £10 per day for the average 2,000kcal requirements required by an adult. That is cheap, particularly for convenient food that some would say is tasty and requires no cooking, no preparing, no washing up – zero skill or effort required.

Let's say that the cost of cooking and preparing food at home from raw ingredients was comparable, and a day's provision could be covered by £10. But what this mainly overlooks is the time (and skills) that such a meal would take for the requisite shopping, peeling, washing, preparing, cooking, serving, cleaning up and putting away – at least a couple of hours in total each day. Time is money, and if you set aside two hours each day, seven days a week, for food procurement and prep, that's 14 hours. Even at minimum wage (£10.42 at the time of going to press), that's £146 a week. You could therefore say that someone could save money by eating CRAP food as this 'time-free eating' would enable £146 in potential wages. For many, it's a no-brainer, while for others, it's a Hobson's choice, because they have three jobs already trying to get by, and don't have time for two hours shopping, cooking and clearing up each day.

As an aside, if you are cooking for a family of four, you could eat well on your £40 per day budget, and the labour could be shared by everyone, so this torpedoes the eating healthily is expensive argument for families. Cooking is a health behaviour associated with higher-quality diets. In one study, where people were invited to attend a 24-week weight-loss group, the participants were randomised into either actively preparing a weekly meal as part of a hands-on lesson (the cooks), or observing a chef prepare the same meal (the audience). While both groups saw significant improvements in healthy eating, the cooks lost significantly more weight at six months compared with the audience (7.3% vs. 4.5%)[69].

I am a great advocate for everyone learning the basics of cookery. But, of course, this was removed from the school curriculum many years ago due to the cost of running the kitchens and probably another dodgy dossier produced by health and safety zealots, terrified over the prospect of young people cooking (utensils of mass destruction). This choice to take the path of least resistance was deemed to be more important than the health tsunami that we are now dealing with. Instead of teaching young people how to convert low-cost produce into tasty high-quality food, some doughnut in the education department thought it would be better to display to students a few food labels on their shiny interactive whiteboards and call it 'food technology'. Now, that's much tidier and easier to deliver, isn't it?

An equally important dimension to this debate is the wider implication of a society that fuels its citizens on ultra-processed foods. While this CRAP produce is cheap at the point of purchase, when you consider the cost that this food has on the environment, the ecology, the economy and in terms of human health, then this is the most expensive food on the planet. In the words of George Monbiot in his book Regenesis[70] (the most important book I have ever read): "Food has to be cheap enough to feed people in poverty, and yet expensive enough to support people who grow it". If I may be so bold as to make a suggested amendment, I'd add the word 'Good' at the beginning of his sentence.

In summary, make your peace with food. I've spoken a lot about the negative aspects of CRAP food, and it is important that you reduce to a minimum or eliminate such junk from your diet. However, don't concentrate on the negative aspects of what you're not supposed to eat, but try to focus on the positive, delicious and nutritious varieties of food that you are going to eat. See food as your ally and not your enemy. Consider the wonderful health-giving properties that many foods have and feel good about bringing them into your everyday meals.

Other influencers of weight

Sleep

Planning weight loss without considering sleep would be as absurd as preparing for skydiving without contemplating safety.

The less you sleep the more you eat, and not just because you have more time to eat (which is implicated as a cause). Moreover, even moderate sleep deprivation results in heightened appetite, a preference for sweet and fatty foods, frequent snacking and a low consumption of vegetables. These appetite and dietary 'fatigue preferences' are driven by both increased desires for such foods, and hormonal changes to the hunger satiety signals that control food intake.

Mirroring the increase in obesity levels over recent decades has been a reduction in sleep in developed countries. For instance, from 1965 to 1999, data from the USA show a 72% increase in the prevalence of short sleep (less than 7 hours), while over roughly the same time period (1971 to 1999) there was a 52% increase in the prevalence of obesity[71]. Furthermore, adequate sleep continues to fall, with only 35% of American adults reporting eight hours of sleep in 1998, and only 26% in 2005[72]. Remarkably, most sleep deprivation in the developed world is voluntary, with FoMO interfering with sensible bedtimes for far too many people.

Social jetlag (SJL) is a recent term which refers to the discrepancy between biological time controlled by circadian rhythms, and social periods which are dictated by obligations and choices such as work, screen time and socialising. The proliferation of artificial light, 24-hour TV viewing, gaming, streaming and the multitude of social media and online interactive sites promise that you never have to be lonely or bored or sleepy ever again. Instead, opt to be permanently entertained or distracted, and rather than being sleep deprived, you can now be socially jetlagged! The problem, however, is that severe SJL is associated with more junk food and higher odds of having overweight or obesity, and, no doubt we will learn in time, a multitude of other health problems.

A search for the word 'sleep' in my Endnote programme (8,000 weight and nutrition-specific scientific references) returned 145 results; a clue to the strength of the relationship between sleep and weight. The evidence from most of the work undertaken into this relationship points to eating too much rather than reduced activity as the primary cause, but this is not to say that fatigue has no role in the relationship.

On top of the increased frequency and volumes of food consumed, it is known that with inadequate sleep comes poorer food choices. Even when calorie consumption is the same, sugar levels in the diets of sleep-deprived people are higher than in those with adequate sleep. When tired, the brain instructs us to eat more, and the emphasis on sugary foods ensures the brain will get its glucose to compensate for the fatigue of sleep deprivation. In a nutshell, sleep-induced fatigue brings on a hungry, sugar-craving, frequent-snacking state, to help the brain to cope.

In one study that closely monitored ten healthy people, a two-week reduction in normal sleep duration led to an average increase in energy intake of more than 300kcal each day, a half-kilogram increase in body weight, and an 11% increase in visceral fat volume[73]. A recent journal article put it bluntly in the title of their paper: 'Why Nutrition Professionals Should Ask Their Patients About Sleep Habits'[74].

Short sleep's ability to scupper any weight-loss attempts was further demonstrated in an experiment published in the *Annals of Internal Medicine*[75] which showed how a lack of sleep curtails the normal protection of lean mass, leading to a lower metabolic rate. So, it can be said that poor sleep not only leads to weight gain, but it also works to keep you overweight. This was confirmed when researchers showed that just by increasing the slumber time of sleep-deprived overweight people, they reduced their daily food consumption by up to 270 kcal, resulting in weight loss of up to half a kilo[76].

Most living organisms have a body clock that regulates body systems relative to the daylight hours which we translate into time of day. Known as the circadian clock (or circadian rhythm), it is guided primarily by light and temperature, rhythmically regulating hormones, energy metabolism and growth. A 'master clock' in the brain coordinates these natural rhythms and, it appears ever more likely, that long-term disturbance of the circadian rhythm leads to disruptive consequences for the hormones and metabolic processes regulated by these recurring patterns. For instance, leptin is mainly produced during the sleep phase in humans, and leptin resistance (a hallmark of people living with obesity) is thought to be one of the consequences of circadian dysfunction brought about by sleep disruption.

As light diminishes, the brain releases melatonin, making us feel sleepy. If, however, we are exposed to light at night, this can affect melatonin release, with excessive night-time artificial light muddying the transition, for our brains, from day into night. Under such circumstances, the changes in circadian rhythms lead to consequences including disrupted hormonal patterns and potential weight gain from altered eating patterns. Even exposure to very dim night-time light is sufficient to alter circadian rhythms, and regular unnatural light cycles are increasingly associated with obesity and metabolic syndrome.

Most people are familiar with the idea that eating late at night is not good for weight control, and this may well be due to the way we process food when asleep. However, another probable relationship between late-night meals and weight is the interference with sleep patterns of late eating, inducing fatigue and leading to more eating and more sugar consumption. The consensus is not to eat meals later than 7-8pm.

Shortened sleep and sleep disruptions also bring about fatigue and daytime drowsiness, and just one poor night's sleep leads to a more sedentary pattern the following day[77]. As if to reciprocate, being sedentary takes its toll on your sleep quantity and quality[78], another vicious cycle. Somewhat ironically, exercise and physical activity banishes lethargy and fatigue and gives us more energy, probably by helping us to relax and sleep better, thus reducing daytime fatigue and helping to break the poor sleep/sedentary day cycle.

Weight and sleep therefore share a well-established inverse relationship: more weight equals less sleep, and more sleep equals less weight. The question is, once again, which is the causal direction in this relationship? To date, studies have been unable to conclusively determine this, but while being overweight creates a number of known sleep disruptions, it appears that it is poor sleep leading to weight gain that is the causal direction favoured by most people in the know.

Screens and sleep

The negative relationship between screen time and sleep is well established, but a causal direction has not been established. Is it because people that spend too much time on their screens voluntarily deprive themselves of sleep? Or is it that they do go to bed on time but the excessive screen time, particularly late-night viewing, acts to interfere with sleep once in bed? Or is it that those that don't sleep well reach for a screen during the night? I spotted this recent study[79] and thought 'Bingo, here's the answer!' The authors looked at the data for 31,000 people and concluded that longer screen time led to shorter sleep. However, I was dismayed to see their final sentence: 'and vice versa!' Therefore, we still don't know what the directional relationship is, but suffice to say, you have a 50% chance of improving sleep if you reduce your screen time!

Alcohol and sleep

Alcohol interferes with sleep architecture and disrupts REM sleep. If you have had a lot of alcohol the night before, even though you may have slept for eight or even ten hours, you probably won't have had the right pattern of sleep and you will most likely have missed out on REM sleep, and therefore you will not be sufficiently rested or refreshed. This is why, after a big session, even if you sleep in till midday the next day, you still feel tired for the rest of the day and then sleep like a baby that night.

Stress and sleep

I'm guessing you are not surprised to hear that stress is also in the mix when it comes to sleep disruptions. Inadequate sleep, emotional stress and weight gain are uncomfortable bedfellows, negatively impacting each other. Both sleep deprivation and weight gain lead to heightened stress, and then stress returns the compliment by making you more overweight and disrupting your sleep further, establishing an antagonistic triad of emotional stress, fatigue and weight gain.

Sleep and aging

In older people, sleep curtailment is also strongly linked to weight gain and the reasons for this are no different to those of younger people. As sleep disturbances are more common in older people, this perpetuates the myth that reduced sleep is a normal part of aging, but it is not, and planning and making appropriate preparations to ensure you are getting adequate sleep applies from cradle to grave.

Obstructive sleep apnoea syndrome (OSAS)

OSAS is on the increase in line with obesity and metabolic syndrome. It is more common in men, but many women also suffer this difficult and distressing condition. The causes of OSAS are complex but where it is driven by excess weight, the mechanics involve fat deposits in the upper respiratory tract narrowing the airway. Together with a decrease in local muscle activity, this results in recurrent partial or complete pharyngeal collapses during sleeping. These changes lead to cessation of breathing for between ten and thirty seconds, which in some cases can happen hundreds of times each evening. This causes a decrease in available oxygen, leading to tissue hypoxia, oxidative stress and inflammation, the main contributing factors to the resultant cardiovascular diseases.

Planning to improve sleep

Feeling well rested and energised is a prerequisite before even considering substantial challenges such as lifestyle changes. In fact, I'd say that many people totally discard notions of change, simply because they don't feel they have the energy to succeed – they never make the starting blocks. Rather than try to tackle why they feel this way, most soldier on and deal with each day as it comes. It's OK, I get it, life is busy, it's tiring and it's often so full of clutter that it's hard to think where the time and energy will come from to even think about change, let alone set about significant alterations to the way that we live. Rest assured, it is the same for most people from time to time, and no one has a monopoly on being busy or tired or feeling overwhelmed. However, perhaps a few changes to bedtime schedules could make a world of difference.

The routines that we adopt around bedtime, like most other aspects of our lives, are largely optional. We have developed night-time patterns that we assume are working for us, but are they? Taking a close look at your sleep plans could pay dividends in helping you to achieve the things in life that are important to you. First, consider your normal sleep duration (hopefully it is around 7.5 – 8.5 hours, which seems to be optimum for humans). If it's not around eight hours, think about some manageable targets that would move you closer to the ideal. Try to have a regular bedtime and, if possible, aim to get up at the same time each day to help with the overall sleep/wake cycle. This usually works OK for weekdays but can go awry at weekends (as can many other plans), but try to avoid huge swings between weekday and weekend patterns. If you feel that your sleep routines could or should be improved, some of the most frequently suggested ideas from the vast evidence base on the subject are listed below.

Avoid eating late

Again, if possible, foster a 'dinner time' pattern where you aim to have dined and cleared up by a certain time (preferably before 8pm) so that you can allow adequate time for food digestion and relaxation before bed.

Get out more

If possible, outdoor activities are the best for promoting sleep because daylight has a big effect on melatonin production and the circadian rhythm. However, all exercise and physical activity is proven to promote better sleep and aid rest, so be as active as you can, just make it outdoors if possible.

Stimulants

Stimulants (nicotine, caffeine, alcohol etc.) should be curtailed if possible as they will all interfere with sleep in one way or another. Caffeine after 4pm is not advisable for people that have sleep difficulties – experiment with decaf. For men, caffeine can play havoc with the prostate (I speak from experience), which is far from conducive to a good night's sleep.

Manage stress

If you are feeling stressed, do something about it! Start by developing a stress-reduction plan and be proactive on things such as prioritising and organising difficult tasks. Don't start stressing over worries before bedtime, either make a list of things to do about it tomorrow, or just forget about it and let sleep find the solution.

Learn how to relax

Experiment with mindfulness techniques or meditation and relaxation practices to calm the mind just before bed or while in bed. Refer to the section on Mindfulness for more.

Avoid bright lights

Bright light, particularly blue light, tells the brain it is daytime, shutting down melatonin production. Computers and phones emit a lot of blue light, and if you must use them late at night, then consider a pair of blue light filtering glasses or switch on the blue light block on your device.

TV, gaming and screens

Playing Call of Duty just before bed might not be the best sleep preparation, but I'm guessing most people don't need to be told that. But if falling asleep is problematic, consider avoiding screen viewing in general at least one hour before bed (this includes TV). Try a good old book (though perhaps not one as stimulating as this one!).

The sleep chamber

The key is cool, quiet and dark. Give some thought to how you can make your bedroom more conducive to sleep. Blackout blinds, heating control and even ear plugs if there is a lot of noise. Some people even say that furniture arrangement and room tidiness are factors in helping them to doze off. Advocates of Feng Shui suggest not adopting the 'death position' with your head pointing north, but superstition is not something I subscribe to.

Bed, mattress and linen

Take a look at your sleeping apparatus, is it up to the job? Are your pillows and mattresses sagging, misshaped or discoloured? Be sure they are supportive, clean, allergen-free and comfortable. Is your bed linen clean and inviting? If your snoozing tackle is getting on a bit, a valuable investment may be to make some upgrades.

Bladder watch!

If you have problems with excessive night-time urination, then experimenting with drinking more fluids earlier on in the day and reducing intake after 7pm may be worthwhile.

Pre-sleep routine

Sleep routines start before you get into bed. Aim for appropriate relaxing or calming activities an hour before bedtime, if possible. If you have difficulty falling asleep, try doing something relaxing such as reading or listening to soothing music. Some people find that getting up and going to another room helps.

Power napping

If you are not shift working, if possible, try to avoid sleeping during the day, but if you must snooze, then try to limit this to half an hour.

Exercise

Regular exercise and outdoor activities are perhaps the best way of improving sleep, including dramatically reducing the time it takes to fall asleep, outperforming most sleep-enhancing drugs. Obviously, though, don't do an hour of high-intensity exercise just before bedtime!

Take away message

The body of evidence linking poor sleep and weight gain is categoric[80]. Poor sleeping is also related to a host of other negative health consequences, all of which dramatically undermine our life expectations and aspirations. Behavioural solutions rather than pharmacological ones are, for most people, the best way forward, and you shouldn't overlook the importance of sleep if you are setting out on a weight-management plan. Experiment with sleep-enhancing strategies and try not to make lots of changes all at once. By introducing changes gradually, you can zone in on those that have the biggest effect. However, for some people, nothing seems to work and, in this case, seeking professional help may be the only answer.

Advertising

Being exposed to regular food cues increases intake, and modern living is accompanied by ubiquitous advertising, typically for unhealthy and ultra-processed foods, much of which is targeted at children who are assumed to be customers for life. Back in 2008, TV-based food advertising in the United States accounted for virtually half of all commercial messages on children's programmes, amounting to eleven ads per hour, most of which are for highly processed unhealthy food. The powerful corporations behind this relentless persuasive marketing know full well that TV advertising is particularly potent when aimed at children.

A recent study that looked at an advertising ban on calorific, refined, appetising and processed (CRAP) products over the London Underground network showed that reduced exposure to such adds had a positive effect on purchasing, with fewer CRAP products being bought (and therefore consumed) by Londoners during the advertising ban[81]. However, despite the enormous detrimental effects that CRAP exerts on a population, the corporations that sell it try all they can to maximise sales. When TfL enacted their ban, this was robustly challenged by industry respondents who deployed a range of strategies during the consultation period. They exaggerated the costs and downplayed the potential benefits of the policy, warning of negative economic consequences, and questioning the evidence for the ban (but without offering evidence for their own position). To further influence policy in this area, the commercial actors also applied to join the London Child Obesity Taskforce and invited its members to their events. They closed ranks to amplify their arguments, and some even raised the potential of legal challenges[82]. The behaviour of big food today reminds me of a piece I read many years ago about smoking...

Big Food similarities with Big Tobacco?

In 2009, Kelly Brownell of Yale University wrote a paper in which she examined the perils of ignoring history. Entitled 'Big Tobacco Played Dirty and Millions Died. How Similar Is Big Food?'[83]. Brownell set out how, in December 1953, the CEOs of the major tobacco companies met secretly in New York City. Their purpose was to counter the damage from studies linking smoking to lung cancer. A year earlier, *Reader's Digest* (then the American public's leading source of medical information) had printed an article entitled 'Cancer by the Carton'[84]. After it appeared, cigarette sales plummeted for two years.

The tobacco industry's response was to publish 'A Frank Statement to Cigarette Smokers', paying 448 newspapers to print it on January 4, 1954. The statement included the signatures of the nation's top tobacco executives and assured Americans that: "We accept an interest in people's health as a basic responsibility, paramount to every other consideration in our business". Every other consideration, that is, except for profit, it would seem.

The 'Frank Statement', however, was a charade, and the start of a fifty-year campaign to mislead people about the devastating effects of smoking. Industry documents from the time showed the duplicity of its executives that tried feverishly to avoid the damaging perception that their products were dangerous, which, if accepted, would surely lead to lost sales, and legislative, regulatory and legal actions that would decimate their companies, and with that, of course, their own wealth and status. As Brownell wrote:

> "A half century of tobacco industry deception had tragic
> consequences. Since the 'Frank Statement', approximately 16 million
> Americans have died from smoking and millions more have suffered
> from debilitating diseases ranging from emphysema to heart disease.
> Had the industry come clean in 1954 – matching deeds with promises
> – many of these deaths would almost certainly have been prevented.
> No one knows how many in total as this is just in the US."

In her article about Big Food, Brownell went on to highlight that the food industry today is under scrutiny for producing products that damage health. She showed how it also faces legislative, regulatory and legal threats that could erode profits and disrupt growth. Restrictions in food marketing practices are now commonplace and certain products are banned in schools, and measures such as taxing high fat/sugar products are either reality or part of the national debate in many countries.

There are, of course, differences between CRAP and tobacco as substances. Selling cigarettes to children is illegal but kids can buy highly sugared potent stimulants in powerful caffeinated fizzy drinks anytime they want. Tobacco is accepted as being addictive but eating or food addiction is far from accepted by the authorities in almost all countries. The case against tobacco was targeted at one product produced by a few companies, but for food it is a far more complex supply web. Brownell points out:

> "The tobacco industry had a 'playbook or 'script' that emphasised personal responsibility; paid scientists who delivered research that instilled doubt; criticised the 'junk' science that found harms associated with smoking; made self-regulatory pledges; lobbied with massive resources to stifle government action; introduced 'safer' products while it simultaneously manipulated and denied both the addictive nature of their products and their marketing to children. There are striking similarities in the way that the food and tobacco industries have responded to public mistrust. Food companies have issued their own versions of frank statements, stating their concern with the public's wellbeing, and pledging to make changes to benefit public health."

Brownell concluded that because obesity is now a major global problem, the world cannot afford to repeat history, in which industry talks about the moral high ground but does not occupy it. Fourteen years on, very little has changed and since then millions more have died from eating too much CRAP. Seems like we are content to accept the perils of ignoring history.

Oxidative stress and free radical damage

A feature of modern life is our increasing exposure to free radicals which disrupt our natural oxidation/reduction (redox) balance and cause oxidative stress (OS). Free radicals are unbalanced atoms – they have a missing electron and become charged particles known as ions. As with all things, free radicals want to be balanced, thus they try to retrieve the missing electron by scavenging one from something nearby. When exposed to free radicals, candidates for this armed robbery include cells, tissues and organs. Thus, free radicals damage all living things that they encounter.

Subsequently, oxidative stress is implicated in several diseases including diabetes, neurodegenerative disorders, cardiovascular diseases and various cancers[85]. It also transpires that OS is strongly implicated in fat cell production, eating addiction, sleep, stress response, genes, the microbiome, insulin, ghrelin and leptin secretion, inflammation, adipokine production, and disruption to appetite regulation by affecting the hypothalamus (the crucial energy regulator in the brain). Therefore, it appears that free radical damage is incriminated in all the key contributors to obesity[86].

Free radicals can enter the body from external sources in the form of pollutants, alcohol, tobacco smoke, solvents, pesticides, certain drugs and exposure to radiation (including strong sunlight). An important part of health management involves avoiding exposure to too many free radicals by taking sensible precautions. But free radicals also have a role in maintaining optimum health and are the primary ordnance in our immune armoury. Produced in immuno-defensive cells, free radicals such as hydrogen peroxide are used to annihilate invading pathogens, infiltrating them, and literally ripping their molecules apart. (Mr Trump, if you are reading, this is the body's very own disinfectant, so there really is no need to drink any.)

In our cells, the marvels that are mitochondria convert the energy from our food, but in the process they produce free radicals as a by-product. Ironically, most vulnerable to oxidative stress are the mitochondria themselves, presumably because of their proximity to these powerful oxidizing agents. The problem is that if you run out of mitochondria, you run out of energy – a very bad situation. Therefore, to counter this, each cell has what are called peroxisomes positioned next to the mitochondria, which release antioxidants to quench free radicals by donating the missing electrons. To ensure our peroxisomes always have a supply of antioxidants, we rely on a good diet consisting of lots of fresh colourful plant foods which is the origin of most of our antioxidants. So, eat up your fruit and veg, it all makes sense now!

Here are a few interesting facts about mitochondria that I think will enrich your life:

- They are of separate evolutionary origin to all our other DNA, being derived from bacteria kidnapped and engulfed by the early ancestors of our human eukaryotic cells that somehow worked out that these little miracles could produce energy.

- Mitochondria are only inherited from the mother, as the fathers' mitochondrial DNA in the sperm cell, self-destructs at the moment of fertilisation.

- If you track back the maternally inherited DNA in our cells, all humans have a theoretical common ancestor – 'Mitochondrial Eve', living around 200,000 years ago.

The research scientist Tobore O Tobore, an expert in the effects of oxidation on the body, strongly believes that oxidation brought about by overabundance of reactive oxygen species (ROS – another name for free radicals) plays a critical role in food addiction and is both a cause and mediator of obesity. Tobore also suggests that ROS play a direct role in building new fat cells, thus rendering obesity and metabolic syndrome more difficult to combat. Furthermore, if Tobore is right, a healthy diet including lots of fresh plants will assist in the treatment of food addictions and obesity[86]. Mr Tobore O Tobore, thank you for your most valuable work.

Drugs with obesogenic effects

There are many prescribed drugs that will lead to weight gain, covering a variety of conditions. The most common are psychoactive drugs such as anti-depressants, anti-psychotics and treatments for conditions such as schizophrenia, anxiety and bi-polar. For people living with mental health disorders, while at the same time trying to manage their weight, this can bring considerable additional and unwelcome stress. With the added burden of their medication compounding matters, this presents an enormous challenge for people at a time when they are often at their most vulnerable. Drugs that are prescribed to alleviate other disorders such as beta blockers for hypertension, corticosteroids for inflammatory conditions and those for allergy, hay fever and epilepsy, are all highly likely to increase weight for the sufferer. There are many more over-the-counter and prescription drugs that are implicated in significant weight gain, and you should always consult your doctor or pharmacist to see if there are effective alternatives where weight gain is not a side effect. I believe that in the face of the current obesity epidemic, health professionals should be acutely conscious of the drawbacks of prescribing medication to overweight people that is likely to lead to further weight gain.

Viral obesity – fact or fiction?

There is a link between obesity and viral infections in animals, in particular exposure to adenovirus-36 (AD36), seemingly causing weight gain, with canine distemper and scrapie also implicated. In the laboratory, when human fat cells were populated with stem cells, and half of them were exposed to AD36, the stem cells in the infected tissues differentiated into adipocytes, where they remained unchanged in the uninfected tissues, revealing that the virus causes an increase in the number of fat cells [87]. A recent review of the evidence of viral agents and human obesity found that, while not conclusive, viral agents as a causal link cannot be ruled out[88]. However, considering these viruses have been around for thousands of years, it appears unlikely they are causing the obesity pandemic.

Alcohol

Alcohol provides 7kcal/g and then, of course, there are the other calories that accompany each drink typically in the form of sugars. Five pints of beer are likely to deliver 900kcals, and a bottle of wine is about 625kcals, both of which are going to have an impact if you are drinking this amount frequently. A splendid resource for those interested in how their drinking may be impacting their weight is the Drink Aware site at www.drinkaware. co.uk. Here you can use all manner of interactive tools to calculate calories and units based upon your own consumption. And if you want to cut down, there are lots of helpful and up-to-date resources, as well as a chat function and a newsletter.

The scientific community is currently undecided on the relationship between alcohol and excess weight, with some studies finding that heavy drinkers are more at risk, others finding moderate drinkers have a stronger relationship with overweight, and some finding no relationship. Overall, the majority of cross-sectional studies since 2005 have demonstrated that frequent light to moderate alcohol intake does not seem to be associated with obesity risk, but that heavy or binge drinking probably does. Some commentators interpret these statistics as a suggestion that heavy drinkers are less likely to adopt healthy lifestyle patterns and that this is why the link is stronger as consumption rises, rather than the calorie contribution of the alcohol.

Micro-nutrient deficiencies

Most approaches looking at diet and its relationship with weight focus on intake of macro-nutrients. However, the micro-nutrient content of the diet is not inconsequential, as vitamins and minerals are involved in a myriad of homeostatic and metabolic processes that regulate body weight. In a 2020 study[89], researchers compared the micro-nutrient intake of 20,000 random people against their weight and waist circumference. The results showed that calcium, magnesium, potassium, copper, zinc and iron (beneficial) intakes were negatively correlated with weight (more dietary minerals, less weight), whereas sodium and phosphorus (deleterious) were positively correlated (more minerals, more weight). The strength of association increased in line with the volumes; in other words, a higher quantity of negative minerals in the diet meant a heavier person, and likewise with the beneficial minerals – more minerals meant proportionately leaner people. This can be interpreted in two ways: are the minerals impacting body weight, or is the amount of minerals in our diet (beneficial or deleterious) simply a proxy measure for how healthy our diet is? Probably a bit of both.

Environmental pollutants

Environmental pollutants have already been mentioned as potential contributors to global weight gain. The authors of a 2021 report cite various examples, and among them are endocrine-disrupting chemicals (EDCs) and increased ambient temperatures in our homes[90]. Endocrine-disrupting chemicals (EDC) are synthetics that contaminate humans through contact with the likes of food packaging, pesticides, detergents and plastics, with us all exposed to thousands of them every day. Currently, there is strong evidence to show that EDCs have a robust effect on obesity, impaired glucose tolerance, gestational diabetes, reduced birthweight, reduced semen quality, polycystic ovarian syndrome, endometriosis and breast and prostate cancer[91].

According to WHO, "Even a small dose can have a strong effect, and cause effects decades after exposure, or even skip a generation and appear as defects in our descendants"[92]. Obesogens, as they are also known, can interfere with homeostasis and thereby increase the susceptibility to obesity. The most sensitive time for obesogen action is in utero and early childhood, and weight gain is one effect, through either epigenetic alteration or hormone disruption, that can lead to a permanently increased number of fat cells. Recently, EDCs have been shown to be accidentally entering our food, and are ubiquitous in highly processed food packaging. While EDCs appear convenient, governments should be seeking to ban them, as their current policy of leaving it to consumers' 'choice' is just plain nonsense.

Ambient temperature

Humans seem to prefer to live in a 'thermo-neutral environment' in ranges between 20°C and 32°C, and this is because ambient temperature influences metabolic rate. However, following the proliferation of central heating over the last forty years or so, temperatures inside UK homes have risen on average by 5°C. In one study, a 24-hour increase of 6°C (from 16°C to 22°C) led to a reduction in metabolic rate of 167 kcal[93]. While it is unlikely to be underpinning the obesity pandemic, warmer homes may just be another low-level contributor to expanding waistlines.

Eating out

In the UK, the total number of food outlets almost doubled between 1980 and 2000[94]. The proliferation of fast-food outlets near home, work or along commutes, leads to greater consumption of takeaway food, and such clusters are now referred to as 'food swamps'. Of course, the more takeaway food that you eat, the heavier you become – a dose-responsive relationship. Clearly, meals sold in fast-food outlets are far from healthy, and more than 95% of all items on both UK and USA menus were found to have high levels of at least one nutrient of public health concern (fat, sugar or salt) in a 2022 study[95].

A study published in 2019 In the 'BMJ', 'A bit or a lot on the side'[96], looked at over 1,000 dishes for starters, sides and desserts served in twenty-seven major UK restaurant chains, with the objective of seeing which of these 'extra' dishes exceeded 600kcal (the recommended maximum for a main meal). The average was 488kcal for starters, 398kcal for sides and 431kcal for desserts, with 26% of starters, 22% of sides and 21% of desserts exceeding 600kcal. Therefore, one in four starters and one in five sides and desserts in

UK chain restaurants exceed the recommended energy intake for an entire meal. When eating out, it's safe to say, meal accompaniments provide 'a lot on the side'!

While on the subject of 'fast food', eating too fast wherever you are has long been known to be a correlate of higher weight (but no one knows the causal direction). A study that recently caught my eye suggested that one hotdog will shorten your life by 36 minutes[97]. By studying 5,800 edible items, researchers at the University of Michigan estimated the effects on lifespan of different foods, and, unsurprisingly, hot dogs didn't fare well. If right, this doesn't bode well for Joey Chesnut, the world's champion hot dog eater, who astonishingly somehow managed to consume seventy-six hot dogs (including the bread bun) in ten minutes. During his gastrocidal life, Chesnut has gobbled around 20,000 hot dogs, which, according to the study I saw, will relieve him of one year and four months of his decadent existence. I suppose the imprudent Mr Chesnut could always switch to burgers!

Anomalies

A 'Western lifestyle and diet' is often cited as the cause of obesity and there is overwhelming evidence to support this. However, according to www.worldpopulationview.com, North Korea has a 40% higher obese population compared to the far more Westernised population of South Korea. If I was to have a guess at explaining this anomaly, I'd say North Koreans are probably quite a bit more stressed than their Southern relatives, and they are certainly controlled to some extent by cheap alcohol subsidised by the government (which is not a bad strategy to subdue a population). But I'm sure it is a lot more complicated than that.

Social, economic, culture and community

For someone locked in a battle with their weight, it may seem odd to think about the social, economic, cultural and community drivers of weight, and how this has any relevance to their current predicament. But these influences will have great significance both for their journey into weight gain and the likely continuance of any weight-related trends. Therefore, to navigate a way out of this complex maze, the imperative of fully understanding these matters cannot be overstated.

Socio-economic status

Socio-economic status (SES) is linked to health, and measures of SES use variables such as education, income and occupation – education is the most stable variable over time. SES has long been a strong predictor of weight at the population level in most developed countries, although recent work in the US shows that the divide between obesity rates in high compared to low SES groups has narrowed significantly over the past three decades[98], and it is likely that this reflects trends across other developed countries. However, despite this, there is still a well-established socio-economic gradient linking obesity and low levels of education, income and deprivation, and this relationship is much stronger in women and children than in men.

This association works both ways, in that low SES predicts weight gain, and being overweight confers social, educational and employment bias, lower incomes, and reduces opportunities for relationships, marriage and social inclusion. A lower income reduces some access to healthy food choices as well as to expensive forms of active recreational pursuits. Disadvantaged neighbourhoods have fewer affordable, healthy, fresh foods, fewer green, open spaces and more fast-food outlets and reduced walkability due to safety concerns. Therefore, for both the individual and the community, the link between weight and SES becomes an entrenched inequality.

Take a moment to examine the age-related charts below that plot income against BMI for men and women. Notice how there is no clear pattern (black arrows) in the first chart representing males, and contrast this with the female chart showing a significant social gradient in every age group, where those in the first quintile (lowest income) are more overweight than those in the fifth quintile (most affluent). It is worth taking a moment to consider this relationship and why you think that it differs between men and women.

When I have discussed this difference with students in the classroom or clients during weight-loss meetings, some themes that emerged have favoured the fact that lower-income jobs for men more often include significant manual labour compared to jobs for women at the same SES level. These discussions also elicit the view that women are far more likely to judge and compare themselves against other women in their social circle or at work, based upon their body shape or weight. For men, they say, that when they get together, the competitive undertone may well turn to their golf handicap or one rep max bench press, and most men would no sooner judge another man by his midriff than they would by his haircut.

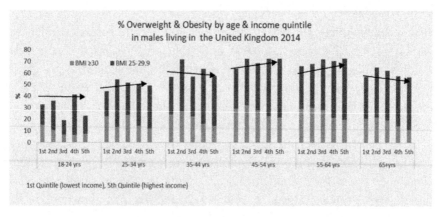

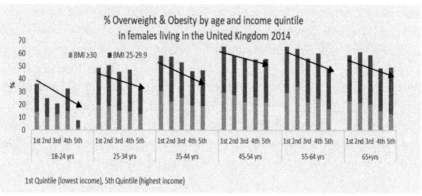

https://www.worldobesitydata.org/ accessed March 2019

If this is the case, SES for women becomes a self-perpetuating cycle, because if you are in a low SES group, more women in your immediate circle will be overweight and therefore little or no pressure applies to lose weight (in fact, it may well be that over time there becomes an inherent obligation to remain overweight). However, as SES increases, more pressure comes to bear to conform to the thinner aspirations and appearances of the more affluent group. In this case, perhaps weight is simply a barometer reflecting life's competing priorities, because people will always assign available time, thought and resources to those things that have the highest priority.

Some argue that declining economic resources make weight control more difficult, but by contrast, discrimination theories argue that it is anti-fat discrimination in hiring and in marriage that sorts heavier individuals into lower-income households. In 2022, researchers from Arizona examined this in their paper entitled 'Deprivation or discrimination?', which compared the two competing theories. They scrutinised the relationship in 27,000 women from South Korea and the US between BMI and SES, divided into two groups: (1) currently married and (2) never married. They found for married women that those with the highest SES had the lowest BMI, but not among never-married women, who may have had higher SES alongside higher BMIs, which points strongly towards weight discrimination in marriage as a key cause of the reverse gradient (more affluent males not choosing overweight women as marriage partners). The researchers dismissed deprivation and anti-fat discrimination in labour markets as causing the link between overweight and income[99].

International comparisons

In 2020, the WHO published its European Regional Obesity Report[4] in which it listed the fifty-three countries included, from wealthy economies such as the UK and Germany, to some of the poorest nations on Earth, such as Tajikistan and Uzbekistan. WHO Europe region is the perfect data set to study social, economic and cultural influences on weight, due to its diverse populations, agricultures and governance, while maintaining reasonable geographic relevance.

The two most striking aspects of the data are the gender differences with respect to the economic prosperity of each country and its inhabitants, and the fact that no country escapes the scourge of weight gain. From Turkey, with two-thirds of its population overweight or living with obesity, to the leanest country in the region, Tajikistan, which still has approaching half of its people overweight or obese. Confounding factors include issues of culture, social norms, resources, agriculture and food availability. Therefore, any trends or comparisons between countries are very difficult to explain. However, some constants can be seen, and generally, in wealthier countries, poorer women are more likely to be overweight compared to affluent women, but in poorer countries it is wealthier women that are likely to be heavier.

The economic status of country and gender trends

A comparison of obesity rates between men and women shows that, in less affluent (LA) countries, more women are living with obesity than men, and in affluent countries (AC), more men are living with obesity than women. It seems, therefore, that personal economic hardship and or living in a low-income country for women promotes obesity. For men, while the link with personal wealth is weak, affluent countries almost always have more obese men than women.

LA Country	% of population obese	of these men	of these women
Eurasia	22%	38%	62%
Azerbaijan	20%	40%	60%
Armenia	20%	42%	58%
Uzbekistan & Kyrgyzstan	18%	42%	58%

AC Country	% of population obese	of these men	of these women
Germany	23%	56%	44%
Sweden	21%	55%	44%
Denmark	20%	57%	43%
Switzerland	20%	57%	43%

Notice the split between the rate of men and women living with obesity is remarkably stable in both poor and affluent countries.

When data was pooled from the forty-two years of collection, an interesting trend appeared. What the graph to the left shows is that overweight and obesity continue to rise for both men and women. However, a couple of interesting nuances arise. The gap between the number of overweight men and women is widening, whereas the gap between men and women living with obesity is narrowing and is on track to reach parity in the next ten to twenty years. Could it be that, as countries raise themselves out of poverty, more men become obese than women? The take-home message is that the prevalence of both overweight and obesity in men in this vast multicultural socio-economically diverse region is growing more rapidly than in women.

Other gender-related trends in obesity occur elsewhere in the world, and they can start from an early age and progress into adulthood. For example, in Israel, significantly more boys and men are overweight than girls and women[100], whereas in neighbouring Arab countries girls and women are heavier than boys and men[101]. Importantly, body weight is a non-medallion trait – that is, it is not inherited from one parent or the other as a dominant allele and passed down from mother to daughter or father to son. Therefore, it is far more likely that it is the social and cultural influences that explain gender difference in population weight rather than genetics.

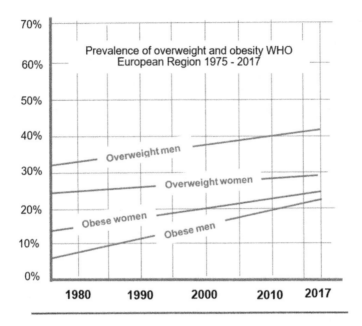

Other socio-cultural influences

Further evidence for the social and cultural influence on attitudes to weight came from a 2013 study conducted in the US, which reported that black women are more satisfied with their bodies than white women. The authors suggested that the 'buffering hypothesis' of black culture protects black women against media ideals that promote a slender female body type. Following on from this, as expected in this study, black women reported lower perceived weight and higher attractiveness than white women, despite themselves having a higher body mass. A key finding was that white women had a negative relationship between BMI and attractiveness, whereas for black women, BMI and attractiveness were unrelated[102].

It is also now apparent that sexual orientation has an impact on weight status, showing a surprisingly binary divide. While lesbian, bisexual and gender non-conforming birth-assigned females have an increased prevalence of obesity compared with straight females, gay and non-conforming birth-assigned males have a lower prevalence of obesity when compared with straight males[98]. This is another important gauge of the significance of social variables and their strong influence on how our weight is expressed.

The examples set out above show how complex the social, economic and cultural influencers of weight are, as well as how powerfully and intricately they are woven into the economics, resources, governance, political landscape and agricultural fertility of a country. I said earlier that I have not come across two people with the same backstory to their weight, and it looks like this applies equally to any two populations. No country escapes the link between social economic status and the weight of its citizens (particularly for women and children), but how this impacts people in each country is probably down to the social norms of that country.

I hope this has helped to shine a light on many of the complex influencers contributing to weight, and that it may help you to consider better your own experiences, and to help you understand your weight in the context of your social, economic and cultural circumstances.

Successful weight-loss strategies

Having considered some of the things that promote weight, it seems only fair to have a foray into the things that people have said have helped them to lose weight. Over the years, I've noted the successful strategies that people have used to manage their weight, and you will probably be familiar with most, if not all, of these common-sense disciplines. I list them not as a prescription, merely to draw your attention to what has worked for others. Also, I think what I take from this is that having some structure about how you go about things and adhering to certain self-imposed life guides, seems to be very helpful for a lot of people. Here are the ones that were most frequently fed back to me as being successful or were commonly reported in the literature:

If maintaining weight loss is your aim (which it presumably is), the most important one to start with, which has been continually mentioned to me and replicated in countless studies, is regular exercise. This is the one marker that identifies success more than any other. Other important strategies that are hailed by successful losers are:

- A healthy weekly shopping order – always have lots of the right kinds of food in the house.
- Always have a sensible breakfast (but many successful losers disagree).

- Monitor your weight more than once each week.
- Commit to an exercise routine and make it part of your life.
- Avoid CRAP foods.
- Eat more fruit and vegetables.
- Control your portions.
- Be aware of food labels and calorie values.
- Make good use of social supports such as family and friends or online groups.
- Choose a food ally and commit to sharing your insights and supporting each other when temptation calls.
- Value food and learn and enjoy cooking.

Researchers examined the weight-loss behaviours of over 6,000 people on a commercial weight-loss programme that had on average lost 24.5 kg and maintained the loss for over three years. Their motivations for tackling their weight included: health issues, appearance, mobility and social prompts. The three core themes helping with maintaining a lower weight were memories of negative experiences, poor health consequences and concerns about how they used to look. The condensed advice from these 6,000 people was: 'Perseverance in the face of setbacks, consistency in tracking progress and weight, and focusing on the positivity of reduced weight, which included improved confidence, pain reduction, enhanced mobility, better fitness, improved body image, better general health, and more positive mental health and outlook on life'[103].

The National Weight Control Registry (www.nwcr.ws) is a US initiative for people that have maintained at least 30 pounds (14kg) of weight loss for one year or longer. It was established in 1994 by Rena Wing, PhD., from Brown Medical School, and James O Hill, PhD., from the University of Colorado, and is the largest prospective investigation of long-term successful weight-loss maintenance. The NWCR was developed to identify and investigate the characteristics of individuals who have succeeded at long-term weight loss and is tracking over 10,000 people to establish successful strategies. The average female weight is 145lbs (66kg), while for men it is 190lbs (86kg), and members have lost an average of 66lbs (30kg) and kept it off for 5.5 years.

Some of the most common strategies used are:

- 98% modified their food intake in some way to lose weight.
- 94% increased physical activity - average of one hour/day (most choose walking).
- 78% eat breakfast every day.
- 75% weigh themselves at least once a week.
- 62% watch fewer than ten hours of TV per week.

Technology

Technology can assist some people in achieving their health and lifestyle goals, and for the techie-minded, the use of wearable devices can be a good option to help improve long-term physical activity and other change targets. Smart scales for some have great benefits and come with a host of useful features. Most include body composition measures and indicate fat mass compared to lean mass, which I think is really helpful. The latest machines are highly compatible with smartphones and fitness apps, and most now come with a free app that automatically synchronises for daily monitoring and tracking. As it is proven that digital self-monitoring of physical activity and diet is effective in supporting weight loss in adults these do seem like good support options. But techie devices are not for everyone and if you are not comfortable with technological widgets, perhaps it's best to stick with traditional scales.

Another popular strategy for many of my clients was to adopt the primary discipline of eating only when sitting down. This simple 'rule' has many virtues. You can't eat on the hoof when there are many tempting high-calorie foods around. You are not allowed to keep testing foods that you are cooking or clearing away. Lounging does not count as sitting, so no sofa snacking. Sufficient people told me about this to make it worth mentioning to you for consideration. In an unruly food world, rules help.

Intermittent fasting for weight loss

Fasting, which is a time related voluntary cessation of eating, has been around for a long time and millions of people regularly fast for health, or as part of their faith. For a great many people, intermittent fasting (IF) is a way of life which they are comfortable with and accustomed to. In terms of the reputed health benefits of IF, the premise is firmly rooted in our ancestry as hunter-gatherer scavengers, where food supplies were far from predictable, and life revolved around a cycle more akin to fast to feast. The continued calorie overload of modern life disrupts circadian rhythms, profoundly affecting metabolic systems, and it is suggested that feeding/fasting cycles are an excellent antidote to reset these overloaded biological controls[104]. There seems little doubt that we are more organically suited to this pattern of eating.

The notion that frequent eating (three meals every day plus regular snacking) is far from optimum, is entirely logical. There is a growing body of evidence that suggests anything you can do to let your insulin-producing beta cells rest, and keep your insulin levels low for longer, will have considerable beneficial effects. Buettner[105] noted: "The body appears to need snack-free time to recover from high-calorie events, such as a typical Western meal". Recently, scientists discovered that mice bred to produce half the normal amount of insulin stayed lean on a 'junk diet' while normal mice became obese. It appears that the regular low-insulin conditions brought about by IF could help to return insulin to healthier levels for longer periods through the day, causing fat cells to burn energy rather than store it.

In a separate experiment, scientists at the Salk Institute found that mice fed a junk diet for eight hours followed by a sixteen-hour fast maintained a normal weight, where a second group that ate the same amount, but spread over twenty-four hours, became obese and suffered from high cholesterol, high blood sugar and other obesity-related ailments. Without an extended break from feeding, the mice appeared unable to process all the fat, cholesterol and glucose they had consumed, and therefore stored rather than burned it. Furthermore, the benefits continued even when fasting was temporarily interrupted by unlimited snacking during weekends, a regimen particularly relevant to human lifestyle[106]. This supports the IF version of Time Restricted Eating (TRE).

TRE restricts the hours of feeding between set times each day, typically only allowing eating between 11am and 7pm, thereby imposing a sixteen-hour fast each day. In animals, it appears that it is the disruption to circadian rhythms that interferes with weight regulation, however, in humans, it is still unclear if it is this or simply the calorie restriction practically imposed by TRE that affects weight loss[107].

With respect to fasting for weight loss, there are several methods (and many other variations that are not mentioned here):

- **Alternate day fasting:** normal eating one day followed by fast or, more typically, considerably reduced calories the next day.

- **5-2 fasting:** involves normal eating for five days followed by two days of fasting or calorie-reduced days.

- **Time-determined fasts:** a weekly set period of fasting between twenty-four and forty-eight hours.

- **Time-restricted fasting:** shortens the amount of time available for eating, for instance between the hours of 11am and 7pm.

My wife and I tend to favour a weekly forty-hour fast (time determined) where we stop eating after a final meal around 7pm on Wednesday evening and then break our fast on Friday lunchtime around 1pm, whereupon we bask in the pleasures of a lovely walk down the river Thames with our four-legged companion, Monty, followed by a much-appreciated lunch at the Boaters in Kingston, or the Anglers at Teddington lock. What a pleasure! Our routine is to allow unlimited water and tea and a very small amount of vegetable juice during the fast, though it's entirely up to you how to go about it. The main thing is, if you wish to try fasting, then find a method that suits you and your lifestyle, so that you can maintain it as part of your way of life. There is no right or wrong way to fast providing it severely restricts calories over the fast period and it is not harmful. Fasting, if done properly, should help to keep your waistline trim and will lead to significant metabolic benefits. I'm also a great believer in periodically resting the liver.

A quarrelsome subject

Fasting for weight loss would regularly crop up at group meetings, or while I was teaching. It was frequently a hot topic as long ago as twenty years past. Typically, someone would ask, "Alan, what do you think of fasting for weight loss?" To which I'd say, "Actually, I'd like to know what *you* think of fasting for weight loss?" And they might respond:

> **Student:** "Well, I've tried it, and it was hopeless, really hard, and I didn't lose any weight. In fact, if anything, I put weight on because I constantly felt hungry and then went berserk when the fast ended. Also, the feeling of denial was just too much".
>
> **Me:** "I hate fasting for weight loss!"

The next person in the group may say something along the lines of:

Student: "Actually, it works for me. Once I got used to it, I could manage OK. I think it helps me in several ways, and it does fit with my spiritual beliefs. I feel stronger for it, and I also think it has a cleansing effect on my body and mind. I do think it is a good way of managing my weight, and it definitely does help me."

Me: "I love fasting for weight loss!"

Many people I have spoken to find adherence to intermittent fasting easier than continually watching what they eat. They say that, psychologically, intermittent fasting suits them because they are not faced with the same eating dilemmas every day: "On non-fasting days, I eat what I want, and on fasting days, I just don't eat, no turmoil or choices to make!" This is backed up by science. Functional magnetic resonance imaging (fMRI) of the brain shows how sensory factors such as the sight, smell, palatability and availability of food can increase appetite to such an extent that it overwhelms innate control mechanisms, a phenomenon described as 'hedonic hunger'. Fasting is therefore one way of removing irresistible temptations. IF also has at least comparable – and typically better – weight loss and body fat reduction benefits than traditional continuous dieting. Many fasters report making better choices on non-fasting days facilitated by the discipline they have learned through fasting.

Fasting is not suitable for everyone, though, particularly young people or those with a history of disordered eating. Women who are pregnant or breastfeeding should also avoid fasting and those with medical conditions such as diabetes should first consult their doctor or specialist health carer. However, on balance, if none of this applies to you, I believe that IF may be a good option for long-term weight management and improved metabolic health, which is well supported in the literature[108]. As a weight-management plan and lifestyle habit, it strikes me as entirely feasible. TRE and IF may provide long-term solutions for people that struggle to manage their weight by trying to juggle food choices every day, and I would certainly say this would be an option worth trying for those looking for an alternative to permanent food-watching.

Insight 1: Orientation

Insight 1: Orientation

Earlier (on page 16), I asked you to consider where you currently are on the lifestyle continuum (LC), and this was the start of your journey. The LC represents a self-assessment of how you feel about your life, the behaviours and choices that you are making at this moment in time, and the impact that this is having on your perceived general wellbeing. It is a snapshot of the reality of your world, based upon events and actual happenings as you observe them and as they happen in real time. Now is the time to delve a little deeper into your thoughts and beliefs about yourself.

As you move from light contemplation through to intense and detailed reflection about each of these questions (and your responses), you will refine and develop your ideas and beliefs until they become crystal clear in your mind. Don't skimp on this, which is a core aspect of your learning; take a couple of hours, a day, a week, a month, a year, if necessary. If each insight takes less than half an hour, you've probably not given them sufficient thought or provided enough detail. Be very specific and try not to generalise. Keep in mind what you have said about your current position on the LC as you consider the next steps. Grab your notebook and take time to answer the following questions.

Body dis/satisfaction

Evaluating, acknowledging and coming to terms with where you are on the body dis/satisfaction scale is a good place to start. Everyone reading this book will be starting from their own place along the spectrum, considering not only aesthetics, but also functionality, vitality and health. There will be those who think about the state of their avatar and feel desperate and depressed about their situation; they have fought for so long with their weight and they just can't see a way out. Others may feel they have just let things go recently, and perhaps just need a little motivation and a few nudges in the right direction to get back on track, but are, on balance, happy and satisfied with their body.

Give it plenty of thought, and write in words your view of your body, and of course your weight needs to be a central consideration. If you think it would be helpful, rank it from 1 – 10 (1 is low). Detail exactly how you feel using appropriate words and be specific about any body parts or areas that are particularly relevant to why you feel the way that you do. The idea of this exercise is not to make you feel depressed or upset (but it may); the point is to develop discrepancy between actions and wants, and to support your decisions for the future. More about this later.

It may be that your current lifestyle and behaviour is having an impact on other aspects of your health and wellbeing, independent of your weight. This might include influencing your mental health or interfering with work or relationships. Describe these in a similar way, considering your weight and any related knock-on issues as one. You must be clear about your beliefs and feelings towards your weight and the resultant quality of life impacts in both physical and psychological terms. Sit in a quiet place while you detail your thoughts. Don't move on to the next question until you have fully answered this one.

Why do I believe this?

Now think about why you have just written what you have. If you had to justify your position to an anonymous onlooker, would they take on your point of view as fair and balanced? While it can be an emotive exercise, try to think about facts. For instance, you could write: "My weight makes me upset". But this is insufficiently detailed. What part of your weight makes you upset and why? What specifically is upsetting and when does it most upset you? Does it upset anyone else? Keep going until you are wholly satisfied that you have written down in entirety why you believe your words about your feelings for your weight are true and accurate. Once done, take a break, and have a nice cup of tea… you will have earned it.

How do I want to be?

Next, I'd like you to give some consideration to your ultimate goals, i.e., if we could run the clock forward a couple of years, this is how your life would be if you were to be successful. Firstly, what are your goals? Are they related to weight or size? Do they include activity, agility, functionality, or fitness ambitions? Are your goals related to a condition or limitation that is being affected by your weight? Do your goals involve other people? Do your goals relate to the rest of your life? Think carefully and write down your goals, and don't limit it to "I'd like to be a size 14".

Why do I want to be like that?

This is perhaps the most important of all the questions. If you can't answer this with any meaning or precision, then your prospects of success are slim (sorry about that!). What will it mean to you and what tangible differences would it make to your life if you could achieve your goals and make them last? You need to be honest with yourself and be realistic, think things through properly.

For example, you might think, "If I achieved my weight goals, I might be in with a chance of dating Veronica from the IT department!" I'm not sure that is such a great reason, because if you did lose lots of weight and she told you to bugger off, you'd no doubt hit the Chinese takeaways with vengeance. Also, if you lost weight and Veronica did go out with you, you'd always be fearful that, if the weight returned, she wouldn't stick around. In my view, you'd be better off asking her, "Hey, if I lost loads of weight, would you go out with me?" She might surprise you and say, "I'll go out with you as you are, I've fancied you for ages!"

What is my proximity to my goals?

Visualise what your life would be like if you could achieve all your goals and maintain them into the future. How close do you feel to this right now? If you have several goals, rate each of them 1 – 10 (1 is very distant). Don't just use numbers, write down the detail behind your rationale for providing the answers that you have. For example:

> *"I want to be fit enough to walk with the dog for at least an hour every day and not to be breathless and over-heating when I go up the hilly parts of the walk. At the moment, I'm a three out of ten in terms of my proximity to this goal."*

Now read through all your thoughts in this first insight task and take time to consider absolutely and in entirety all the words you have written. Make amends and changes until you are totally happy with your view of things. Perhaps type them up or write them out neatly and keep them close to reflect on over the coming weeks. Complete the above task before reading any further. Take as long as you need and revisit it lots of times until you are utterly sure it is clear, and it is the truth.

You are not going to act on any of this just yet, that will come later. Before that, you need more time to prepare and to understand how weight loss works. For now, just clear your head and take sufficient time to think about your words. How deeply you take into consideration these questions and how comprehensively you answer them will greatly influence your prospects of success.

Genetics and epigenetics

"Genes load the gun and environment (lifestyle) pulls the trigger."

George Bray, 1998

If parents were to ration their genes when they had children, which is what happens (50% each), you'd probably refer to this as a 'generation'. The link with body weight among generations was noted one hundred years ago[109], and despite considerable subsequent research, factors that affect weight heritability are still poorly understood. Genetics, the complexity of which seems to know no bounds, influence everything about us, and the expression of our weight is no exception. Genes definitely influence the differences in weight between individuals living in the same environment, however estimates as to the strength of this influence range rather unhelpfully from 20%-90%[110]. First, let's take a close look at genes, which are made from strands of DNA.

DNA and genes

DNA stores its information as a code made up of four chemical bases, represented by the letters (A) adenine, (G) guanine, (C) cytosine and (T) thymine. The sequence of these bases holds the key to how organisms are built and how they function. These DNA bases pair together along with sugar and phosphate to form nucleotides, which align into two long spiral strands – the famous double helix. The double helix resembles a ladder where the bases are the rungs, and the sugar/phosphate molecules are the side frames. The double helix contains one gene from each parent, known as alleles. Two identical alleles and your genotype for that locus (location on the chromosome) is homozygous; two different alleles, and your genotype is

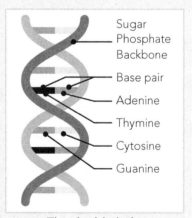

The double helix

heterozygous. Alleles are either dominant (they appear to be optimum for the role) or recessive (they may be damaged or sub-optimal), with the dominant allele generally being the one expressed ('turned on'). The total combination of alleles makes up our 'genotype', which therefore refers to our general genetic characteristics based upon the sequence of genes we inherited from our parents.

Genes are a specific section of DNA, anything from 500 letters to over two million! They encode traits, that is, they produce the most important materials for life, proteins, the building blocks of life and the foundation of all hormones and enzymes, critical for chemical reactions and bodily control. From the twenty amino acids used in humans, every protein that we need can be made. Amino acids are folded to create complex three-dimensional protein structures, the shape of which is specific to their role. The instruction for this feat is woven into the DNA sequence of the gene, transcribed into RNA, and translated into the structure of a protein in a feat of unimaginably intricate biochemical origami.

Genes bundle together in their hundreds or thousands and are coiled tightly to fit into one of the twenty-three chromosome pairs. Genes with similar functions are found together in chromosomes such as those for eye colour, hair colour, height and skin tone. Although every cell contains the full set of around 23,000 genes, only about one-tenth of them are expressed, or 'turned on' in any particular type of cell (because specific cells need only particular proteins).

Eye colour is a classic example of a fixed genotype, where the allele is either brown or blue. The brown allele is dominant and the blue allele is recessive, therefore if the child inherits two different alleles (heterozygous) then they will have brown eyes. The brown allele is dominant because brown eyes are optimum for vision (darker irises reduce reflection within the eye, cutting glare and improving contrast discernment). For the child to have blue eyes, they must be homozygous for the blue-eye allele (they inherited one blue allele from each parent).

Interestingly, the theory regarding the proliferation of the less-efficient blue eye suggests that, following a random genetic mutation and consequent alteration to eye pigment, for someone in a world where everyone had brown eyes, having blue eyes rendered you very special –

your mating advantage took a huge leap forward! How this happened to two people simultaneously to make a child homozygous for blue eyes (so it could be passed on) requires a staggering set of coincidences.

Evolutionary development requires such random gene mutations (known as single nucleotide polymorphisms [SNPs]), and it has been calculated that these occur in three out of every 1000 cells or embryos. Such a mutation will confer either a benefit to that individual organism, in which case it is likely to proliferate in the population, or a negative effect (more likely) in which case it is unlikely to become widespread and established in the gene pool. Over a period of around four billion years, this random game of chance has delivered us from primitive single cells in a primordial swamp somewhere on Earth, to the highest-order organism in the known universe. The magnitude of this happenstance is barely comprehensible.

Genetic influence on weight

You only have to examine geographical differences to realise that the concept of inherited susceptibility to weight gain is a valid one. The top ten most obese countries are all in a tiny part of the world in the South Pacific. The percentage of inhabitants in each island living with obesity is: Tonga (77%); Cook Islands (70%); Tuvalu (62%); Nauru (61.0%); Niue (61%) Kiribati (57%); Samoa (56%); Palau (55%); Marshall Islands (53%); and Micronesia (50%)[111]. There can be little doubt that some people are more genetically inclined to gain weight, and weight and body shape are no doubt heritable, but to what extent?

Everyone has come across significant family resemblance between parents and their children, and it has been proposed that children with two parents living with obesity have an approximate 80% risk of becoming obese compared to 20% in children with two lean parents[112]. But how much of this is genetic and how much is behavioural is not resolved to any satisfactory conclusion. It is the delicate interplay between our genes, environments and behaviours that is the key to weight, and to all our health outcomes for that matter. The goal for researchers is to untangle this complex relationship and establish the relative contribution of each, but that is proving tricky.

The environmental changes over recent years have led to an explosion of weight gain across the globe. Therefore, while genes confer the potential for weight gain, it is the environmental factors that are driving the obesity pandemic. There can be no sharper example of the interplay between genes and the environment than in the Pima Indians living in Arizona. Eighty years ago, the obesity level and prevalence of metabolic diseases were very low within the tribe, but after the Second World War there were dramatic changes to their environment. The introduction of a Westernised diet and loss of traditional lifestyles led to a dramatic obesity (and diabetes) epidemic within the tribe. Pima Indians, it transpires, have a strong genetic predisposition to weight gain and diabetes, which is expressed only in the presence of a Westernised lifestyle[113].

Thrifty genotype

Around sixty years ago, the 'thrifty genotype' hypothesis was proposed by James Neel[114]. Thrift, meaning sparing use of available resources, in this case refers to the efficiency with which energy is used in the body – metabolic thrift. Over millennia, genes that protect against famine have been incrementally favoured and established as a characteristic of the gene pool for all of humanity. For our early and recent ancestors, the ongoing scarcity of food and the frequency of famine would ensure the thrifty genotype's continuation and proliferation in the gene pool. Neel figured that those whose genes were selected and arranged with the potential to store more body fat in times of plenty, were most likely to survive the inevitable (cyclical) famine. Similarly, they would be more energy efficient and frugal in the use of their internal fat stores during periods of food crisis.

The thrifty genotype theory was tested on rats with the assumption that a thrifty genotype (obese-prone rat) would have a survival advantage in a food-restricted environment. Two modified rat genotypes were used: obese prone and lean prone (where each had been genetically modified to express genes for fatness or leanness). Each rat type was exposed to prolonged low food intake and high wheel running; a procedure that leads to eventual starvation. The results showed that although identical in initial body weight, the obese-prone rats better maintained blood glucose and fat mass, and survived twice as long and ran three times as far as their lean-prone counterparts[115].

The thrifty genotype hypothesis is generally accepted as an explanation for genetically inherited susceptibility to weight gain. An obese-prone genotype provides a big survival advantage when food supply is inadequate, but in the context of calorie-copious contemporary living, overfeeding an organism that has been programmed over tens of thousands of years to thrive in an energy-sparce environment leads to profound metabolic derangements, the consequences of which are bleak.

Phenotype

So now we know about the 'genotype', and that not all genes are 'expressed'. It is only your 'switched on' genes that represent your 'phenotype'. The mechanics of this are complicated, but basically the body changes our gene expression to reflect prevailing environmental circumstances. The sum of all these 'chemical marks' is known as our phenotype, and it is entirely unique to each one of us. Even identical twins, as they grow and develop, will start to become more and more individual, especially if they are living apart, as differing environmental exposures will alter each of their phenomes.

Therefore, the phenotype relates to an individual and their expressed genes, partly because of inheritance and partly a result of the environmental experiences that they encounter. So we can see that genotype is fixed, while the phenotype is malleable and is 'influenced' and constantly changing due to environmental and lifestyle factors. Some of the gene expression 'influencers' with the greatest authority include nutrition, climate, air quality, toxins, disease, physical in/activity and stress.

The 'thrifty phenotype' hypothesis states that the growth of the foetus is programmed by its early life nutritional environment, which confers certain metabolic characteristics on the individual (phenotype) resulting in profound effects on health and weight in later life. For instance, malnutrition during the first trimester of pregnancy, affects the growth rates of different tissues (nutritional thrift), acting to alter organ function. The purpose of this is to build a thrifty offspring who is adapted for survival in poor nutritional circumstances.

The Dutch famine of World War II was the result of the Nazi blockade of food to over four million people in the densely populated Northern Provinces of the Netherlands. Fifty years later, this led to the epidemiologic observation that children born to mothers who were in the early stages of pregnancy during the siege and subsequent famine, were at significantly increased risk of cardiometabolic disorders in adulthood. Thus, when food is scarce, the foetus can make changes to be able to subsist on lower levels of nutrition to better survive the anticipated famine when they emerge. These changes include permanent structural alterations of organs, altered behavioural responses and changes in gene expression[116]. These initial findings led to a new understanding that early-life environmental conditions can cause changes in humans that persist throughout life.

This genetic gift for gene manipulation to help survive famine achieves the objectives of the genes, which is to improve mating prospects to enable the genes to proliferate – the only thing they are interested in; genes don't give two hoots for you, the host! But this is no gift, it's a loan, and it must be paid back in full. Hypertension, poor insulin secretion, insulin resistance and obesity are the repayment dues. These invariably result in premature death for the gene carrier, but the genes achieved their goal, and probably got passed on... that's all that matters to them.

If, however, during pregnancy, the opposite occurs and too many calories are consumed, this signals an abundance of food to the foetus and the genes will respond accordingly. This time, the response of the foetus is to build extra fat cells to cater for the excess available energy it expects and to make good use of it by storing it away for the next inevitable famine. The extra fat cells are permanent and will be a feature for life. They will demand (through the instructions in their genes) that they always be fed, and the obedient appetite machinery will react accordingly. The genes have once again remodelled the instruments at their disposal to cater for the prevailing environmental conditions and confer a mating advantage for their host living in a time when extra food is available. However, even genes are (probably) not omniscient, and, should the cyclical famine not materialise, then we are all aware of what the future holds for that person now carrying the extra biological luggage.

Genes implicated in obesity

Geneticists have documented a number of genes that can be statistically associated with human obesity, but it is apparent that there is not a single gene responsible for the current pandemic of obesity, with each suspect gene making only a small contribution. One gene in particular (known as the FTO gene) has attracted a lot of attention, and studies find that people carrying it were on average 1.2kg heavier and faced a 30% higher chance of obesity. Those with both FTO genes (one from each parent) were on average 3kg heavier and carried a 60% greater risk[117].

In another study that looked at the effect of exercise on the reduction of fat mass in a twenty-week endurance training programme, those with two FTO alleles lost less body fat than other study participants, with the researchers concluding the FTO genotype influences the body fat responses to regular exercise. But the FTO variant is surprisingly common, with two-thirds of European or African descendants and one-third of Asians carrying at least one allele, which means that very many people are in the 'slightly higher risk' category.

Genome wide association studies (GWAS) have found many gene mutations related to body weight, but their effects are very small. For example, a large GWA study (that cited 482 authors!) found that ninety-seven gene mutations with the strongest associations with BMI explain only 2.7% of weight variance[118]. A later study, hailed as a breakthrough, then identified 1,000 mutations associated with BMI, but even all these variants together only accounted for just 6% of the variance in BMI between people. It appears the effect of genes on weight may not be the critical determinant that has been previously proposed.

Family, twin and adoption studies

Before the human genome was decoded, family studies offered the only possible way to estimate the role of genetic and environmental factors involved in the variability of weight. These old twin studies estimated (but by no means established) the genetic contribution to weight and led to the huge variability mentioned earlier.

Family studies work on the premise that heritability and gene sharing is governed by family proximity in the following order: identical twins; non-identical twins; parent/child; siblings; first cousins and so on. Twin studies are therefore powerful instruments in that both types of twins (identical and non-identical), from conception, share their environments. That is, they share the same womb for the same period, grow up in the same household, share the same family environment, and are of the same socio-economic status. This presents a unique opportunity to impartially assess the gene/environment effect.

Adoption studies (using twins) provide a further model for examining how genes respond to new or novel environments. For example, weight similarities between adopted children and their biological parents (living in two separate households) emphasise the role of genetics, while correlation between non-related (adoptive) children with non-related parents and siblings is evidence of the role of the family environment.

In other study designs, researchers compare monozygotic (identical twins – one sperm one egg) against dizygotic twins (two sperm, two eggs, producing regular siblings born simultaneously) and evaluate weight similarities. Monozygotic twins are essentially identical at the gene-sequence level, whereas dizygotic twins share only half their genes. When reared simultaneously in the same environment, the difference between weight similarities of identical twins and non-identical is likely to be genetic.

Thirty years ago, a study examined a sample of 540 adults classified as thin, medium, overweight and obese, and found a strong relationship between parents and their natural children, but no relation between the weight of adoptees and their adoptive parents[119]. A few years later, the same researchers examined data on 673 sets of identical and non-identical twins, with just under half of the sample pairs of twins separated and living apart. They found that, even when put into completely remote environments, the twins would, to a degree, track each other's weight and that their weight comparisons correlated only slightly less than the twins that were living together[120].

In another study, seven pairs of adult male identical twins completed a three-month diet and exercise programme. The result was a seven-fold variance in the difference in weight change between pairs than within pairs[121]. Similarly, fourteen pairs of very overweight identical twin children were subjected to twenty-eight days of a very low-calorie diet (400kcal/day). The result, thirteen times more variability between pairs than within pairs[122]. What these results tell us is that it is genes that are deciding how much weight will be lost. In the same way, overfeeding studies using multiple sets of twins show that body weight responds similarly to overfeeding, within rather than between twin pairs, illuminating the genetic effects of overeating[123].

On the other hand, a 2010 study examined fourteen identical adult twin pairs for weight (with at least a 5kg weight difference). Their food intake was recorded using the incontrovertible doubly labelled water (DLW)§ method, and accelerometers were used to measure physical activity. Despite claims from the overweight twins that they lived the same lifestyle as their lean twins, data from the DLW and accelerometers proved that there was a significant difference in food eaten (averaging 760kcal/day more) and that they had undertaken half as much physical activity (averaging 429kcal/

§ The doubly labelled water (DLW) technique is the gold standard for measuring energy expenditure. The subject is given a dose of water enriched with the stable isotopes deuterium (H2) and oxygen 18 (O18) and urine samples are collected to measure the disappearance of these isotopes. From this total energy expenditure can be calculated with a high degree of accuracy.

day less). Despite their identical DNA sequences, it was different lifestyles causing the weight differences. The authors concluded that "Obesity is associated with eating more, snacking more and choosing less healthy foods, and exercising less at high intensities"[124].

Other indicators of the importance of environmental exposure include the fact that identical twins rarely die of the same cause. In fact, as they age, twins become more and more different, and the importance of environmental exposure becomes apparent. Furthermore, monozygotes with identical genes when reared apart can differ in height by as much as four inches, despite having identical genes for maximum height potential.

As global weight gain continues, and being a healthy weight becomes a minority pursuit, perhaps the concept of genetic vulnerability gradually loses its validity. The question ought not to be "Why are so many people overweight?" (that's apparent) but rather "How are some people remaining lean in our obesogenic world?" The increase in weight over the past fifty years points squarely at the increased availability of CRAP food and, to a lesser degree, a reduction in physical activity in Westernised societies. Evidence for this comes from the marked increase in BMI seen in migrants (including first second and third generations) who move to a Western society, compared to their leaner countrymen who stay at home[125].

The importance of behavioural choices was reaffirmed when researchers from the Lausanne University Hospital assessed whether genetic background and/ or dietary behaviours were most closely associated with weight and waist circumferences. From the sample of over 3,000 people, they concluded that there were no associations between genetic risk and BMI, with no significant gene-diet interactions found. It was dietary intake that was responsible for the waist circumferences of their middle-aged cohort[126].

Recently, work on the gene/environment susceptibility relationship has shown that people with the highest genetic risk of metabolic disease and obesity benefit the most from lifestyle strategies that are proven to protect against such diseases. A large study of UK participants showed that a healthy, plant-based diet offered significantly more protection to those with the highest risk, compared to those with the lowest risk[127]. Genes therefore confer the potential for obesity and lifestyle diseases, but it is our environments and how we interact with and respond to them that determines the outcome.

A recent genetic study that looked at the relationship between unhealthy lifestyles and the risk of death from all causes, found that: "unfavourable lifestyle behaviours predicted higher rates of death independent of genetic risk."[128]. In other words, genes may make you more susceptible, but even if you have Rambo-style genes, unhealthy lifestyles will still trump your golden genotype.

Staying with the environmental theme, researchers from Holland tested the idea that people living in an obesogenic environment, choose less-healthy options, because that is all that is available. If this is the case, then it is assumed that simply changing the food environment will lead to more healthy snacking. To test this premise in real life, 'The urban snack project' selected 'hotspot locations' for unhealthy snacking, and developed an appealing affordable, healthy snack, with attractive branding, to be despatched from a small food truck. They found that, despite people's appreciation for the snack, the food truck, and the branding, the locals didn't buy the healthy snack[129].

In terms of the impact that exercise and physical activity can have on susceptible genes, a cross-sectional study set in London followed 970 adult female twins. The outcome: that physical activity was the strongest independent predictor of total-body fat, even for those with a genetic predisposition to being overweight[130]. This was confirmed in 2010, when a study examined data on 20,000 people living in Norfolk and concluded: "Our study shows that living a physically active lifestyle is associated with a 40% reduction in the genetic predisposition to common obesity"[131]. Similar studies have shown that an active life can blunt 'obese' genes by up to 75%[132]. Collectively, this data proves the importance of exercise in combatting obesity for people with susceptible genes. Once again, the mechanism is not necessarily through the calorie value of the workouts combatting overconsumption, but more the impact it has on the genes.

Inherited behaviours

The genetic association with obesity conjures ideas of biological factors or physical traits that incline the body towards gaining weight through homeostatic or metabolic mechanisms. Scientific enquiries in this field examine the physiological determinants of genes: energy efficiency, fidget factor, glycaemic control, lipid accumulation and so on, to make a genetic case for weight gain. This is understandable – as obesity manifests in the body, it makes sense to search for clues in that area. However, often overlooked is the influence of genes on behaviour and the way our brains behave. The ways in which we think are likely to have a much more profound effect on our weight compared to the way our stomach, fat cells, liver etc go about their business. This offers promise, as our brains are far more plastic than our bodies.

By way of example, personality traits such as conscientiousness, self-control and impulsivity are all heritable, as are such things as mood, depression, and educational attainment, all of which are closely linked to weight. Genes also influence personality characteristics such as motivation, diligence, ambition, work ethic, relationship with exercise, and, crucially, appetite, snacking and preference for certain foods. Consider the collective impact this may have on weight (and other health outcomes), and it appears that the psycho-behavioural impact of genes far outweighs any physiological effect.

When it comes to lifestyle choices, the question is: what leads one person to be motivated to exercise, to buy and cook healthy foods, and invest time and resources into healthful activities, while another person has little or no motivation to do any of these things despite knowing full well that it would be of significant benefit to them? Are their genes telling them to sit on the couch, to do what feels best or eat what tastes nicest, or has their upbringing paved the way for a lifetime of preferred lifestyle choices? How much of our behaviour is nature, and how much is nurture?

Where siblings are concerned, I've heard parents many times state that: "One child is hard working and studious, always does all his homework and will also help around the house. His brother/sister, on the other hand, is lazy and disinterested, never lifts a finger and always needs to be pushed to do schoolwork. But we have brought them both up in the same way!" I'm sure you have your own examples of within-family differences in behaviour.

Proposed in 2007 by the late Professor Jane Wardle, behavioural susceptibility theory (BST) theorises that genetic susceptibility to weight operates via food preferences and appetite mechanisms[133]. A person's desire to eat at the sight, smell or taste of palatable food is known as food responsiveness. Satiety responsiveness refers to eating only when hungry and stopping when sated. These two traits appear to be at the core of BST. If you are highly food responsive, ubiquitous and aggressively marketed CRAP foods are designed and destined to make you overeat. Those with weaker satiety signals are more likely to overeat in response to larger portion sizes and multiple opportunities to eat, which, let's face it, represents most of the

Western world! Therefore, people inheriting avid appetites and a penchant for calorific foods or frequent snacking are the ones susceptible to overeating in obesogenic environments, explaining why those with the strongest susceptibility have the greatest weight gain.

Summary

There is no doubt that genes are a considerable influencer of weight, and thrifty genotypes will always face the greatest challenges in a given environment, and it seems to me that this is driven by Wardle's behavioural susceptibility theory. But, for genes to express their tendency for encouraging weight gain, this relies on making decisions and choices that favour excess calories in, and limits calorie expenditure. We no longer live in a world where calories are sparse and hard work is required to acquire energy, which keeps everyone lean, and therefore it is the preferences and behaviours that now create the risk of weight gain.

Environments are frequently blamed for poor health, and this is understandable, and the difficulties of living in areas of high deprivation are apparent to all. But, as lifestyle is simply a summary of the choices that we can make in any given environment, I prefer to think of the concept of 'environmental lifestyles'. While genes will influence the difference between the weight of individuals living in any given environment, the more powerful force will be the adopted lifestyle within that environment.

Studies that use validated measuring techniques (DLW and accelerometers), nearly always find the differences between the weight of related and non-related people, down to the simple calorie equation, those who eat the most and move the least are typically heavier. All of this points to the effect that genes have on our behaviours and the choices that we make around food and activity as the influencers of our weight. If this is the case, then it really changes nothing, because if you are overweight and you want to permanently lose weight, then you must change your behaviour, same back then, same now.

If as Jane Wardle suspected, behavioural susceptibility to food cues, or weaker satiety signals are a problem for you, then recognising and accepting this and understanding the genetic basis (rather than I'm weak willed, flaky etc) is needed. In this case, good planning and organisational skills and a structural approach to change are vital. The key question here is: What is the more powerful force in my life, the pain of my weight or the inconvenience of being organised? More on this in the chapter on change.

From this we can gather that for those with a genetic susceptibility to weight gain, life will be more difficult in an obesogenic environment, just as people with a susceptibility to respiratory problems will suffer more, living in places with poor air quality. To put it another way, genes interacting with the environment explains why one smoker gets lung cancer and another doesn't. However, the reason that there is so much lung cancer in the world is due to the number of people that smoke, not for any genetic reason. Equally, the reason that there is so much obesity in the world is due to the volumes of CRAP that people eat.

It is a fact that everyone is dealt a genetic hand of cards at birth. For some, this can lead to resentment at what people see as an unfair burden that they must carry throughout life (my mum's overweight, my gran was overweight, my sisters are overweight and so are my kids). People will often use this perceived 'poor hand' to abrogate their responsibility to make the right lifestyle choices, and things get progressively worse. However, while we start life with a set hand of cards, ultimately it is how we play those cards that really matters. Obesogenic environments do make many choices difficult, but seldom impossible.

Finally, dwelling on our gene inheritance serves no purpose. Thinking about your genetic inheritance in negative terms is defeatist and probably outright wrong in any case. Think not about the gene sequence, but gene expression. Genes are malleable, we have just seen how we can influence and change how they work and how they impact our weight and health, relative to the environmental choices that we make. We can change our behaviour and we can change our gene expression, and we have seen the major impact that exercise and physical activity has on our genes. Just maybe, the big fellah upstairs when he dealt our hand, slipped in a couple of wild cards to help us out.

Nutrigenomics

An area that has gained much attention lately is nutrigenomics – the science of personalised nutrition, or more correctly, the relationship between nutrients, diet, and gene expression. It is clear now that diet alters biological function by interacting with genes, switching them on or off. The principle behind nutrigenomics is that each of us, by nature of our differing genomes, is likely to have an optimum diet, also meaning that many people may have diets that are counterproductive or sub-optimal to their needs.

If you are unconvinced by the power of food to fundamentally alter organisms and the gene level, then look no further than a beehive. In there, you will observe the sterile worker bees that toil day after day until they turn their stings up after just a few weeks. Contrast this with the queen bee, who lives for years and unbelievably lays up to 3,000 eggs each day. But they are genetically identical organisms that only differentiate into two entirely different life forms because the queen eats royal jelly, whereas the worker bees get nectar and pollen. Clearly, the royal jelly contains nutrients that provide genetic instructions to unleash the 'queen genes'.

Not only is it the individual nutrients, but the whole composition of our diet that will affect the genome, including the macronutrient balance of carbohydrates, proteins and fat and the micro-nutrient content of vitamins, minerals, and phytochemicals. Also, we must consider the quality of the food that we are eating, the way that it is grown, stored, and transported and the effect that this has on its biological value. The collective effect of the foods that we eat over the years (as well as the inter-generational effect of our parents' and grandparents' diets before us) will have a profound influence on all aspects of our health and longevity. In this way, we ought to think of food, not only as providing immediate nourishment for our day-to-day needs, but as biological information that guides our genes to determine our fate (and that of our progeny) in relation to health and longevity, and probably a whole lot more.

I have no doubt that nutrigenomics will very quickly become a commercial behemoth, feeding off the worried well and those with money to burn. For all we know, it could unlock decades of healthspan for some people, but for it to be successful, you must eat what you've been told to eat, and therein lies the problem. From years of working in and around health and wellness I've learned that most people, broadly speaking know what is good for them and what is not, but as you know, knowing what to do, does not always translate into action. For most, I suspect that nutrigenomics will be another ephemeral 'influencer' fad, that makes some insipid yet glamorous YouTuber very rich. If there is anything to take from nutrigenomics, I would say that it is evidence of the omnipotence of our diets, and hopefully it's just another nudge to help us to make better food choices, which of course we already know we should be making.

Weight and wellness

"The epidemic of non-communicable (lifestyle) diseases is an educational failure not a medical failure."

Bailey, 1989

Health is like friendship, you only realise its value when it's lost, and so when I first started writing this section, I felt obliged to detail all the accompanying maladies that overweight people might encounter, to help them to change. Fortunately, I came to my senses and realised the futility of such a catalogue as a catalyst for weight loss. Therefore, rather than banging on about how lethal this disease is or how horrible that one is, I thought it would be more helpful for people to learn why too much fat in the body causes problems. However, I have included a section about metabolic syndrome and diabetes as these are most closely related to weight.

In years gone by, corpulence for most was economically inaccessible, and a substantive girth advertised status and wealth. People even selected their physicians based upon their rotundness! But make no mistake, carrying too much fat has its consequences, one of which is the impact on health. Nearly 2,500 years ago, Hippocrates noticed the medical consequences of excess body fat, and, as Professor David Haslam observed in his excellent medical history of obesity[134], Hippocrates noted:

"It is very injurious to health to take in more food than the constitution will bear, when, at the same time one uses no exercise to carry off this excess."

Hippocrates believed it was a poor diet and lack of movement that was causing excess weight some 400 years before Christ was born. His wisdom on this matter pre-empted the landmark findings of a 2003 study that determined that being very overweight (BMI > 40) is expected to reduce life expectancy, on average, by up to nine years[135].

I have always struggled with the idea that being fat is a disease. Of course, I recognise that if left unabated, runaway weight gain will inevitably lead to a deterioration in health, but I'm still not convinced that crossing the BMI > 30 threshold automatically denotes disease. Medicalising obesity serves only to diminish the importance of the primary drivers of weight gain, which are social, environmental and culturally based, or just a result of learned life routines. Medicalisation of excess weight places the onus instead in the hands of those wearing latex gloves, a problem for which a tablet or a scalpel is the only long-term solution. As a strategy, this has spectacularly failed to date, and I believe (as do many doctors), that this lack of medical success will endure.

However, as if to highlight my ignorance in these matters, the American Medical Association recognised obesity as a disease in 2013 (of course they did, medicalising obesity brings it into their domain), and two years later a disease burden study estimated obesity to be one of the five most important risk factors for disability-adjusted life years (in 1990, it was not in the top 30)[136].

Why is sickness more prevalent as we get heavier?

To answer this question, we must start with the fundamentals, which means examining the vessels that hold our fat. Fat cells (adipocytes) first develop during late gestation in humans (between the second and third trimesters), with further fat-cell expansion between nine and eighteen months of age (termed the 'adiposity rebound'), and then finally at the onset and throughout puberty. By early adulthood, fat cell numbers are largely determined, with the average, healthy-weight adult having around 30 billion of them. The fat mass acts mainly as a silo for energy storage, but also as an insulator to prevent heat loss, as a barrier against dermal infection, and as a protective cushion against physical external shock.

Fat cells are unique in their potential for continuous and seemingly limitless growth, leading to enormous variability. For example, fat mass can account for as little as 3% of total body weight in elite athletes or as much as 70% in people living with severe obesity. For other tissues (organs, etc), size and volume are tightly controlled (except, that is, for muscles, which can also change dramatically – just ask a bodybuilder – although if heavy lifting is withdrawn, much to their chagrin, the big muscles soon disappear, and therefore muscle mass too is controlled).

If weight gain started in childhood, the danger is that many more fat cells are likely to emerge; twice, thrice, or more at the point of adulthood. But for people that were a healthy weight as a child, and then gained weight in adulthood, they may have no more fat cells than an average-sized person (their cells just got bigger). The problem is that, from a weight perspective, it is disadvantageous to have more fat cells than we need, and there are two primary reasons for this. Firstly, once inflated, adipocytes are instructed to preserve their precious cargo, and react to weight loss by secreting chemical messengers called adipokines, which send a powerful signal to the brain slowing metabolic rate and calling for more food. Therefore, more cells = more adipokines.

Secondly, larger fat cells produce more leptin, sending a stronger signal to the brain that energy stores are full and you should eat less, and if you have fewer cells with more lipid in them, this will produce more leptin. Therefore, the same amount of lipid (fat) stored in fewer fat cells has a greater appetite-suppressing effect than fat stored across many fat cells. This is why our fat is now referred to as the largest endocrine organ in the body, uniquely in control of its own destiny. Taken together, these control systems explain to me, at least, why people that were not overweight as children generally lose weight more readily than those that were.

The amount of fat that we carry therefore depends both on the number of fat cells and their size (the amount of lipid they contain). In early life, as BMI increases, both metrics rise – larger and more numerous fat cells. Once in adulthood, cell turnover maintains a relatively constant number of fat cells in an average-weight person (although experimental work in rats shows that new fat cells can form throughout life if overfeeding continues). Losing weight significantly reduces fat volume, but the number of fat cells remains unaltered[138].

Typically, in adulthood, weight gain is the result of fat cells expanding, but there is a limit as to how big they can become (how much lipid they can store). When they are full, new cells must be created to take up additional lipid, because, when fat cells become engorged, they become dysfunctional releasing chemicals that lead to inflammation and a myriad of associated pathologies. Bulging fat cells also leads to lipid leakage from the safe confines of the adipocyte, causing fat accumulation in organs such as the liver, pancreas, heart and vasculature, in fact in most places[139, 140]. It is primarily this leaking of fat into the organs that brings about the health consequences of being overweight.

The emergence of new fat cells (over and above existing numbers) may therefore offer some protection, as the new 'healthy' fat cells alleviate the stress on the overwhelmed adipocytes, which makes perfect biological sense. So, building more fat cells is one way of keeping fat in safe storage, and staying metabolically healthy. However, because most people continue to get heavier throughout life, these new fat cells ultimately become lipid-laden themselves, and we literally end up with an even bigger problem. In short, as we overeat, the fat cells get sick, and then the body gets sick as a result. Cardiovascular disease has been described as the "collateral damage" of fat-cell dysfunction[141].

I hope that this explains why those that were overweight as children find it more difficult to lose weight than those that were a healthy weight during childhood. However, this is not to say that weight loss will be impossible. By way of an analogy, people that are five feet three inches tall will have more difficulty playing basketball than those who are six feet ten, and that is just a fact. But short people can still play basketball, and you may wish to type "NBA legend Tyrone Curtis Bogues" into YouTube to see the power of belief and determination in the face of tall obstacles.

Metabolic syndrome (MS)

MS is a precurser to the major mortal diseases of modern society, including diabetes and cardiovascular disease (CVD). MS is characterised by several abnormalities which, like type 2 diabetes (T2D), are primarily driven by a genetic predisposition compounded by a Western lifestyle. The estimated prevalence of MS in Western countries is staggering, with approximately one-third having MS, one-third having one or more components of MS, and only one-third being free of all major characteristics of MS[142]. Although there is no internationally agreed description, generally, two of the ailments listed below in addition to an expanded waist circumference is a positive diagnosis for MS:

1. High blood pressure.
2. Irregular lipid profile (high [bad] cholesterol and high triglycerides).
3. Insulin resistance & or glucose intolerance (both precursors to type 2 diabetes).

A large waist circumference is the chief predictor of metabolic syndrome and the primary driver of the other metabolic abnormalities. Diabetes, stroke, high blood pressure, coronary artery disease and malign heart enlargement are far more likely with an enlarged waist circumference compared to an increased BMI[143]. This is because an expanded waist is a proxy measure for fat accumulating inside the peritoneal cavity where our vital organs reside, enabling the fat to 'seep' into the besieged organs and cause havoc.

Cardiovascular disease is still the biggest killer in the West, and as MS is a clustering of the main CVD risk factors, it presents a perilous situation. Men with MS are 90% more likely to die of CVD than those without. It is also cardiovascular complications that blight people with diabetes, ultimately causing death in most cases. Insulin resistance (IR) is implicated in most, if not all, of the features of MS[144] and, as we will see, in T2D also. If you are resistant to insulin, you must produce more, and as insulin promotes weight gain and encourages hunger, this leads to even more weight gain. The greater fat mass leads to a downturn in physical activity (which is independently related to most components of MS[145]) and exacerbates IR. Both of these promote further weight gain, lower levels of movement, and accelerate the underlying metabolic disturbances; it's a vicious cycle. Subsequently, the only successful approach to reversing MS is weight (waist) reduction and a sustainable increase in physical activity. Moderate to high-intensity exercise (if tolerable) appears particularly effective[146].

Diabetes

The strongest link between genes, the environment, and disease in humans, relates to our most essential metabolic function – blood sugar control. Malfunction of this bedrock of mammalian life is catastrophic and, if untreated, it will eventually prove fatal.

Diabetes has been around for a long time. The Ebers papyrus (1550 BC) describes a polyuric state that resembles diabetes. The word 'diabetes' was first used by Aretaeus of Cappadocia in the 2nd Century AD, stemming from the Greek meaning siphon. Mellitus is Greek for honey. As the name suggests, a recognisable feature of diabetes mellitus is the expulsion of sugar from the body. It is a complex condition, but considering the bond between diet, lifestyle, weight and glycaemic control (of T2D), everyone with an expanded waist should at the very least be cognisant of the basics, and I hope these next few pages will accomplish this.

Diabetes is a condition in which there is long-term raised blood glucose concentration caused by a lack of the hormone insulin (insufficient production and/or inaction of the hormone). This is because insulin is needed to shuttle glucose from the blood and into cells where it can be burned for energy or safely stored. However, without effective insulin, sugar accumulates in the blood and the cells are deprived of glucose, and so fats are increasingly used for energy production. But the consequence of fat metabolism in the absence of glucose is the production of ketones and excess acidity. In extreme conditions, this can result in ketoacidosis and diabetic coma.

Type 1 diabetes (T1D) occurs more often in childhood or early adult life (but age is not a limiting factor). It is an autoimmune disorder, typically triggered by a random viral infection, leading to the (accidental) destruction of the insulin-producing beta cells of the Islets of Langerhans in the pancreas. This results in absolute insulin deficiency, requiring lifelong insulin injections. T1D occurs mainly in people with a genetic predisposition (known as a susceptible haplotype) and is not related to lifestyle or weight.

Type 2 diabetes (T2D) is usually a disease of middle or older age, and it is by far the most prevalent form of diabetes, accounting for around 90% of all cases. It is T2D that is most strongly linked to weight and lifestyle, although there remains a significant inherited aspect to T2D. Because of the strong association with weight and lifestyle, T2D is the most pertinent type of the disease to discuss in this book.

Prevalence

Globally, T2D is increasing exponentially, and aside from the distress that living with diabetes brings, sufferers are twice as likely to die from heart disease or stroke than those with normal blood-sugar control. Diabetes UK estimated that, across the country in the year 2020, three and a half million people are detected diabetics with a further half a million diagnostically oblivious to their condition. Together, that is 6%, or one in every sixteen people, and your likelihood of developing diabetes is five times higher if you are black or Asian[147]. T2D was first reported in children more than 30 years ago as an anomaly when cases were extremely rare. Today, the routine diagnosis of T2D in children follows a global trend.

Areas of high social deprivation see greater prevalence and poorer diabetic health outcomes for its residents. Mortality rates for people living with diabetes in the poorest postcodes are 2.3 times the national average, compared to 1.3 times in the wealthiest areas[148]. Life expectancy is reduced on average by ten years in those with T2D, and, at the point of diagnosis, half have already developed significant complications. In the UK, over 100 amputations each week are attributable to diabetes.

Progression of diabetes in the UK	
Year	Prevalence
1940	200,000
1960	400,000
1980	800,000
1996	1,400,00
2004	1,800,000
2010	2,800,000
2020	4,000,000

(Diabetes UK website, accessed June 2021)

Global cases of diabetes

Half a billion people are living with diabetes worldwide, which means that over 10% of the world's adult population now have the condition, with the pandemic expected to rise to 700 million people by 2045. There is a large variation in the prevalence of T2D between countries, ranging from 31% in Pakistan, to 0% in Togo, which is in rural Africa. Diabetes rates have traditionally been very low in rural China, but the rapid urbanisation of China is seeing a dramatic escalation in diabetes, currently at 12%, representing one in five of all people with diabetes on Earth. South Asian countries (India, Pakistan and Bangladesh) have a high diabetic percentage, which is continuing to increase as urbanisation and Western diets permeate these traditional farming societies. In America in 2021, around 11% of the population were living with diabetes; that is 35 million people, compared to Europeans where the average across countries is around 6%. Astonishingly, half of all people around the world living with diabetes are undiagnosed[149].

Highest total number of diabetics (in millions) are:

- China   141m
- India   74m
- Pakistan   33m
- USA   32m
- Indonesia   20m
- Brazil   16m
- Mexico   14m

Diabetes mellitus consists of many different subgroups, with the two largest labelled type 1 and type 2 diabetes.

Pathophysiology of T2D

T2D involves two failures that restrict glucose entering cells:

1. Insulin resistance (cells no longer respond properly to insulin).

2. Deterioration of insulin production in the beta cells of the pancreas.

As both aspects are progressive and worsen as the disease advances, full-blown diabetes occurs when the body requires more insulin (to overcome the resistance), but pancreatic insulin can't keep up and falls below requirements as the beta cells gradually perish. At the time of diagnosis, beta-cell function is normally reduced by about 50% and continues to decline. There has been much debate as to whether IR or beta-cell depletion is the primary defect, and the central question of which precedes the other remains unanswered. In fact, the contributions of IR and beta-cell dysfunction vary considerably among diabetics, with genetic and environmental factors contributing to each.

Blood-sugar control

In non-diabetics, blood glucose concentrations are maintained within narrow limits, balancing the three main pathways which are: glucose released from the liver, intestinal absorption of glucose from food, and large-scale glucose uptake into muscles and fat cells. Following a meal, nutrients are sensed by the intestines, pancreas and brain, which relay signals to the muscles, liver and fat, and then back to the brain, to develop a coordinated response. After immediate energy requirements have been satisfied, any remaining glucose is stored as glycogen (in the liver, 20%, and muscles, 80%) and fats slip seamlessly into the adipocytes. During fasting, these stored nutrients are released back into circulation for use by all cells.

This balancing act is driven by: Insulin acting in the presence of circulating glucose (following a meal), and glucagon, the dominant hormone during fasting or continuous exercise. They work together in concert, each in turn opposing the action of the other, enabling harmony.

Insulin

The pancreatic Islets of Langerhans were discovered by Paul Langerhan and are so named because they sit distinct from other cells in the pancreas (Islets from the Latin for 'Island'). They can sense blood glucose, and following a meal, when glucose levels spike, the pancreas responds by releasing insulin from the beta cells within the islets. Insulin then acts on target cells elsewhere in the body (muscle, fat and liver) to tell those cells to stop doing what they were doing during the fast, and now, following the meal, start to:

■ *Skeletal muscles* – take up circulating glucose and store it as glycogen.

■ *Liver* – stop releasing glucose, instead take it up and convert it into glycogen (and store it).

■ *Fat cells* – stop releasing fats, instead absorb fats and glucose (convert glucose to lipid and store it).

■ *Pancreas* – stop producing glucagon.

■ *All* – stop using fat as an energy source and start using sugar (there is lots of glucose about and this body only has limited storage capacity for glucose, but it can store virtually unlimited fat. If push comes to shove in the future, we can ask the liver to convert fat back into sugar).

Glucagon

When blood glucose is low, such as during fasting or sustained exercise, insulin production dramatically falls, and glucagon is secreted from the alpha (α) cells of the islets. Glucagon has the opposite effect of insulin, acting to deliver the following messages:

- Liver – release glucose so that organs that rely solely on glucose (such as the brain and kidney) have enough to function.
- Fat cells – release lipids into circulation for general energy supplies.

Let's eat!

Let's now apply the theory to practice and eat a large bowl of pasta (carbohydrate is the main nutrient of concern when considering how diabetes works). Ten seconds after swallowing our food, it is where we crave it – in our stomach. The stomach brings in water, digestive enzymes, and hydrochloric acid (not for carbohydrates, mainly for protein) and mixes it into what is known as a chime. After a short while, the liquid chime containing the long chain or complex carbohydrates slowly empties from the stomach and the intact carbohydrates are released into the small intestine.

In the intestines, the gradual action of amylase (the enzyme responsible for carbohydrate digestion) acts to break the long chains into ever shorter strands known as polysaccharides, disaccharides and, finally, monosaccharides (glucose). At this point, glucose is absorbed through cells in the intestinal wall and quickly enters the blood, whereupon our primary fuel source can now be delivered to every cell in the body. Following a carbohydrate-based meal, glucose quickly builds in the blood, upon which our bodies must swiftly switch from famine to feast mode. To start this process, glucose must first penetrate the beta cells of the pancreas to trigger the insulin release. The beta cell's 'glucose sensors' ensure that the correct amount of insulin is secreted relative to prevailing blood-sugar levels. Insulin is released and quickly enters the blood, binding to target cells such as hepatic (liver), adipose (fat) and myocyte (muscle), instructing them as set out above.

After all the nutrients from the meal are absorbed and in storage, or in use as an energy source, insulin concentrations fall away to form a low residual background level (to ensure that cells can always shuttle some

146

glucose). Glucagon is now secreted from the alpha cells of the islets in the pancreas, and this hormone enables the release of the stored nutrients, until the next meal.

Insulin resistance

As previously stated, fat, liver and muscle cells require an insulin signal to take up glucose, which is why they have insulin receptors on their surface, constantly 'listening'. Unfortunately for people living with T2D, not only is their insulin production diminished, but the target cells become 'deaf', which is known as insulin resistance. Therefore, following a carbohydrate meal, while some insulin is released, its action is ineffective, and the large amounts of glucose unlocked from the food are restricted from entering the major target cells, leaving the majority circulating in the blood.

Hyperglycaemia (high blood sugar) is a toxic situation, and if the body cannot 'push' glucose into cells, it has just two options: convert sugar to fat and store it (although its ability to do this is limited) and/or, filter sugar out of the body via the kidneys and get rid of it in the urine. This requires a lot of water, resulting in large losses of fluid, explaining the insatiable thirst and frequent urination for people living with diabetes. The removal of large amounts of sugar in this way also explains the rapid weight loss that can accompany the onset of T2D.

In the early stages of the illness (before the pancreas fails), persistently elevated insulin combines with endlessly increased blood glucose, and it is these maladaptations that are implicated in insulin resistance (causing a reduction of insulin receptors at the cell surface and increasing inflammation within the cell, which further inhibits insulin signalling). As with most biological systems, if you overload them with stimulus, they decrease their response.

Thus, a vicious cycle ensues: more glucose in the blood, requiring more insulin, resulting in less sensitivity, requiring more insulin. The pancreas cannot keep up and eventually fails; type 2 diabetes is the only outcome. Through the action of IR, obesity causes diabetes and diabetes causes obesity, and here's how. If sugars cannot be transported from the blood to the muscles (because they are IR) this will lead to fatigue and lethargy (another classic symptom of diabetes), resulting in a downturn in physical activity. As muscle activity maintains insulin sensitivity in the largest organ in the body (the muscles), a sedentary life accelerates T2D. Furthermore, with less movement comes lower amounts of sugar burned in the muscles, leaving more to be converted into fat and stored around the body. More fat, more IR, more IR, more fat; another intractable vicious cycle.

Drivers of T2D

The rising incidence of T2D mirrors the obesity pandemic and the growing forces of modern, urban societies and their powerful obesogenic environments. Clues to this are evident in the fate of immigrants from South Asia moving to the West, who swiftly develop higher rates of diabetes than their new host populations and that of their indigenous people living back home. This firmly points to environmental lifestyles compounding an underlying genetic susceptibility.

Although obesity nearly always causes insulin resistance, not every person with a BMI greater than 30 will go on to develop diabetes, which is largely dependent on genetics. The common genetic risk variant for T2D relates to insulin secretion and pancreatic beta-cell failure, which is necessary for the development of diabetes[151,] because a healthy pancreas can keep up with the demands of severe insulin resistance. The take away message: excess fat is a powerful trigger for beta-cell failure in genetically susceptible individuals.

Even taking the genetic aspect aside, weight and waist circumference are the two greatest risk factors for T2D. The risk increases by three times in overweight people (compared to those with a healthy weight), rising to seven times for those with a BMI higher than 30, and twelve times for BMI higher than 40[152,153.] It is entirely obvious, then, why weight loss reverses the underlying metabolic abnormalities of T2D and, as such, improves glucose control.

Previously, T2D was considered a progressive lifelong disease (worsens over the years) requiring ever increased medication. However, recently it has been shown that remission of T2D (non-medicated normalisation of blood sugar for 3 months) can be achieved through diet alone. A loss of 15% of body weight can be sufficient to put T2D into remission in most cases, an outcome that is not attainable by any available medication[154] . Furthermore, benefits extend well beyond glycaemic control, improving CVD risk, quality of life and psychological health.

People living with T2D appear to be intolerant of sugar and starch, and the adoption of a low carbohydrate diet has the dual effect of waistline reduction, and normalisation of blood sugar[150,155]. But much less attention has been paid to meat consumption. Eating red and processed meat is an established dose responsive risk factor (higher consumption - greater risk) for cancer[156] and cardio-vascular disease[157]. However, more recently, meat consumption has been proven to increase the risk of T2D[158].

These findings have somewhat put the cat amongst the pigeons, as most people currently believe that it is a high carbohydrate diet driving T2D. But the recent data on meat consumption are clear and unequivocal. For instance, a recent Australian study examined impaired glucose tolerance (a reliable marker for both pre-diabetes and full-blown T2D) in over 9,000 women, comparing meat eaters to those on a plant-based diet. Their results showed a diabetes prevalence of just 1.2% for those on a plant-based diet, compared to meat eaters, where their incidence was 9.1%[159a]. A further report that studied over 700,000 people, found those with the highest consumption of both processed and unprocessed red meat, increased their risk of T2D by 27% (processed red meat) and 15% (unprocessed red meat)[159].

The mechanisms driving this link are still unclear, but there is a suspicion that it is the increased BMI of meat eaters that may be the causal link. In which case, this brings us back to the nutrient overload hypothesis. What is clear to me from all of this, is that T2D (and more importantly, the damaging complications) is not inevitable, and there are at least two dietary avenues open to people living with T2D, one of which is likely to hold the key - only they can find that key. Those options are a plant-based diet, or a low carbohydrate diet. Critically, each should be accompanied by significant weight loss if it is to prove to be the silver bullet that people are seeking.

Furthermore, both a very low-calorie diet (VLCD) or bariatric surgery (which restricts calorie intake) independently puts T2D into remission in the majority of cases within days, before the person has lost any meaningful weight. The suggestion, therefore, is that it is the prolonged calorie overload rather than the resulting obesity that is causing the problems.

Proof of this came in a ground-breaking paper in 2011, when scientists tested their hypothesis that both beta-cell failure and insulin resistance can be reversed by dietary restriction of energy intake. They enlisted eleven people with T2D and put them on an eight-week, 600kcal-a-day diet. After only one week, blood sugar normalised, liver glucose output improved, and liver fats reduced dramatically. The first-phase insulin response and maximal insulin response became normal at eight weeks, which are key indicators that glycaemic control is optimal. The researchers said that normalisation of both beta-cell function and liver insulin sensitivity was achieved by dietary energy restriction leading to decreased pancreatic and liver fat stores. They concluded that the abnormalities underlying T2D are reversible by reducing dietary energy intake[160].

Furthermore, it was reported at the Diabetes UK Professional Conference 2021, that calorie-restricted diets followed by gradual food reintroduction may not only lead to remission of T2D, but also normalise cardiovascular disease risk and heart age. The DiRECT study, co-led by Prof Roy Taylor of Newcastle University, has shown that people that achieve rapid weight loss via a calorie-restricted liquid diet can achieve and maintain diabetes remission, with a 'clinically useful' reduction in cardiovascular risk assumed to follow[161].

Summary

Therefore, it looks like it might not be the obesity per se that promotes T2D, but the chronic calorie overload that simply overwhelms the body and leads to fat accumulation around the vital organs. Take away the constant overload of calories (required to maintain overweight and obesity) and for most people, this puts their diabetes into remission, reversing their diabetes by reducing IR and restoring beta-cell function, thus normalising blood-sugar control.

You will no doubt have guessed that I'm not going to offer any dietary or exercise advice for the successful management of metabolic syndrome and diabetes, because as you rightly know: "telling people what to do, diminishes the prospect of change". However, a summary may be helpful.

The increased damage to the vascular system of a person living with diabetes means that the benefits of healthy eating are greater. A healthy diet will provide vitamins, minerals and antioxidants to resist further oxidative stress on the vessels, as well as bolstering immune function by enabling swifter repair of tissues and repulsion of invading pathogens (infections can be more threatening to people with diabetes). Healthy eating will also help weight management, normalise blood pressure, improve lipid profile and ameliorate lipotoxicity (damage to blood vessels, liver and pancreas from elevated fats). Regular exercise will have the effect of reducing insulin requirements through an increased uptake of glucose and improved insulin sensitivity. A prolonged reduction in carbohydrates is likely to put most T2D into remission and, in some cases, has led to a total cure[155a]. If you are living with diabetes, before making any significant lifestyle changes, you should first speak with your GP or diabetic health professional and discuss your intentions.

Psychological impact of weight
Stress

A very strong link exists between stress and excess weight, which happen to be two of the greatest health threats associated with modern societies. It is a fact that people suffering long-term stress (signified by elevated levels of the stress hormone cortisol) have expanded waistlines compared to people who are not stressed[162]. Obesity and chronic stress are both extremely prevalent, and according to the American Psychological Association, in 2022, more than a quarter of US adults say they're so stressed they cannot function![163]

The human stress response evolved to help us in dangerous situations, invoking a cascade of hormones in a well-orchestrated and near-instantaneous physiological change of state. In our distant past, the level of threat required to trigger this adrenaline-fuelled superpower would often be life-threatening, leading typically to either 'fight or flight'; each involving a considerable physical act. Were you unfortunate enough to find yourself wandering around the plains of central Africa 100,000 years ago, you may well have been stalked by one of several predators partial to a bit of human flesh. This could have been giant hyenas, cave bears, lions, eagles, snakes, other primates, wolves, sabre-toothed cats and maybe even giant predatory kangaroos! As Rob Dunn puts it in his entertaining and enlightening article 'What are you so scared of?', "Back then you weren't so much the big man as the Big Mac!"[164].

When confronted with danger, the senses (primarily the eyes, ears and nose) send data to the brain's emotional processing centre the amygdala for interpretation. If danger is confirmed, an instant distress signal is despatched to the hypothalamus which acts as a command centre that coordinates the fight or flight response. The hypothalamus sends signals (via the adrenal glands) to increase heart rate, respiration and blood pressure. Alertness and senses are heightened, nutrients for energy are released, as are coagulants to reduce haemorrhage and analgesics to deal with pain. All in all, quite an astonishing transformation, all happening in the blink of an eye. So fast, in fact, that it enables the body to respond quicker than the information can be processed. This is why a bursting balloon, if unexpected, makes you jump out of your skin, but, if you see it coming, it simply doesn't have the same effect.

As the initial rush of adrenaline subsides, a secondary wave of hormones, including cortisol, maintains systems on high alert until the threat is over. Cortisol has several effects on the body, one of them being sugar craving (to replenish depleted stores used to run away from the giant carnivorous kangaroo!). After the event, the parasympathetic nervous system (the brake) returns things to normal, and cortisol, residual adrenaline and other hormones dissipate from circulation.

The stress response has helped humans to fight off or run away from threats for millennia. However, contemporary stressors are psychological, such as worrying about paying the bills or the stress of having a jerk for a boss! But irrespective of the source of the stress (life threatening or just worrying), we have a similar hormonal response, which is why your heart rate quickens when you open your monthly utility bills. In the context of contemporary stress, instead of fighting or running to burn off the concoction of compounds coursing through our veins, we simply sit there feeling anxious and agitated; we want to run away from it all, but realise the futility of that, so instead we have a beer and try to forget about it.

Over time, repeated activation of the stress response damages the body, leading to problems such as high blood pressure, vascular damage, central obesity and metabolic syndrome[165]. A further problem with stress (or perceived stress) is that we often attempt to relieve or cope with this altered state by using substances or behaviours that are considered pleasurable such as smoking, drinking alcohol, using recreational drugs and comfort eating. These behaviours also partly explain why the psychological consequences of chronic stress include anxiety, depression and addiction.

Some people exercise to manage stress (very wise), but most people exercise less, because being sedentary is more rewarding in the short term and, when you are stressed, you seek rewarding behaviours to soothe the self. However, the perilous combination of frequent stress and the accompanying soothing behaviours is a sound formula for an early demise.

Eating in response to stress has two forms: appetite (energy based) and hedonic (reward-based). As stress alters appetite and increases reward-based eating, this leads to eating in the absence of hunger, and a tendency to select more fatty, sugary, salty foods, to boost reward. The net result is an increase in total calorie intake and, by default, skewing the balance of the diet towards the unhealthy end of the scale. To make matters worse, it has been shown that when rats are given a high-fat diet, their stress hormones increase, which illustrates how stress and calorific, refined, appetising and processed (CRAP) foods combine to create a self-perpetuating cycle, each feeding the other.

It is not known why stress affects eating (some people eat less), but for those that eat more, elevated cortisol and its relationship with appetite and the hormone insulin are suspected as the link. Cortisol also slows metabolism, as researchers from Ohio State University showed when they compared people's perceived stress against their metabolic rates and found that, on average, those reporting one or more stressors in the twenty-four hours prior, burned around 100 fewer calories than non-stressed people. The research team suggested this could theoretically result in a 5kg weight gain in one year[166].

Stress also interferes with brain performance and, in particular, executive function, which refers to the higher cognitive processes that enable planning, forethought, self-regulation and goal-directed action. Thus, it is easy to see how the skills and disciplines required to lead a healthy life in unhealthy surroundings can be quickly blown off track. For some, more than anything, stress-related impaired executive function would be the one thing that most negatively affects weight and de-rails other health-related life goals.

When money worries arise, stress is never far behind. The financial hardships of living with obesity were highlighted in a recent US study that found populations with the greatest number of overweight people had the highest bankruptcy levels. The researchers noted the link between weight and chronic health issues (medical expenditure being a major cause of bankruptcies in the US). Furthermore, obesity is consistently linked with lower wages, discrimination and unemployment, which clearly contribute to the association[167]. Another grinding vicious circle involving weight gain, money worries and stress!

Internalisation occurs when a person blames themselves for their predicaments, which, where weight is concerned, can lead to compounding behaviours such as binge eating, reduced exercise activities, poor body image, low self-esteem and social isolation[168]. And so the vicious cycle starts: weight gain, stigma, stress, elevated cortisol, sugar craving, binge eating, less exercise and more weight gain, reduced self-esteem and more stigma – another example of a self-propelling downward spiral, in this case, weight-related stress and stress-related weight[169].

Trauma or acute stress in childhood can lead to weight difficulties in adulthood and there is an established link between both prevalence and degree of weight gain in people that suffered trauma or adverse events as a child[170]. Post-traumatic stress disorder (PTSD) in adulthood is also associated with weight gain, which has been proven in war veterans[171] and in people exposed to other highly stressful situations such as survivors of the World Trade Centre disaster[172]. Clearly, both acute and chronic stress play a role in weight gain.

In summary, chronic stress is a very high-risk situation for weight gain, and this appears to be a bi-directional relationship. Stress defies our attempts at weight loss, with multiple conflating pathways generating potent forces resisting our health- and weight-related ambitions. This effect is most likely led by sub-optimal executive function which de-rails our best-intentioned lifestyle plans. Stress induces overeating, comfort eating and poor food choices, it promotes fatigue and reduces energy and enthusiasm for physical activity, and it increases alcohol consumption and interferes with sleep. If you were to ask me to come up with a cast-iron plan for weight gain, I'd probably just cut and paste those last few sentences.

If you consider stress to be a contributing factor in your weight (I'm guessing that you are not alone), then rather than thinking of a weight-loss plan right now, you may first want to think about a stress-loss plan. I'm no expert on stress relief, but I do know that lots of people have told me that self-care strategies like regular, enjoyable exercise, meditation and mindfulness techniques have helped them immensely to reduce and manage their stress, which has in turn enabled them to make progress in their health-related behaviours. One thing that I do know, is that you can escape vicious cycles by invoking virtuous circles!

Weight stigma

Weight bias refers to negative weight-related attitudes or beliefs, expressed as stereotypes, prejudice and discrimination towards people because of their weight. The stigmatic power of obesity was exposed around thirty years ago when studies with children found they would prefer to be friends with other youngsters depicted with missing limbs or eyes, and with any disability rather than obesity. As adults, people said they would prefer to be blind or deaf themselves, or have any disability, rather than live with their obesity[173].

People living with weight are greatly stigmatised and face more prejudice than any other social group. They are viewed as lazy, weak-willed, stupid, lacking motivation and self-discipline, and uninterested in their health[174, 175]. One study found that frequent exercisers regularly discriminate against and even dehumanise people living with obesity[176]. The irony is that they don't see that their victimisation drives overweight people to take less exercise. These negative stereotypes lead to mistreatment, teasing and humiliation, and are reported to affect employment, wages, educational opportunities and healthcare services.

Weight discrimination leads to increased stress and more negative emotions, which coexist with existing health pressures and reduced quality of life. Collectively, this promotes greater anxiety, excessive worry, fear, apprehension and physical symptoms such as fatigue, heart palpitations and tension. Anxiety can be general, or manifest as panic or stress disorders and phobias, which can be a direct result of societal bias and discrimination. These adverse psychological conditions aggravate a stress pathway already under pressure, and lead to additional weight gain.

Weight bias starts with others, but if perpetuated, can become internalised, known as weight self-stigma. This leads to self-devaluation and a sense of shame, guilt, self-blame, poor self-worth and a sense of inferiority[177]. In one study, participants described the impact of obesity on their self-identity and used language such as "ugly", "freak", "hate", "blob" and "disgust"[178]. Furthermore, internalised self-stigma confers a higher risk of psychosocial trauma, greater depression, binge eating and poorer weight-loss treatment outcomes for those affected[179-181]. Therefore, it is right to say that, where it is tolerated in society, weight stigma perpetuates obesity.

Remarkably, healthcare professionals and family members can be the most frequent sources of weight bias[182]. For example, despite the fact that nurses in the UK have higher rates of overweight and obesity than the general population[183], they can be culpable when it comes to treating people less favourably due to their weight[184]. Overweight people sense these pervasive stereotypes in healthcare and, as a result, are less likely to complete recommended cancer screening and more inclined to avoid future care[185]. A desperately sad and grossly unfair outcome.

In the workplace, employees with obesity are perceived as having lower supervisory potential, lower self-discipline and worse personal hygiene. They are less likely to be seen as suitable for public-facing sales positions and as having lower promotion prospects compared with average-weight peers[186].

There are countless examples of weight discrimination, and one stealthy form is the differing views that people form towards successful weight reducers, depending upon the methodology of their weight loss. For instance, if people are thought to have lost weight via surgery, they are thought of more negatively than people that lost weight through diet and exercise. In other words, you didn't have the moral fibre to make the right choices, so you had to take the easy option! Such opinions extend to employment decisions, where weight loss resulting from surgery is not valued by prospective employers[187].

If there was a surgical procedure to cure alcoholism, or gambling addiction, or drug addiction, would people take up the same pious standpoint? "You are not entitled to that surgery because it's your fault, no one makes you drink, gamble, or inject the heroin, why should I spend my taxes on fixing you?" Would anyone in their right mind judge a cancer patient differently, based upon the treatment that they received?

As I have stated, I believe that a good deal of obesity is underpinned by eating toxic CRAP products, and food compulsion and addictions. On top of this, I suggest that many more adults are now living with obesity because, when they were children, they were exposed to an obesogenic home environment for all their formative years. In my view, such circumstances make weight control through traditional conscious control very difficult. I would say that it displays ignorance in the extreme to discriminate against and stigmatise people in such situations.

Sadness and depression

Subjective wellbeing (SWB) and health-related quality of life (HRQoL) are closely related to happiness, and as such will have a bearing on mental health. Sadly, people living with obesity report lower levels of SWB and HRQoL and this is particularly the case for women, those of prime working age, and people with a higher level of education[188]. Depression has a negative impact on BMI, which is another bi-directional relationship, and the link between weight and mood disturbances is slowly being unravelled.

One line of enquiry is the inflammatory aspect of being overweight, which interferes with metabolic and vascular functions, with insulin and leptin resistance and hypertension all viewed as key risks for developing depression and anxiety. For some depressed people, engaging in behaviour that makes them feel guilty is part of a cycle of depression. The worse they feel about themselves, the more they are inclined to do things that make them feel bad about themselves. It is this dysfunctional thinking that can lead to more episodes of binge eating, making a bad situation a whole lot worse.

Raising the issue of weight

For healthcare professionals reading this book, I would ask that you consider the work of Hughes et al[189], who, in 2021, set out to investigate the perceptions, attitudes, behaviours and potential barriers to effective weight-management care in the UK, using data collected from 1,500 people with obesity. This was considered alongside the views of healthcare professionals working in the field. They found that, of the 47% of patients who discussed weight with their health carer, it took on average nine years from the start of their struggles with weight until a discussion occurred. The health carers reported that about two-thirds of the time, it was they themselves that initiated weight-related discussions, mainly raised due to concerns about weight-related comorbidities. For those not raising conversations about weight during a patient interaction, they cited lack of patient interest (72%) and low motivation for patients to lose weight (61%) as reasons to avoid such a conversation.

This contrasts with the claims of patients, who said they would support discussions about weight with their doctor or nurse, providing it is in the context of better health[190]. They also reported raising the issue of weight 50% of the time, confirming that most people with obesity (85%) assumed full responsibility for their own weight and subsequent weight-loss challenges. Following such conversations, patients reported a variety of emotions including feeling supported (36%), hopeful (31%), motivated (23%) and embarrassed (17%), and this highlights the importance of an empathic and understanding approach to weight discussions, irrespective of who initiates the conversation.

A 2021 review on the same subject found that health carers were reluctant to discuss weight due to a lack of confidence in treatments, and in their patients' ability to make changes, as well as the stigma and awkwardness of raising the subject of weight. Many healthcare professionals believed that overweight and obesity were not medical issues, and instead belonged in the domain of wider societal responsibility. They also believed that weight was not a priority, and that other behavioural interventions, including those relating to smoking, often took precedence[191].

It is also my experience that most healthcare professionals feel uncomfortable discussing weight with their patients, primarily because they have little confidence in the available treatments, or the dismal success rate of dieting. Many consider that 'common obesity' is not a medical issue, but recognise it is the weight related illnesses that they are managing. This is why, in my view, non-medical, community-based behavioural-change services are so desperately needed, so that healthcare professionals feel that they can raise the issue of weight and that they have a remedy at their disposal that will have a reasonable prospect of making a difference for their patients.

Longevity

Frame your mind to mirth and merriment, which bars a thousand harms and lengthens life.

William Shakespeare

The mean lifespan in the UK is around eighty-one years, with women living about five years longer than men, which is about the average for Europe. When UK records first began 180 years ago, life expectancy was around forty years, and so the lifespan of Brits has doubled in this short time, which is remarkable if you consider humans have walked the Earth for 300,000 years. Currently, if you live in central Africa, you will be in the minority if you pass the grand old age of fifty-four, whereas in Japan you can expect to survive two-thirds longer and become a mid-octogenarian.

Presently, in industrialised nations, around one in 6,000 become a centenarian and one in five million make it to 110.

Forecasting life expectancy is important but problematic. Relying on past mortality trends is unreliable because of temporal fluctuations in 'lifestyle epidemics'. In 2021, Dutch researchers projected life expectancy for eighteen European countries considering the impact of smoking, obesity and alcohol, and of the lifespans of forerunner populations. They project that life expectancy in these countries will increase, on average, from eighty-three years for women and seventy-eight years for men in 2014, to ninety-three years for women and ninety-one years for men in 2065[192]. So, despite our best attempts to degrade ourselves, we seem to be on track to get even older before we end up on the wrong side of the grass.

However, the assumption that most people want to live longer is unsound. For a start, what does living longer actually mean? Longer than what? Longer than our parents did? Longer than our neighbour? If you drill down into the concept of longevity, it turns out that most people are disinterested in lifespan, and are more concerned with healthspan, one definition of which is: 'The period of life spent in good health, free from chronic diseases and the disabilities of aging'[193]. While medicine relentlessly pursues the goal of extending lifespan, most people would prefer an extension to their healthspan.

However, health is not a binary state – either good or bad – but in constant flux, sometimes good, sometimes not so good, making healthspan a subjective term. But this is fine, because if you perceive yourself to be in good health, then you are – it's entirely relative to your personal circumstances at any time. Therefore, it is the pursuit of extending healthspan that should occupy the minds of both the individual, and perhaps more pertinently, those pulling the levers at the national morbidity and mortality management machine.

The goal of eternal youth took a significant boost when, thirty years ago, Cynthia Kenyon of the University of California showed that altering a single gene in worms (C. elegans) doubled their life span and kept them more active. Since then, much work has been undertaken on human durability, although a lot of it is based upon data obtained from various animal models. Some of the more intensive studies have centred on diet, calorie restriction and, more recently, intermittent fasting to defy the actuarial tables.

Calorie restriction

Calorie restriction (CR) without malnutrition is shown to enhance longevity and healthspan and ameliorate conditions like diabetes and dementia in non-human organisms including fish (what about that? It turns out fish can get dementia![194]), rats and mice[195, 196]. It's not entirely known how CR works to protect health and longevity, but it probably involves shifts in metabolism, alterations to the microbiome, lower oxidative stress (slowing free-radical production), less inflammation, better insulin sensitivity and changes to the endocrine and nervous systems[197, 198].

This idea (that less food equals greater life/healthspan) is not new. In 1935, Clive McCay at Cornell University extended the average lifespan of rats from three to four years by cutting their calorie consumption by around 30%, which also resulted in a more youthful life and fewer late-life diseases (one-third of the calorie-restricted rats simply died of old age)[199]. Other studies have found similar effects. These geriatric-rodent revelations prompted some people to explore and adopt a variety of micro diets, hoping they will do for humans what was achieved in rats and mice under experimental conditions. Micro diets are very meagre (sometimes liquid) diets of around 500 kcals/day promoted through various books and magazines. Of course, they lead to rapid and considerable weight loss, but the proponents of such diets also make a host of other wild claims, few of which are backed up by long-term studies in humans.

However, some say there may be significant disadvantages to micro diets, such as, for women, amenorrhea and risk of osteoporosis, and for all, potential reduction in the ability to withstand stress, injury, infection or exposure to extreme temperatures. To date, though, none of these drawbacks have been proven in humans or animals in controlled studies. When CR is applied to our closer relatives, monkeys, the results to date have been mixed, with one study showing no longevity benefits and only marginal metabolic improvements[200]. On the other hand, a twenty-year study at the Wisconsin National Primate Research Centre found at the point that 50% of control-fed monkeys had died, only 20% of the CR animals had perished and CR delayed the onset of age-associated pathologies such as diabetes, cancer, cardiovascular disease and brain atrophy[201].

While this is all well and good in other species, the question is, would it have the same effect in humans? Several studies have shown metabolic benefits in humans adopting CR[202-205] and one would be forgiven for assuming that this would lead to increased healthspan and lifespan. To try to answer this, in 2020, scientists took an in-depth look. Their extensive investigations determined that moderate CR (12 – 18% reduction in calories) in humans could improve longevity and decelerate natural expected aging (primary aging) and reduce numerous markers of disease risk (secondary aging). They concluded that moderate CR did not induce any negative factors, such as reducing quality of life, increasing appetite, or interfering with memory, suggesting it was tolerable, safe, and did not compromise cognition[206]. Interestingly, it is still unknown if the effect is general to all calories consumed or specific to the decrease in protein consumption, a concept that has recently gained many supporters.

If CR in humans proves to be an elixir of youth, it will rely on people reducing their food intake by between 240 – 360kcals every day for the rest of their lives. Maybe over time, people do adjust to these lower calorie values and modest daily food shortage becomes more manageable as appetites adapt accordingly, in which case, perhaps CR may have legs.

Intermittent fasting for longevity

New diets have recently emerged as alternatives to continuous calorie restriction, to improve health using an alternative to the implausible option of permanent dieting. The most popular is intermittent fasting (IF), involving adjusting feeding timings or frequency to establish periodic bouts of fasting or energy restriction for twelve hours or more. IF has shown benefits equal to or above continuous calorie restriction, including reduction in disease and slowed aging. There is a growing body of evidence that such regimes improve health and longevity if undertaken for extended periods[207]. In rodents, both fasting for twenty-four hours every other day or twice weekly extends lifespan up to 30%, independent of both total food intake and weight loss[208]. Other emerging strategies that show promise are those that seek to reduce protein intake, with some arguing that this is key to slowing the aging process[198].

The key to longevity

It's one thing when something works in a lab using rats, fruit flies or worms, but it's quite another when it works in humans (either biologically or practically) and is validated by a study that follows them for decades. Therefore, if we are looking for proven strategies for longevity, we ought to look at what has actually worked in people over decades or even hundreds of years (an observational longitudinal study).

People residing on the Japanese Island of Okinawa are, collectively, the oldest living people on Earth. Remarkably, in one village alone (Ogimi), they have fifteen centenarians strutting their stuff (one in 200 compared to one in 6,000 elsewhere). On top of this, of the 3,000 villagers in Ogimi, over 170 are in their nineties, which vindicates the stone inscription at the entrance of the village that reads: "At 80, you are a mere youth. At 90, if your ancestors invite you into heaven, ask them to wait until you are 100, when you may consider it!"

The diet of the people of Okinawa is rich in high-antioxidant, brightly coloured plant foods such as fruits, seaweeds and a variety of vegetables, all of which are thought to be anti-aging. They eat more fish than meat and consume significantly lower amounts of sugar than others in Japan. Their staples are nutrient-dense and calorie-sparse – quite the opposite of a typical Western diet. An interesting island 'rule' is to only eat until you feel 80% full, following the ancient local wisdom of rejecting overeating. It sounds like Okinawan weight wisdom is all that we need.

Longevity is not just about a good diet, there are other important factors such as social practices, an active life, and of course genetics (longevity runs in families). A feature of life on the island of Okinawa is the close bonds formed through the social and emotional connections encouraged between all residents. Social structures known as *moai*, are informal groups of friends and newcomers that meet regularly to pursue shared interests. Importantly, the fruits of the collective moai labours are then pooled and their contributions are shared with others who may need support. Social support is extremely important; it leads to a reduction in psychosocial stress, promoting better executive functioning and facilitating the development of healthy habits[209].

In a typical industrialised society, aging carries a social stigma and negative stereotypes portray older people as senile, frail and of little use to society. Aging is often framed as a degenerative process leading to illness and death, proven to negatively impact older people and accelerate their decline. However, in Okinawa, society is structured so that older residents retain purpose, or *ikigai*, which, according to Okinawans, is 'the core of one's true nature'. They believe that pursuing one's ikigai gives life meaning, maintains positivity and connects you with nature and those people that you care for and that care for you. As importantly, ikigai keeps you active mentally and physically.

To illustrate the value of considering aging in a positive way, Becca Levy, professor of epidemiology and psychology at Yale University, studied optimistic expectations for old age. Her work (which has been replicated elsewhere) shows that those with positive outlooks for old age (for instance associating it with wisdom, rather than decrepitude) had better health decades later, were much more likely to recover fully from a disabling injury and had a lower risk of Alzheimer's. Basically, people with the brightest beliefs about aging lived seven and a half years longer than those with the most negative views, which astonishingly trumps low blood pressure, low cholesterol, a healthy weight, and abstaining from smoking, and exercising regularly[210].

On the strength of all of that, I'm currently planning the first global octogenarian rodeo festival. Events will include bareback bucking bronco trials, barrel racing and wild bull riding. I've got plenty of years ahead of me to polish up my steer-wrestling skills, which I intend to make a clean sweep of when I'm finally eligible. For those with animal hair allergies, there will be complimentary side events such as consuming 300 Carolina Reaper chillies in the shortest time, and, of course, several weight categories for bare-knuckle boxing.

Human lifespan continues to extend, and longevity increased by more in the last century than for the combined 300 millennia that Homo sapiens have walked the Earth. By 2050, the number of people over the age of sixty-five is expected to reach 1.6 billion, which will constitute one-fifth of the world's population and as much as one-third for the population of Europe[211]. Many people see that as a problem, but I don't. If you consider that, while certain physical attributes and some mental agility is lost in older age (such as reaction times and working memory), other cognitive functions continue to build, including executive function and complex problem-solving. Together with experience, expertise and accrued life skills, this makes the seventy-plus generation our greatest custodians of wisdom. The key, then, is looking after yourself and keeping your avatar in good working order, so that you can continue to marvel at life, while at the same time disseminating your accrued wisdom for the benefit of all.

Healthy weight in older age

The resilience of youth is legendary. It applies as much to carrying excess weight as it does to all the mishaps that befall most naive saplings. But young people can be excused for carrying excess weight because much of child obesity is in my opinion at the discretion of parents. However, as we age, I can't help but think that we ought to learn to avoid the pitfalls and mistakes that have blighted us in the past. In the words of GK Chesterton: "The follies of men's youth, are, in retrospect, glorious compared to the follies of old age". Over time, weight takes its toll, and as each decade passes, a comparable measure of overweight will have a proportionally far greater impact on the body and mind of an older person. Consider now setting your stall out to enter your latter years free of the burden of excessive weight.

It is currently argued that living with a high BMI reduces life expectancy simply because this accelerates aging. Excess weight is known to affect longevity through DNA degradation, shortening of the telomeres, systemic inflammation, and general functional declines, all of which make us biologically older than we chronologically ought to be. The proponents of this idea suggest that obesity and aging are two sides of the same coin[212].

Carrying some extra weight during mid-life may, on the face of it, seem like a good idea, and I have regularly heard the erroneous belief that it will protect you from frailty in later life. This is because we associate frailty with thinness in later years. But frailty markers are primarily, shrinking, weakness, exhaustion, slowness, and low physical activity, and frailty is associated with both being overweight and underweight. One study followed 1,100 people for over twenty-two years and found that being overweight during mid-life increased the chances of frailty in later life by over a third, compared to healthy weight participants. For those that were living with obesity during mid-life, their increased risk of frailty was an astounding five times greater! The researchers concluded: "Development of frailty may start in mid-life, and obesity is one of the underlying causes."[213]

Longevity summary

In conclusion, if it is many more health years that you are seeking, then it looks like it's the same old (boring) message: eat a variety of healthy foods, avoid the CRAP, don't overeat, stay active and keep socially engaged. Sounds like a pretty good life to me! Add no smoking and only moderate alcohol to that list, and it could give you over a decade of extra life and healthspan[214]. As a bonus, you might also want to toss in the wise words Charles Dickens when he said: "Cheerfulness and contentment are great beautifiers and are famous preservers of youthful looks".

Gut microbiota

We are what 'they' eat!

In what is the most beautiful and intimate example of symbiosis on Earth, the 100 trillion micro-organisms, from thousands of different species, that coexist as an ecosystem in the human gastrointestinal tract, is emerging as one of the key indicators of human health. Mostly bacteria, but also including fungi and protozoa, the gut microbiome consists of *lactobacillus* and *bifidobacterium* groups (each of which has hundreds of sub-species) and yeasts such as *Saccharomyces boulardii*. Enormous interest surrounds this ground-breaking field of human health, with the microbiome now considered as a virtual organ of the body, influencing our phenotype and health.

To illustrate the complexity of this system, the human genome consists of about 23,000 genes, whereas the microbiome has over 3 million genes[215]. Furthermore, there is a little-understood viral component to the microbiome, known as the virome, which, it is postulated, acts to manage the abundance of certain bacteria by infecting and destroying them when they become overpopulated.

There is a unique heritable aspect to the microbiome. Pre-birth, the digestive tract of a baby is thought to be sterile (few microbes – although this is still debated). However, as the infant emerges from the womb, trillions of micro-organisms transfer from mother to child. Following this seminal event, breastfeeding becomes the important vehicle for developing diversity of the child's biome, and up to 80 million bacteria are transferred via breast milk each day[216]. However, the mechanism by which intestinal bacteria translocate from the gut to the breast is unknown. Gut diversity in the infant increases up to the age of around thirty months, when it becomes not too dissimilar to that of an adult.

It is becoming apparent that 'seeding' a healthy gut microbiota at birth and during early life may prove to be an important cog in the sophisticated machinery required for a lifetime of good health. This is why a simple remedy for new-borns arriving by C-section that have bypassed the microbial exchange of a vaginal birth, is the swabbing of the neonate with gauze that has been pre-incubated in the vagina of the mother to mimic the natural transmission of microbiota to the child. If the body has the answer, why look elsewhere?

In terms of the transmission of the biome from one host to another, humans are the main reservoir of healthy intestinal bacteria, and exchanges occur readily between individuals. Both commensal (healthy) and pathogenic (disease potential) intestinal bacteria are primarily transmitted between hosts through the faecal-oral route. Once bacteria become airborne (for example, through flushing a toilet or using a shower), viable bacteria can disperse around a room. Bacteria are abundant on surfaces that have been touched by human hands. The presence of these intestinal-associated bacteria, together with poor hand-washing procedures, provides a reservoir for bacteria in the built environment that have the potential to transmit to humans – this can be both good and bad.

Humans make physical contact through socially accepted behaviours such as hand shaking, hugging and kissing. The frequency and intimacy of these actions increase as an individual interacts with a close family member or friend compared with a stranger. Thus, there are several different social and cultural factors that contribute to the transmission of our intestinal microbiota. In other words, our healthy gut bacteria enter the body in the same way pathogenic bacteria do, and gut bacteria spread both locally and globally through their human hosts. Other animals can also transmit bacteria to humans and vice versa, and therefore, treating livestock with antibiotics has escalated antibiotic-resistant strains of bacteria in humans[217]. Avoiding antibiotic treatment may not be possible if you are ill, however it is possible to reduce your exposure by cutting meat consumption or adopting an organic diet.

In a healthy person, an extremely diverse population of gut microbes coexist in balance and harmony. However, the microbiome can become disturbed because of illness, poor diet, antibiotics, or chemotherapy, for example, all of which can change the multiplicity of micro-organisms present, whereupon normal interactions are disrupted. This typically leads to a reduction in biodiversity and the system loses its strength and resilience, a concept known as 'microbiota dysbiosis'[218]. Consequently, the now-distorted products and interactions of the microbiome (the metabolome) produce a knock-on effect downstream, which is most likely to manifest as a metabolic disturbance and/or ill health[219].

A damaged microbiota

The microbiota is largely stable once established, however there is still uncertainty about how it is restored following depletion or disruption when it is most vulnerable to opportunistic harmful bacteria occupying a niche previously filled by a beneficial species. It is thought to be unlikely that the colony returns to exactly the same state as before being compromised.

Certain things can negatively impact the microbiome, such as smoking, unnatural food additives and some artificial sweeteners (which can affect the insulin sensitivity support offered by the biome), which is ironic, as many people with diabetes and metabolic syndrome use artificial sweeteners misguidedly to aid their condition. An extreme consequence of an imbalanced biome is the production of amine oxides, which can lead to atherosclerosis and cardiovascular disease[220].

Antibiotics don't impact human cells because human cells are eukaryotes and antibiotics are designed only to disrupt the fundamentally different prokaryotes (bacteria, for instance) by damaging their cell wall or foiling DNA replication. Therefore, antibiotics are extremely effective at protecting us against the prokaryotes that cause many of our contagious diseases. But in 2016, Martin Blaser described antibiotics as a four-edged sword[221]. The first two edges are the benefit to the individual in treating their infection and to the community by preventing the spread of disease. The third edge was noted in 1945, when Alexander Fleming warned of the danger of antibiotic resistance in his Nobel acceptance speech. The fourth edge is only now being realised, and it is the cost that antibiotics exert on our health via the collateral damage on our intestinal microbiota. Certain other drugs such as anti-acids, metformin, anti-depressants, and laxatives, as well as chemotherapy, are also harmful to the microbiome.

One very real problem for many people is that if the good guys are killed following illness or drug therapy, then before the body has time to repopulate them with the natural pro-biotics transferred from other hosts, harmful bacteria can take their place, secreting inflammatory products and causing intestinal problems. Under such circumstances, treatments that replace missing health-promoting microbes and 'repair' the microbiota are emerging. Medically supervised pro-biotic treatments can now relieve symptoms of ailments of the lower digestive tract, including Crohn's disease, inflammatory bowel disease, ulcerative colitis, antibiotic- or chemotherapy-associated diarrhoea and some food allergies.

Where the biome of an individual has been damaged beyond natural self-restoration, faecal microbiota transplantation (FMT) is showing a lot of promise. During FMT, the stool from a healthy individual is collected (screened for pathogens) and then transferred directly into the colon of the patient. This results in a sudden restoration of favourable microbiota, which would not be achievable through natural transmission alone. The next big 'bio-medical bonanza' could be 'live bio-therapeutics', which are products that contain viable and highly diverse mixtures of micro-organisms from healthy individuals that can be taken orally by others. This may (or may not) overcome some of the natural reluctance of patients to undergo FMT. Either way, as an investment opportunity, I'd say: "Get your money on this shit!"

Globally declining microbiome health

Western lifestyles and diets are altering the intestinal microbiota at a population level. Recently, it was observed that traditional rural hunter-gatherer societies that eat no processed food and do not commonly use antibiotics or disinfectants have a more diverse intestinal microbiota that includes bacterial species now missing from Western populations. This study indicates the importance of preserving the 'treasure of microbial diversity' present in traditional rural communities worldwide[222].

Of course, as the local and global conservation of the microbiome relies on healthy bacteria being endemic in the population, any widescale decline in diversity could have a dramatic population-wide effect. For example, the consumption of a high-fat, low-fibre diet, which is typical of Western populations, has been shown to cause the extinction of intestinal bacteria if the diet is consumed over several generations[223]. Furthermore, excessive use of antibiotics can have similar effects, with some microbial species never recovering[224].

Such a loss of microbiota diversity in Western societies coincides with an increase in autoimmune diseases and allergies, particularly in children[225]. Originally termed the 'hygiene hypothesis', it has long been observed that the children of families that keep pets suffer fewer atopic diseases than those who don't[226]. I'd say equally as significant are the (paranoid) trends of constantly disinfecting surfaces and excessive use of fancy-smelling room sprays in a quest to render the home a scented sterile tank. At the same time, the continued use of antibiotics to treat children could lead to an escalation of cases of inflammatory bowel disease, asthma and obesity in later life[224].

Pre-biotics, pro-biotics and syn-biotics – what are they?

Diet is primarily responsible for modulating the abundance and variety of micro-organisms in the gut, providing there are no other confounding factors. However, it is now being claimed that the gut biome can also be enhanced by consuming commercially produced live micro-organisms, known as **pro**-biotics, usually added to yoghurts, or taken as food supplements. **Pre**-biotics can also be bought as supplements and are the 'foods' that micro-organisms feed on to promote growth, which usually consist of some indigestible carbohydrates and fermentable dietary fibre. **Syn**-biotics are a mixture of pre-biotics and pro-biotics. It is estimated that the global pro-biotics market will exceed \$65 billion by 2024[227].

As the benefits of a healthy microbiome attract more attention, pro-biotic claims are now appearing on all sorts of products including fruit juices, cereals, and even cosmetics. A Google search for pro-biotic pet food returns over eleven million results! Producers claim all sorts of benefits, including relief from constipation, eczema, obesity, depression and even brain fog. We have seen this nutritional gold rush previously, most notably in the case of vitamin and mineral supplements, whose sales in the early part of this century reached ridiculous proportions, despite the general medical consensus that, for most people, they are completely unnecessary, and in some cases dangerous. Pro-biotics are now the new vitamins, but experts say that, at best, the benefits of these products are wildly exaggerated and, at worst, they simply don't work. But people do like to take a pill!

In 2016, researchers from the University of Copenhagen published the results of their systematic review testing the hypothesis that taking pro-biotic supplements changes the diversity of bacteria in the colon. The faecal samples in the studies that they reviewed revealed no evidence of an impact of pro-biotics on colon microbiota in healthy adults[228]. Another study that looked at claims that pro-biotics enhance the balance of appetite hormones also found this to be false[229].

If you are still not convinced, before you dash out and start buying these magic capsules of bio-health, I would consider the body of evidence that suggests they have little benefit to already healthy people, as there are two primary problems:

1. There is currently no accepted consensus on what a 'healthy' microbiome is, which may turn out to be as individual as our fingerprints.

2. The strains of pro-biotics found in commercial products may not survive the highly acidic environment of the human stomach which can reach a pH as low as 1.5. Even if some did survive and reach the large intestine, there would be so few, that without the right nutritional surroundings, they would not thrive and preferentially alter your internal ecosystem.

Be warned, the science is a long way off deciphering this extremely complex field, and due to the diversity of the micro-organisms and the complexity of the cohabitation of these creatures, the commercial approach of proposing this or that individual beneficial species is probably just guesswork. It's rather like suggesting that to improve your condition you could eat either a badger or an earwig.

Microbiome and diet

We consume micro-organisms in each meal. While it is not known how many of the ingested organisms go on to populate the gut, both fresh water and food are important vectors for incoming bacteria and other gut-dwelling organisms. However, the key message is that species that thrive in one dietary environment will perish in another, so a healthy microbiome relies on dietary diversity. The microbiome is malleable, subject to environmental exposures, and it is believed that nurture is more influential on the biome than nature, with long-term diet being an important influencer.

Far more attention has been dedicated to the microbes in our faeces than to the microbes in our food. Research into consumed microbes has tended to focus on the species which cause disease, or those which are thought to confer some "pro-biotic" health benefit. In 2014, scientists wanted to know more about the effects of ingested microbial communities, and how this varies from diet to diet and meal to meal[230]. To learn more, they characterised the microbiota of three different dietary patterns: 1) the average American: focused on convenience foods, 2) US Department of Agriculture (USDA) recommended: emphasising fruits and vegetables, lean meat, dairy and whole grains, and 3) vegan: excluding all animal products. Microbial analysis showed that the USDA meal plan had the highest total amount of microbes at $1.3 \times 10(9)$ per day, followed by the vegan plan at $6 \times 10(6)$, and lastly the American plan at 1.4 × 10(6). To put these figures into perspective, the difference between the USDA diet and the American diet is a thousand times more (i.e., ten million to ten billion).

Fibre

Unlike sugars and other simple carbohydrates, fibre is a plant-derived indigestible carbohydrate that is not absorbed in the small intestine but instead travels intact, to the large intestine. Once there, insoluble fibre helps to cleanse the colon and form a stool, while a subset of fermentable soluble fibre called oligosaccharides are eagerly awaited by gut microbes, which devour them using fermentation. This produces a myriad of short-chain fatty acids (SCFAs) lowering the pH of the colon, which helps aid the survival of friendly organisms and produces a hostile living environment for pathogenic bacteria such as Clostridium difficile.

The resulting SCFAs and other metabolites are thought to be great promoters of health: improving insulin sensitivity and nutrient uptake, which aid the colon in destroying potentially cancerous cells and disarming free radicals in the colon. A healthy microbiota will also stimulate the immune system, degrade toxic food compounds, kill ingested pathogens, and synthesize the B vitamins and vitamin K (the enzymes needed to form vitamin B12 are only found in bacteria). These fermentable forms of edible soluble fibre are now referred to as 'pre-biotics', the sole role of which appears to be to nourish beneficial colonic micro-organisms, which in turn produce valuable compounds for use by the oblivious host[231]. (Oligosaccharides are also in breast milk for the same reason.)

It appears that a threshold consumption of fibre is not only beneficial, but essential. Low-fibre, high-fat diets independently yet synergistically cause degradation of the mucus barrier in the colon (the physical barrier that separates us from our microbial tenants). Just three days of low-fibre diet make the inner mucus more penetrable to bacteria[232] inviting infection and inflammation in the body. Fibre is a key nutrient for a healthy microbiome (read, healthy person) but the discussion around fibre appears to have been overshadowed by the fat versus sugar debate. Forty years ago, Audrey Eyton and the F Plan worked out the importance of getting plenty of fibre in your diet. Not much of the (important) stuff in *Weight Wisdom* is new!

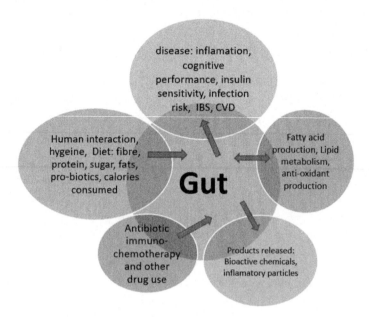

Inputs and outputs of the microbiota

I hear voices in my gut!

It transpires that the gut microbiota is also inextricably linked to appetite, satiety, and possibly body weight. Recently, there have been suggestions that the dietary relationship that exists between the human host and gut microbes might not be mutually advantageous, and that gut microbes may facilitate the consumption of foods beneficial to themselves. This idea, that gut microbes selectively manipulate their host's eating behaviours to increase their own wellbeing, may also, at times, be to the detriment of the host's wellness and fitness. This 'microbial control' is believed to be made possible through their ability to stimulate cravings or preferences for food in the host that benefit themselves and suppress their competitors[233].

This has led to the development of the concept of the microbiota-gut-brain axis. The 'aliens' within, can somehow cross-talk with their host by producing neurotransmitters and SCFAs with neuroactive capabilities[234]. These alter fatty acid receptors, intestinal taste receptors, intestinal transport mechanisms, and satiety hormone levels. They also exert influences on the brain-reward and satiety pathways and produce mood-altering toxins, by hijacking the neural axis that exists between the gastrointestinal tract and the brain[235]. Therefore, when you feel the urge to reach for a cream bun, stop and ask yourself, is this for me, or for them?

Optimising the biome

Carrying too much weight or consuming a low intake of fibre is characterised by lower biome diversity and subsequent poorer health which can be reversed by weight loss and increasing dietary fibre[236]. It appears that the imbalance associated with being overweight, results from some organisms out-competing others due to the prevailing nutrient environment. It must therefore be either excess calorie consumption or dietary composition that compromises the biome and suppresses micro-organism diversity. I'm struggling to see how too much food might do this, so I'm favouring the idea that it is a poor diet that is the common factor between overweight and microbiota dysbiosis.

Bacteria multiply rapidly at body temperature and with the right food. *Lactobacillus* can double every thirty minutes, turning 100 bacteria into over three billion in just twelve hours. Healthy bacteria can therefore quickly become established, provided they have the correct nutritional conditions and that they are not outcompeted by hostile bacteria that have flourished because of years of poor diet, illness, or the proliferation of biome toxins.

The best way to improve biodiversity in the gut is to eat a healthy and balanced diet including many food groups, and focus on an abundance of fresh natural plant foods. Fresh plant foods are the most important because they contain lots of pre-biotic compounds that your gut flora can feed upon. In general, fruits, vegetables, beans, legumes and whole grains like oats, corn, wheat and barley are all excellent sources of pre-biotic fibre. If you are concerned about gluten, rather than abandon grains, seek out oats, buckwheat, corn, flax, sorghum, quinoa, amaranth and millet, all of which are highly nutritious and low or void of gluten. (If you are not intolerant of gluten, avoiding gluten-producing foods such as whole grains will put you at increased risk of heart disease because grains are such an important contributor to vascular health[237]).

Fermented foods like kefir, yoghurt with live active cultures, pickled vegetables, kimchi and tempeh are considered pro-biotic foods because they contain the active live bacteria that are advantageous to us. The most beneficial are those that contain 'the mother'. This is the build-up of yeast and sugars produced during fermentation, which contain nutritional properties, such as acetic acid, citric acid, vitamins, minerals and other micro-nutrients. It will collect at the bottom of the bottle of such products as a cloud or gel-like substance. It contains B vitamins and polyphenols, which are great for health. Since it is already an acidic environment, the bacteria have a better chance of surviving the low pH of the stomach compared to an alkaline product such as a dairy-based pro-biotic.

I don't give dietary advice, but if someone pressed me for a single piece to improve health and weight, I'd say "get more natural fibre in your diet" (that is, if there is not much in there presently). As well as the benefits to the microbiome and protection from vascular disease[238], increasing natural fibre in your diet will require an increase in plant food consumption. In turn, this will boost vitamin, mineral and antioxidant intake, lower the overall energy density of your diet, hopefully displace some of the CRAP in your diet, improve the balance of macro-nutrients and bring more water. I will, however, add a cautionary note, that this dietary change should be gradually introduced – making sudden changes will lead, at the very least, to embarrassing gastric problems!

It is early days for the emerging science of the microbiome, and far more is unknown than is known. I believe that the microbiota is crucial to health and, as such, I would suggest you consider how you can support these little critters to thrive and provide you with optimum protection from disease. I suspect there are many other benefits that we are yet to learn about. As always, I'd say get your (gut) health from your food, unless otherwise advised by someone medically competent in this field. Hippocrates was no fool and was responsible for one of the most-often quoted pieces of food wisdom: *Let food be thy medicine, and let medicine be thy food.*

Exercise and physical activity

"If you don't make time for exercise, you'll probably have to make time for illness."

Robin Sharma

Is it the food or is it the lack of physical activity?

It appears that, for years, the scientific community just couldn't seem to make their mind up about whether the lack of physical activity in our lives was responsible for the obesity epidemic or not. Some research suggests that the downturn in physical activity in recent years has had no influence on the obesity epidemic whatsoever[239], while back in 1995, much was made of the work of two leading experts in the field of energy balance, who, in their empathically titled study 'Obesity in Britain: gluttony or sloth?'[240] suggested that it was our sedentary lives as much as anything that was driving obesity. This self-inflicted fog of war, was music to the ears of the producers of CRAP products, who avidly seized upon the study: "You see, it's not our fault after all, you lot are just too lazy!"

The experts behind this study subsequently conceded that the data for their study "may not have been reliable" and reversed their judgement. Now, while I don't wish to tell these eminent scientists how to go about their business, I think I may have already mentioned the recklessness of relying on what people tell you they eat to reach valid conclusions! The problem was that by the time they changed their minds in 2003 when hauled in front of the Health Select Committee, the damage had already been done, and for a long time, we took our eye off the real problem – the CRAP food.

Had you bought into the conclusion of their 1995 review, having taken the health advice of the time and dutifully gone for your daily brisk half-an-hour walk, what you might not realise is that if, on your return, had you eaten one crumb more than the one-and-a-half chocolate HobNobs counterbalance

(145 kcals), you would now be fatter than before you set out on your walk! The point of course being that increasing levels of activity to try to counter the extreme increase in the consumption of energy-dense foods that we are now devouring, would involve unrealistically high levels of exercise.

Movement and health

Most people living in the developed world are sequentially more sedentary than their parents, grandparents and great-grandparents. And there is no question that the UK population is now far less active than we were decades ago, with this decline set to continue. According to the UK government, around one-in-three men and one-in-two women are not active enough for good health, leading to one in six deaths and costing an estimated £7.4 billion annually[241]. In this section, we will examine the two key relationships between movement and health and movement and weight.

It was over sixty years ago when a landmark study first made the link between physical inactivity and fatal disease. The study, entitled 'Coronary heart disease in London busmen'[242], opened with: "The incidence of coronary heart disease is less in the conductors of London's double-decker buses than in the drivers of the same age. In particular, the 'sudden death' rate of conductors under fifty is one-third of that of drivers". By using information on the size of uniforms, the authors also showed that the girth of conductors was less than that of drivers in all age categories from –twenty-five to sixty-four. After adjusting for things such as smoking and diet, the sole difference between the two was the amount of physical activity required to do either job.

For many people, vigorous physical activity is no longer a regular part of their day, rarely walking briskly, cycling or embarking upon any meaningful exercise and physical activity. Most of our waking hours are now spent in front of screens or engaged in pursuits requiring relative stillness. But, as is now evident, being motionless for prolonged periods (sitting or standing) is toxic. If this is you, depending upon how you look at it, the question is either: 'Am I spending too little time being physically active?', or 'Am I spending too much time being sedentary?'

Movement behaviours collectively include physical activity, sedentary behaviour and sleep, and together they have a profound impact on health, weight and appetite control. Our movement behaviours are subject to change, and it is possible to be active while also having high levels of sedentary time and vice versa. A better behaviour profile (more activity and sleep, and less sedentary time) improves physical and mental health, and results in lower weight, whereas a poor movement profile induces excess calorie consumption and poorer dietary habits[243]. This theory, that exercise and physical activity supports the regulation of appetite by helping the body to re-tune or fine-tune its energy needs and therefore adjust calorie consumption according to needs, is a nice idea that's entirely plausible.

One of the key issues about exercise and physical activity is that it is a lifelong commitment. This is because you cannot accrue the benefits, if you are very active one month and sedentary the next – you are now sedentary once again, and carry all the risks associated with a sedentary life. The good news is that it works the opposite way round too. A recent study has found that, even for those that have been sedentary for many years, if they start to get active, then they quickly achieve the health benefits of someone that has been active for years, particularly if becoming active also leads to weight loss[244].

Movement and weight

This established inverse relationship (the more you move, the less likely you are to die early) also applies to BMI, and those with the highest levels of exercise and physical activity are likely to have the lowest body weight and vice versa. Bolstering this evidence is the proof that people that have lost weight and maintained it spend less time sitting than those that put weight back on[245]. If you are thinking that this is not you, then you may be right, but while population studies may not hold true for everyone, they do for most people. Also, it's worth remembering that exercise and physical activity are independently protective of health, even in the absence of weight loss. Once again, though, the big question is, what is the direction of travel in this relationship? There are several ways you could frame this same question: 1) Does physical activity keep you lean? 2) Does physical inactivity lead to weight gain? 3) Does weight gain lead to physical inactivity?

Despite what I may think about the direction of causality, it may well be entirely individual, and for some it will be low levels of exercise and physical activity that lead to high BMI, and for others the opposite direction might apply. Answering this question for yourself is a vital piece of the jigsaw. Think carefully and consider how this relates to your own circumstances. Pay particular attention to questions two and three above and ask yourself, which of these is mostly true for me? Write down your thoughts in your notebook.

The three most-reported barriers to becoming more active that were noted in a large systematic review of over 50 studies conducted in 2021, were lack of self-discipline/motivation, pain or physical discomfort, and lack of time. Consider your own barriers and be clear on what they are. Each will have its own solution, which, if you give sufficient consideration, you will be able to overcome. Write these barriers down in your notebook. Don't read any further until you have completed this task and you are content with your conclusion. Be very clear about this relationship and how it applies to you, and how it first came about. Be sure of your barriers to change. Don't attempt to change right now, just look deep into your beliefs, and try to gain a good understanding of the situation.

Direction of causality

Now that you have done your own historical investigation into your individual relationship between weight and exercise and physical activity, and hopefully reached some conclusions, it may be worth looking at some of the theories and ideas behind this relationship in a general population. But do bear in mind that there is no universally established route, and as I have said, it is in my opinion likely to be individual (other than in childhood, when I believe BMI dictates exercise and physical activity).

BMI dictates exercise and physical activity

In adults, weight gain impairs aerobic fitness and increases musculo-skeletal difficulties, which eventually make physical activity more challenging. Excess weight makes exercise more strenuous, and temperature control can be a problem in warmer settings. As weight increases, the frequency, volume, duration and intensity of exercise and physical activity all decline, particularly for strenuous activities. There is also evidence to suggest that, as people get bigger, they become fearful of exercise and physical activity[246], which is likely to represent the greatest barrier of all to overcoming weight difficulties. In most cases, this fear is totally irrational, and if this is something that you have sensed, then you will need to examine this fear and resolve to overcome it. The section on behaviour change will assist you with this, possibly by using behavioural experiments.

It is also very apparent that people with weight difficulties exclude themselves from sport and exercise settings due to the frequency of traumatic weight stigma experiences, discrimination, and fear of further stigmatisation. In addition, people with obesity report strategically managing their social relations to avoid stigmatising reactions by others in exercise settings, for example by exercising alone and avoiding social physical activities[247]. Many overweight people report negative comments when they are exercising in public, and for a substantial number this can be a bridge too far and, as such, being overweight becomes a significant barrier to undertaking regular physical activity. This process often starts in early age, and as it takes hold, low levels of physical activity become preferential and acquire the intractable status of 'behavioural norm'. Under these circumstances, undertaking occasional exercise and physical activity requires significant willpower and effort, as it entails resisting the considerable lure of the comforting and familiar feelings of being sedentary.

Exercise and physical activity dictates BMI

Advocates of this view state that by being inactive, we burn fewer calories and therefore leave the door open for weight gain. It is true that people can control their weight through exercise alone, but only if done in high volumes and high intensity every day for at least one hour[248]. But do ask yourself, is this realistic? Will you do this every day for the rest of your life to control your weight? If yes, crack on! If no, don't go there. I'm not convinced by this populist (energy equation) dogma. It may well be that low exercise leads to high BMI, but it is doubtful that the relationship centres around calories.

In my opinion, the most important impact of exercise and physical activity is the effect on brain health. As an explanation for weight gain, the absence of exercise and physical activity is far more likely to leave the door open for a decline in mental health and wellbeing, leading to more episodes of depression and general low mood. Just like feeling tired, feeling down leads to loss of resolve and degraded decisions. Without the positivity, enhanced efficacy and fortitude afforded by good mental health, poorer lifestyle choices are inevitable. Being sedentary is the opening that gives weight gain the foothold it needs, but not because of the fewer calories burned. Regular exercise improves mood and is an excellent therapy for those suffering from anxiety and depression and other mood-altering ailments which can and do lead to comfort eating. For instance, for non-exercisers taking part in a twelve-week experiment, those that exercised for about half an hour each day had significantly fewer bouts of emotional or hedonic overeating than the non-exercising controls[249].

Exercise and physical activity generates feelings of self-efficacy and gives us a sense of empowerment and control over our decisions and direction. I believe that becoming more active provides leverage for change in all aspects of our life. The 'investment' in physical activity acts as a reserve of capital for when more difficult life choices are required. This could well be the greatest effect that exercise and physical activity has on helping humans to remain a healthy weight in a world that promotes chronic overconsumption as the default option. Exercise and physical activity also helps to keep the body strong and avoid injuries, allowing for a more active and energetic life. This enables us to think positively and ambitiously about the things that we would like to achieve both for now and in the future, fostering a positive attitude to life and improved mental wellness. The benefits of physical activity are not therefore simply about calories burned, but more about improving sleep, reducing fatigue, and enhancing mental health.

Without regular exercise and physical activity, there may also be a disruption to our exquisite appetite mechanisms that control energy management within narrow parameters in the body. As we become more sedentary, we become further de-sensitised to this primal homeostatic mechanism. Once you lose control over the core energy-management function and the mechanisms of appetite, the battle with your weight is all but lost. And if you keep ploughing and sowing the same furrow, you will keep reaping the same harvest. The truth behind this directional relationship remains out of grasp for now, but irrespective of which is the preceding protagonist, exercise and physical activity or BMI, one thing is for sure: eventually, it becomes an entrenched vicious cycle.

Energy balance

Despite the well-established link between exercise and physical activity and health, there is still a lot that is unknown about the complex relationship between exercise and total energy expenditure (TEE) – all movement in any one day. It appears logical that increasing daily physical activity (structured exercise or regularly grafting in the allotment) will lead to an overall increase in TEE and assist with the energy imbalance required for weight loss. But recent work has challenged this, advocating instead that undertaking more 'structured' physical activity is likely to be balanced with compensatory additional rest[250]. This idea posits that TEE is controlled within finite parameters for each species, which advocates refer to as 'constrained' TEE.

Scientists have shown[251] that, for people that are currently inactive, increasing physical activity does increase TEE (presumably adjusting upwards to within the set parameters for humans), but in people that are already active,

TEE plateaus as the body adapts to maintain TEE within a narrow range, a finding that is supported elsewhere[252]. For those that value exercise as an essential partner to weight control (count me in), this may at first seem counterintuitive because it suggests that it's pointless getting more active, as you will rest more and the net effect on TEE will be zero. But while this may be true (only for those that are already active), it requires a belief that weight control is achieved by overwhelming calorie consumption through increased exercise and physical activity, and it suggests that the only true value of exercise is to control weight. A strategy and mindset that I'd say is flawed from the outset.

I happen to believe that the calorific effect of exercise has little or no bearing on weight control, and therefore I don't find the constrained TEE theory at all challenging; in fact, I'd guess it's probably correct.

Evolution

Being regularly physically active is requisite for a healthy and balanced life. The reasons behind this are somewhat unclear, but a leading theory stems from the known evolutionary cycle of food seeking, hunting and gathering, followed by feasting and rest. The accompanying pattern of dependent bouts of high and low physical activity shaped and selected our genes to optimise this cycle, and this ancient programming remains intact following thousands of years of human evolution. This pattern of intermittent moving and feeding, subsequently evolved 'thrifty' systems to enable good storage of excess fuel and efficient use of energy to facilitate bouts of intense physical activity, even in a prolonged fasted state. Following a successful hunt, exhausted fuel stores are replenished, the hunter rests and recovers, and the cycle is repeated. Rational observers can appreciate the folly of the modern default cycle, which for the majority, is feast, rest, feast, and repeat!

It is suggested that the presence of a certain threshold of physical activity is needed to ensure that this ancient cycling of metabolic processes continues, so that we don't succumb to the physical decay so common in Western life. Some scientists contend that a crucial mechanism to avoid metabolic collapse would be via regular exercise and maintenance of the physical activity genes, some of which, they say, may be potential candidates for the 'thrifty genes' of our hunter-gatherer ancestors[253]. It's a very compelling reason to regularly exercise.

Humans are very energy efficient

To illustrate this relationship between calories in and calories out (and the futility of trying to manage your weight through exercise alone), I'd like you to imagine jumping on a bicycle, and instead of taking water, take vegetable oil. You may be surprised to learn that vegetable oil has about the same number of kilocalories (8,300/ltr) as our primary modern fossil fuel used for locomotion – petrol (8,600/ltr). While petrol will kill you if you drink it, vegetable oil won't, even though both are oil-based derivatives of energy from the sun.

If you take the most energy-efficient, commercially available internal combustion engine, and put it on two wheels (such as a modern 50cc scooter), then put five litres (one gallon or 43,000kcals) of petrol in it, and mount one average-sized adult on it, at absolute best, they are likely to be able to cover around 150 miles before it conks out. If, however, you took 5 litres of vegetable oil (41,500 kcals) and put an average-sized human onto a bicycle, you might be surprised how far they would travel on one gallon of edible solar-packed fuel.

Pedalling at a moderate speed of 15mph on the flat, such a person would expend around 350kcal per hour. Therefore, they could keep going, theoretically, for around 120 hours on one gallon (41,500 kcals) of vegetable oil, covering about 1,800 miles, twelve times the distance of the most economical form of mass transport that the human mind has conjured since the birth of the industrial revolution – the horse, donkey and camel are also still far more energy-efficient locomotors than the internal combustion engine.

Humans, therefore, are over ten times more energy efficient than the most technologically advanced machinery specifically designed to move us around. We can undertake vast amounts of 'work' from relatively modest amounts of fuel. So, the next time you decide to tuck into an average portion of fish and chips from your local chippy (about 800kcal), remember that, if you wanted to neutralise the effects of this indulgence, simply jump on your bicycle and pick another chippy 35 miles away (for the return journey) and off you go! The exercise will do you good, mind!

While on this subject, there is a novel idea currently doing the rounds. Rather like calorie values on menus in restaurants, the suggestion is that these values should be converted to physical activity calorie equivalents (PACE).

This would be quite fun. Just before you tuck into the salted caramel and whipped cream crêpe, you would catch a glimpse of the menu PACE info: *"WARNING 15 KILOMETER RUN REQURIED!"* Calorie labelling on restaurant menus is becoming more common, and this can only be a good thing. Where this has been looked at, researchers find that, not only is it helpful for diners to choose better options, but it also leads to the introduction of lower-calorie items in those establishments[254].

Exercise and hunger

A lot of people worry that, if they get more active, they will become hungrier and thus eat more and make matters worse, but I'm not inclined to think this way. When I was young, I used to believe that swimming made you hungry – was it something to do with the chlorine? As kids, we would swim with our scout group every Monday evening, and as they would have exclusive use of our local pool, the normal shackles of bathing were off, no bossy lifeguards, and lashings of pandemonium! I always remember, come 9 o'clock, on our way home, impecunious as usual, walking past the chippy was an excruciating torture. By the time we got home, we were so hungry we would have eaten the Lamb of God!

What I had forgotten is that it was a thirty-minute walk to the pool, followed by a one-hour session and fifteen minutes either side for changing etc. Also, it was drummed into us that you mustn't eat two hours before swimming (presumably to stop children throwing up their meal in the pool). Add all of this together, and for an eleven-year-old, five hours without food and a lot of activity in between is going to result in only one thing – perceived starvation. Thankfully, I've since learned that exercise helps fine-tune the appetite, which is just what you need for weight management. Also, swimming in particular does not make you more hungry over the long haul (nor does any other exercise for that matter) and exercise and physical activity are important contributors to helping the body regulate its energy requirements[255].

Many people tell me that they can't find the motivation to exercise, and this is one of their main problems. If this is the case for you, then you need to rearrange your thinking. It is not that you don't have the motivation for exercise, it's just that you have the wrong perception of a relevant exercise for yourself right now. For instance, someone might consider that a thirty-minute potter round the allotment ticks the exercise box for the day, while others are not content until they have smashed out ninety minutes of sweating buckets. I know I'd be quite motivated for one, but not the other, so it is your perception of exercise and what is appropriate right now that matters. If getting in the garden for fifteen minutes seems manageable, then this is your exercise, and if it is enjoyable, you won't need to find any motivation. Keep it fun and within your capabilities, and as you get fitter, you will be able to do more. Gradual increases in duration, frequency and intensity are the key ingredients to success when it comes to exercise.

Exercise recommendations

Research has shown that, where exercise is concerned, routine is very important as it not only helps with adherence but actually leads to more exercise[256]. The UK government's current, well-evidenced advice on physical activity is that each week we should undertake:

- at least 150 minutes moderate-intensity activity, or seventy-five minutes' vigorous activity, or a mixture of both

- strengthening activities on two days

- reduce extended periods of sitting.

If formal exercise is your bag, the current recommendations for weight loss and general health (such as improvement in blood pressure, insulin sensitivity and cardiorespiratory fitness) is moderate-intensity aerobic exercise three to five times each week. Resistance training is also recommended for the preservation of lean mass during weight loss, and to support muscular fitness, physical independence, and improved quality of life[257, 258]. The advice is to vary intensities to include both moderate and higher intensity activities and focus on overall volume of exercise and physical activity[259]. Where higher-intensity activities can be tolerated, this is encouraged.

Not everyone is a fan of exercise, and these people often consider their aversion to exercise as the root of the problem. If this is the case for you, I'd be inclined to remember that a problem is an opportunity brilliantly disguised, and I would say that it just happens that you haven't yet discovered the exercise or activity that, given the chance, you can grow to love. Perhaps most of all, people tell me that the best way to increase exercise and physical activity is to engage in fun, convenient activities that you are likely to want to do more of, and, if possible, those that include family and friends.

Take away messages

■ Food is underpinning our weight, but don't discard exercise and physical activity if you want to be physically healthy and psychologically strong enough to take on the challenge of permanent weight loss.

■ Putting weight to one side, being sedentary will lead to your early demise, sooner or later, one way or another. So, if you don't move much, be prepared to relinquish all your worldly possessions, and make your peace with God.

■ If there was a safe, psychoactive drug that created the same tangible feelings of confidence, optimism, efficacy and positivity that exercise brings, it would fly off the shelves, and I would say it would be the most efficacious drug to date for weight management for both children and adults.

I hope that this section has helped you to see that exercise and physical activity are not optional if you are in the pursuit of attaining and maintaining a healthy weight along with a healthy body and mind.

Insight 2: Awareness

Part 1: Why?

Let's revisit Insight 1, where you took time to self-reflect on your current situation (Where am I now, where do I want to be and why?) Review the notes that you made and take sufficient time to consider them, and, if need be, make amendments until you are fully satisfied that this represents how you still feel about your weight and your future goals and aspirations. The questions were:

1. Where are you right now with respect to your weight?

2. Why do you believe this?

3. How do you want to be?

4. Why do you want to be like this?

5. What is your proximity to these goals?

Now the time has come to dive into the abyss. I want you to think about why you are overweight. I never ask this lightly, and would not expect my clients (or you) to answer it straight away. You must think long and hard and reflect upon all contributing factors for days, weeks, months if necessary. For all of us, our body weight echoes a unique voyage with the resolution woven into each of our life stories. Ultimately, you must understand and accept your own journey, with all its twists, turns and deviations, that have led you to where you are now.

Before you start to think about this in too much detail, let me set out a typical discussion that I would have had with my clients (in this case, a fictitious person – let's call her Tina). Having conducted my initial assessments and got to know Tina over several weeks and built up some trust, I would say something along the lines of:

Me: "Hi there, Tina, lovely to see you again. I'd like to ask you something that I've been meaning to mention but haven't got around to just yet. Tell me, Tina, why do you think you are overweight?"

Tina   (a little taken aback) may say: "Well, I'm not entirely sure, I mean, I don't eat a lot and I try to stay as active as I can. I think it may be a genetic thing, you see my mother always struggled with her weight and my sister is also overweight. I was rather hoping you could tell me why I'm overweight, that is why I paid the £30 assessment fee."

Me: "But Tina, with the greatest of respect, how would I know why you are overweight? I mean, I don't really know you. I certainly don't live with you, and while I'll take your word for what you have reported that you eat and how active you are, other than this passing information, I can't hope to guess as to the real reasons why you are overweight. I know this is a big question, so I think it will be helpful if you can take some time to consider it in full and maybe make some notes each time you think of something new. Perhaps next week, or when you feel ready, we can go through in detail what you have concluded?"

The point of this uncomfortable and rather abrupt discussion is to bring into focus for the client the reality that each of us knows, or, perhaps more correctly, is aware of the circumstances that have led them to this point in their life. This discussion could be about our health, professional performance, personal finances, relationships, or whatever. The problem, of course, is that these backstories are complicated and can be difficult to delve into, or seemingly too complex to untangle, or too overwhelming to consider in a rational way.

Sometimes, the upstream tributaries that have culminated in our troublesome predicaments are too painful or upsetting to dive back into, and so we banish them from the frontal lobes and allow them to drift deep into our vague recollections, consigning them to the folder labelled 'What the hell happened there!?' You may disagree, knowing that you think about your weight all the time – it's never far from your mind. However, don't make the mistake of confusing concerns, anxiety, or dismay about your weight with the very different cognitions that represent clarity, understanding and insight into the cause and continuation of your waistline. You must come to realise the patterns of behaviour, beliefs and actions that are upholding your weight if you are to escape the torment of continually treading the weight-loss path without making the progress you want.

It is a sad fact of life that many people must endure or overcome significant challenges and disadvantages, often bestowed upon them through no fault of their own. These physical stumbling blocks may include obstacles such as chronic health conditions, disabilities, loss of functionality or mobility, or a deterioration in quality of life, and can sometimes be due to a sudden event: 'My mental health deteriorated as a result of a serious car accident!' In such accidental or catastrophic circumstances, there is little that we can do other than to accept what has happened and do our best to deal with our predicament.

Most people will have experienced some kind of physical misfortune in their lives, some will have been minor, and some won't. If your starting point resulted from a sudden event, or series of events, then coming to terms with this and accepting it will be an important step in your journey. Where this is the case, you are probably acutely aware of it, and I raise it simply to prompt you to include any such events and their consequences in your rehab strategy.

It often helps to remind ourselves that we all know someone that finds themselves in a far worse situation than ours. Witnessing others around us that are dealing with great adversity and doing so with humility, helps us to appreciate the blessing that our lives truly are. Use the strength that you see in others to inspire you to bring into focus all the positive things that are in your life. Practice this daily, reflect upon how much you really do have, and nurture a sense of genuine gratitude for your own situation. This is central to our core wellbeing and will provide leverage for our efforts for change.

Thankfully, cataclysmic events are few and far between, and more often, weight issues are a result of a long-term nudging effect, the accretion of small incremental influences over time. Even the ravages of vascular disease that can strike with devastating suddenness (stroke and heart attack), typically result from years of gradual injury and physical insult. Behind each of these complex and intricate causes, there is a critical path, culminating in the current situation. Sorting the causal wheat from the benign chaff is not always easy, but it is vital if you are to emerge with a roadmap to a better place. Because, if you don't know where you're going, you'll probably end up somewhere else!

The purpose of Insight 2, Part 1, is to consolidate your awareness of how your weight situation arose. How and why did you become overweight? You must be completely honest and search long and hard to establish all the facts. Consider absolutely everything, the food, culinary skills, the people around you, the cultures, the social influences, activity patterns, economics, health awareness, parenting, time restraints, habits, personality traits, snacking, your neighbourhood, work influences; you get the idea, just about everything that may have contributed. Awareness means becoming fully conscious of the trodden path. You must seek and find absolute clarity as to the origins of your weight and unravel the intricate web that is your unique story of weight gain. Don't be afraid to speak to other people such as friends, parents and siblings if you think that they can help you to find the truth.

This task involves many hours of reflection and contemplation. It must start with your earliest memories, the first self-realisation that your weight might be an issue. When did you first become aware, and can you remember how you felt about this? What did you think at the time about why you were heavier than others of your age? With the benefit of your current vantage point, what do you think now about your views back then? Does your current view corroborate what you believed back then, or do you think differently now? If you do, make notes on why your views have changed over time.

As painful and difficult as it may seem, this may involve implicating others that you love: "My parents used to let me eat whatever I wanted, whenever I wanted it". Or, "My grandparents used to bring huge bags of sweets every time they came, or each time I visited them". The objective is not to apportion blame, but to find the truth. Without truth, you are lost and cannot continue your journey. Crucially, under no circumstances must you blame yourself, simply be honest and factual, and reality will emerge.

After you have thought about your childhood (if this is where your weight started), you should now think through your life as a young adult and continue through to where you are now. There may be factors that have arisen since childhood that have been equally as impactful on your weight, and be sure to excavate these memories and fully explore them. Think about the same food- and people-related influences, this time in the context of your time between early adulthood and now.

Set aside time in a quiet place to make a start, and if you can spend one hour focusing solely on the task, then you have made a good start. Make a heading in your notebook and make a start: "THE REASONS I BECAME OVERWEIGHT ARE…" Continue to go over things over the next few days, or, if necessary, weeks, and you should start to gain a real awareness of the history of your weight. Keep your notebook handy, and when you recollect something that you think is significant, write it down, reflect upon it and give it sufficient consideration to either rule it out, or include it as one of the contributors to your weight. Keep going until you are sure you have covered all the main issues. As you piece together the contributors to your weight, you should start to feel more empowered and enabled.

Part 2: How?

Once you have completed to your absolute satisfaction the reasons that you became overweight, now you should apply the same forensic approach to the question of how it is your weight difficulties continue to endure today. Why and how is this being perpetuated? Don't skim over this, see it as an entirely separate exercise. Take into consideration every aspect of your current daily routines in just the same way that you deemed how things started. Make a separate list so that you are fully aware of all the valid reasons that you think you are maintaining (or increasing) your current weight.

Above all, don't ever feel negative or guilty about your thoughts and beliefs during this Insight 2 exercise, your findings will hold the key to a better future, and this reflective learning may well be the turning point for you. Detail all the key contributors in a neutral and truthful way, taking time to add sufficient detail so that, if someone else were to read it, they would have a clear picture of your beliefs in relation to your weight.

There is only one acceptable outcome from this task, which is absolute clarity in your mind for the reasons why you became overweight in the first place, and a truthful explanation of the factors upholding your weight troubles to this day. You must feel no shame or embarrassment, nor must you place the blame with anyone; especially yourself. Don't look upon any of this in a negative way or judge your actions or choices harshly, or look to mitigate or justify matters by citing extenuating circumstances. Just seek the truth. This deeper understanding and lucidity surrounding your weight will be your armoury for change. The goal is simply to understand what happened in the past and why the situation is being perpetuated. A sense of confidence will emerge as you learn about the choices that you have made and the habits that you have formed over the years, and why you took these decisions, or why you felt that you had no other options.

Your goal for Insight 2, Part 2, is to be able to ask yourself: "If I had the power to change all of these things, past and present, would I still be overweight"? If the answer is no, then you have completed the task. This is the cause of your weight, and the formula for your holistic restoration. However, I don't want you to think about changing anything right now, you have much further on your journey to travel, and much more to learn before starting the process of change. We have all the time in the world for change. For now, just keep thinking about how you got to where you are now, and why you are maintaining (or exacerbating) this position. You will start to feel positive and even liberated by your revelations if you have completed the task successfully – it is indeed a significant accomplishment.

I can't tell you how important it is to undertake this exercise diligently and in its entirety. Don't just read these pages and then move on to the next pages. This exercise forms the foundations upon which you can reach your life plans and aspirations; don't just spend five minutes, and consign it to the 'WTHHT' folder.

Take your notebook and, on a fresh page, write along the top: **THE REASONS THAT I REMAIN OVERWEIGHT ARE...**

Eating and food addictions

"Please God, make me chaste, but not just yet."

Confessions of St Augustine

Over many years, I have observed with interest the debate about whether or not food addictions exist. I have heard arguments from both sides of the scientific community, each postulating plausible explanations for their positions; the time-honoured scrimmage between two diametrically opposed scientific views. I trust and believe in science wholeheartedly; I understand it to be a search for the truth. However, while the evidence pendulum has swung in favour of recognising eating addictions as real, it is likely to take a while to convince the public and public health officials of the clinical legitimacy of this challenging disorder. This translates into considerable delay in the transition from research affirmation to policy and service provision.

Seeking to disentangle the complexities of human behaviour, randomised, double-blind, placebo-controlled trials, cohort and cross-sectional studies, and studies that review other studies and reviews, all aim to accomplish what is unobtainable – the omniscient evidence base; but even such scientific rigour has its boundaries. On the other hand, the empathic interactions of the talking therapist can transcend all that can be written in scientific code. Which is why listening to what people tell you can, and often does, put health and wellbeing practitioners ahead of the scientific behemoth, travelling at its glacial pace. During many confidential personal interactions through the vector of a trusting client relationship, I have witnessed clarity that scientific trials simply can't reveal: self-identified food addicts make no bones about using food to self-medicate.

I have met far too many people that have confided in me their despair over their food addiction to even vaguely consider that eating addictions are not real. With resounding regularity, my clients have described to me the crushing consequences that being ruled by food has had on their lives. That all-too-familiar journey through use, misuse, abuse, reliance and finally addiction. When an online survey asked nearly 500 members of the public if they thought eating addiction was real, there was substantial support, with over half favouring treating obesity as an addiction[260]. Those struggling with their weight often describe their relationship with certain foods as abnormal and relate well to the concept of food addiction or compulsive eating. Relationship issues with dysfunctional foods may be at the heart of weight difficulties for many people.

I have met people that have lost their careers, their health, their dignity and even their families because of their compulsive eating. They know it is destroying them and burdening the lives of those that they love. They accept that it is ruining them and will probably kill them, but they just can't stop. Perhaps those that deny that eating addictions are real think that these people just lack a bit of moral fibre and should knock up a more appropriate New Year's resolution. If what I have described above is not an addiction, then it is very like one.

From these encounters (and a lengthy investigation into eating addictions), I have drawn only one conclusion: for many people, a compulsion to eat and to overeat even when not hungry has become the controlling factor of their life. The analgesic properties of eating are tangible and for eating addicts, food is the drug of choice. For those on the cusp, using food to self-medicate (for a myriad of psychological issues) is normal and perhaps the entry point for full-blown eating addiction.

Some time ago, a scientific article captured the imagination of the press and was widely reported in the tabloids under the heading: 'Food addiction doesn't exist'. Following years of conflicting points of view, this 'review of reviews' aimed to look at all the published data and draw some conclusions. It turns out that the deductions of the researchers were not exactly what the tabloid headline suggested. The authors of the study determined that, unlike drug addiction, people don't become addicted to the substances in foods, but instead have a behavioural addiction to the process of eating and the rewards associated with it[261].

In other words, not *food addiction* but *eating addiction*. Not substance-based, but behaviour-based. Food addiction, they said, may be used as an excuse for overeating and blaming the food industry for producing 'addictive foods', which, they say, is a way of removing responsibility. Eating addiction, they concluded, stresses the behavioural aspect, whereas food addiction appears more like a process that simply befalls the passive individual. Either way, they concluded that eating addictions are real. A recent study that questioned almost 300 bariatric patients using the Yale Food Addiction Scale, found that 37% were addicted to food[262].

In this book, I do not distinguish between the terms 'eating addiction' and 'food addiction'. Frankly, I'm disinterested in whether people's addictions are with the food or with eating (certain foods). It's an academic point of zero value to the addict. For me, they both amount to the same thing: those suffering from compulsive eating have a real illness and require considerable help to overcome it.

The scientific community seems happy to have reached an uneasy compromise, which is that food does not have any psychoactive or addictive chemicals or compounds, but eating for some does become compulsive. I don't agree with their view about the psychoactive impotence of CRAP edible products (or people would binge on apples, which they don't). In any case, even if they are correct about this, gambling does not have any psychoactive chemicals or compounds, but for some it becomes compulsive and it's accepted to be an addiction, whereas eating addiction isn't. In May 2023 the American Psychiatry Association (APA) presented an application for including food addiction in the Diagnostic and Statistical Manual of Mental Disorders (DSM) as a substance use disorder. With 300 psychiatrists present, when asked if food addiction was a substance use disorder, 98% responded yes.

We need to move on from the sterile debate about whether it is food or eating that is addictive and concentrate on the notion that this is a real illness affecting very many people, all of whom want to escape this condition as desperately as any other addict. The director of the National Institute on Drug Abuse in the USA, Nora Volkow, has observed, "I've never come across a single person that was addicted, that wanted to be addicted".

Compulsive eating may have a far greater impact on population obesity than has previously been considered. In 2013, authors of a topical report noted the neurobiological and behavioural similarities between compulsive overeating and psychoactive drug dependence, and the link between compulsive eating and weight gain. Using the Yale Food Addiction Scale, they examined the impact of compulsive eating on non-diagnosed compulsive eaters. They found that over 5% of the population of Newfoundland may be affected by food addiction, which was strongly associated with obesity and the severity of obesity. Their conclusion: "This means that although individuals may not be clinically diagnosed with food addiction, food addiction symptoms are potentially part of the cause of increased fat mass in the general population"[263].

The similarities between the addictive impact of 'food as a substance of abuse' and other 'classic' drugs is now well documented[264]. Through brain scans, neurologists can accurately identify the brains of alcoholics and drug addicts, and several neurological imaging studies have now shown that compulsive eating produces changes in 'hedonic' mechanisms in brain-reward circuitry like those induced by drug and alcohol abuse.

The commonalities between compulsive eating and drug abuse further extend to mood effects, external cues, environmental availability and the cognitive factors of restraint, ambivalence, and attribution. The conclusion of a similar study was that there is a wide overlap of the brain mechanisms underlying the rewarding effects of foods and drugs, and they say that foods, like drugs, are strong reinforcers[265].

The authors of a study of highly processed foods (HPF) concluded: "HPFs can meet the criteria to be labelled as addictive substances using the standards set for tobacco products"[266]. Such conclusions add to the overwhelming evidence that the interaction between a food-addicted mind and out-of-control consumption is no different to any other substance or behavioural-based addiction.

Researchers in the USA wanted to find out if there was a specific set of traits related to food-addicted people that were overweight. They enrolled forty-six people living with overweight or obesity, twenty of whom met the criteria for food addiction based on the Yale Food Addiction Scale. They were subject to a battery of other assessments (such as those that measure food-enhancing emotions, palatable-eating motives, impulsivity scale, food-craving inventory, and more) which showed that: "Food addiction represents a distinct phenotype within overweight and obesity, marked by greater emotion dysregulation, impulsivity, and cravings…"[267]

Is food addiction new?

As a fourteen-year-old working-class lad growing up in Burnley, Lancashire in the 70s, I regularly bemoaned to my parents that there was nothing for me to do in my spare time. My father promptly remedied this and, before I knew it, I was serving drinks behind the bar at Byerden House working men's club, a place I remember with great fondness; the people I met there I will never forget.

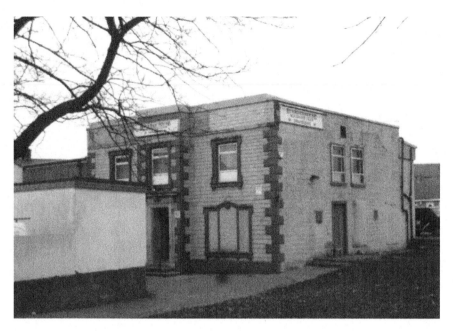

The grim exterior of Byerden House masked the warmth and laughter inside and the welcome extended to all that crossed the threshold.

Saturday afternoon in the games room, to palpable excitement, the highly anticipated event of the pies arriving was an important thread in the fabric of club life: "Pies 'ave come!" Eric would announce. Having let their birds fly, familiar faces from the adjacent Homing Pigeon Club would arrive for this time-honoured ritual. "Pint of Thwaites and a 'tato pie"... happy days!

As I recollect, most people were lean back then, but there were exceptions, and Kevin was one. Kevin liked his pies. Normally, he would have a cheese and onion and a meat and potato, and some days a meat and onion too. Eric would rib him: "Kev has heard of lots of people starving to death, but he's never heard of anyone bursting!" I don't know what happened to Kev, but I do remember him saying to me one Saturday afternoon, "See 'ow some folk can't stop drinkin' or smokin' when they start, well fo' me, it's the same but wi' food". I never forgot that.

One of the clues to the history of food addiction is the practice in the 70s and 80s of jaw wiring, where people would volunteer to have their jaws wired shut in a desperate attempt to 'cure' their food addiction. It would of course lead to weight loss (comparable to bariatric surgery), but weight regain was inevitable as the underlying addiction had not been resolved.

More recently, someone has had a variation on my theme for an oral-weight control device, and while not as elegant a solution, they have constructed a magnetic teeth clamp which has undergone scientific trials, to see if it was efficacious and tolerable. Well, it did work, and in the overweight trials, people did lose 5kg over the two-week period it was worn[268]. But I don't think it's a patch on my theoretical device.

Is it food?

Before delving too far into the science of food addiction, I would like to make an important distinction. In the forty years that I've been working in the field of wellbeing, I have yet to come across anyone addicted to apples, lamb, eggs, cauliflower, tuna, prawns, avocados, mackerel, oranges, blueberries, sweetcorn, strawberries (you get the idea), even though most people would say that many of these foods are truly delicious. Instead, addicts identify the culprits as chocolate, sweets, puddings, high-fat, high-sugar, high-salt foods and takeaways, biscuits, cakes, confectionery, crisps, sugary drinks and so on, products that are CRAP.

Fat in isolation is not very palatable, but adding sugar or salt amplifies the appeal enormously (one of the cardinal rules in processed food: when in doubt, add sugar!) It appears, to me at least, that there are three primary target 'substances' for the eating addict:

- sugar (in its various forms)
- high fat and sugar combinations (sweets)
- high fat and salt combinations (savouries)

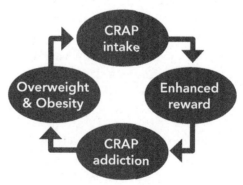

A CRAP vicious cycle

Consumption of CRAP sets up a vicious cycle of eating that interferes with the reward circuitry of the brain. This leads to dependency and addiction, which itself leads to weight gain. The cycle is continually reinforced until it becomes a self-perpetuating torment.

For the eating addict, I consider 'CRAP fixes' as powerful and compelling as any psychoactive drug. One approach to obesity or compulsive eating by some professionals is to suggest moderation. Cutting out food groups (CRAP) for some is frowned upon, as allegedly "it creates a craving". I've heard it from numerous professionals: "A little bit of what you like is good for you!" They forgot to add the essential caveat: "That is, providing you don't have an addiction to it". I wonder how the 'little bit of something is good for you' approach would go down in the treatment of other addictions:

"Hi Frank, instead of cutting out the cigarettes and relying on your vape, I suggest you keep on smoking so as not to crave the fags, but just don't light up too many!"

"Good morning, Cynthia, you need to continue using all the recreational drugs that you currently use, but just consume less or take them more infrequently – maybe just at the weekend?"

"Ronnie, keep using the gambling app and visiting the bookies, but how about just backing the dogs for now?"

Many people fear changing their eating patterns because they think that they won't be able to handle the deprivation. But there are two types of deprivation, that which deprives you by not having something, and that which deprives you of other things by having it. Most people never consider the second type, but it has the most profound importance. The first focuses on the short-term 'instant gratification', whereas the second sees the long game. I would say depriving yourself of happiness, self-esteem, vigour and many more health years trumps the perceived deprivation of the ephemeral gratification of CRAP foods. In psychological terms, this is called 'decisional balance'.

The path to abstinence is difficult and unrelenting; success is a journey, not a destination. As I and many others see it, absolute abstinence is the only salvation for the addict.

Understanding addiction

Understanding the terminology and definitions of addiction will be helpful for anyone that identifies themselves as having a dysfunctional feeding relationship, or who self-diagnoses as a food addict, chocoholic etc. Recognising how the addicted brain works helps to empower people to break the cycle of addiction and support them to avoid relapse. This is an essential step in starting the process that can eventually help them to learn from, and avoid, relapses in the future.

Although current definitions or criteria for drug addiction differ, almost all emphasise the following as factors:

- Compulsion or loss of control.
- Discomfort of withdrawal.
- Positive psychoactive effects.
- Harm or detriment caused to:
  - One's own health.
  - Personal circumstances.
  - Family friends and relationships.
  - Social interactions and functioning.
  - Economic and career prospects.

Addiction differs from 'dependence', which refers instead to a need for a substance to function normally. 'Tolerance' to a substance is when a person no longer responds as they initially did and therefore more is required to achieve the same effect. This is why people with substance use disorders use more and more as their condition progresses.

While addiction as a condition is not disputed, which substances are addictive is. For example, caffeine, nicotine and cocaine's addictive properties have all previously been challenged. Furthermore, addiction is not always an all-or-nothing phenomenon, more characteristically, individuals vary in their vulnerability to the addictive substance or behaviours, and this relates to different genotypes, socio-economic circumstances and inherited personality traits[269].

The contrivance of addiction

Reward-based learning (RBL) is founded upon the principle that the brain teaches the creature to make the most of beneficial opportunities, minimise costs and avoid punishment when choices are presented. RBL guides us through life, improving the likelihood of finding what is valuable while sidestepping threats. Development and refinement of 'reward prediction error' (the difference between predicted rewards and those actually received) continually fine-tunes the system as the brain responds to innumerable stimuli. The theory of addiction suggests that the substance hijacks the brain's reward circuitry, enabling the addiction to take control of RBL.

When we eat sugar, the brain's reward system is activated, signalling pleasure and generating a 'liking' reaction. This teaches us to eat more of it and eat it again and again. We think of sugar as inherently pleasant, but this pleasure does not result from our taste receptors, but instead in the evolved ability of sugar to activate the hedonic (pleasure) pathways in our brains. If, for any reason, sugar could no longer do this, it would still taste just as sweet, but it would no longer be pleasurable. In another example of how the brain learns to move us towards benefits and away from danger, if a sweet taste is 'paired' with a nasty visceral illness such as eating candy floss until it makes you vomit, the person switches from thinking of the food as highly pleasing (unconditioned response) to perceiving it as disgusting and developing an aversion for it (conditioned response).

The brain can learn in more complex ways than by pairing taste with outcome. For example, bitterness typically elicits an aversion, but with perseverance this can be overcome, particularly when paired with a good experience that has a pleasing outcome (such as learning to appreciate fine whiskey with friends). At first, the whiskey always tastes the same (vile to the uninitiated), but the pairing with a pleasant outcome (being with friends and the sensation of intoxication) teaches the brain to allow whiskey to unlock hedonic brain systems. The fact that we can learn to like sour or bitter tastes which, by default, our circuitry is set up to reject, tells us that it's not solely the food substances that provide us with the pleasure, but also the accompanying associations which combine in complex ways to trigger our brain-reward circuitry. Similarly, food aversions can and do happen when the consumption of something tasty leads to a bad reaction or illness. In such cases, the sufferer can go on to develop a total aversion for that food, no longer considering it tasty, but instead regarding it as repulsive.

The phrase 'reward circuitry' encompasses a collection of brain structures that are activated by rewarding stimuli. It is a complex region of the brain responsible for motivation, reward and reinforcement, and it works by using the neurotransmitter dopamine to provide pleasurable sensations to enable the brain to teach itself, guiding us how to respond and how to proceed both for now and in the future. This highly developed brain region is probably the origin of the creation and advancement of civilisation and the epicentre of all human happiness. Dopamine is the source of all our pleasure – more dopamine, more pleasure. Whenever we engage in an activity that the brain interprets as beneficial for us (usually from a survival perspective), such as sex, eating or play, it gives us a squirt of dopamine, which makes us feel good and motivates us to repeat the behaviour. Unfortunately, what the brain has evolved to consider as good for us, often isn't.

CRAP elicits a large dopamine release and, as the degree of pleasure derived from eating equates to the amount of dopamine released, CRAP teaches the brain that this is the nourishment of choice, and keeps us going back for more. The sequence of obsessive attraction to CRAP and activation of the binge cycle after the first bite triggers addiction-like neuroadaptive responses driving the development of compulsive eating.

Continued consumption of CRAP nurtures the binge cycle, which gathers momentum, causing dopamine release to increase in frequency and magnitude, resulting in a lessening of the pleasure derived from dopamine. Subsequently, as seen in both humans and animals, the consumption of CRAP evokes adaptive changes in the brain resulting in a neurochemical blunting of responses to rewarding stimuli, driving further food-seeking behaviours to overcome this reward resistance. This is how CRAP hijacks the brain, and in particular the dopamine system. The addictive potential of CRAP is now well-established[270].

As stated, overeating is likely a compensatory response to the reduced pleasure perceived, because of 'reward blunting' by excessive indulgence on CRAP. Eric Stice, a senior scientist at Oregon Research Institute, comments: "The weakened responsivity of the reward circuitry increases the risk for future weight gain in a feed-forward manner. This may explain why obesity typically shows a chronic course and is resistant to treatment."[271] Compounding matters further is the available evidence showing an inverse relationship between body weight and the number of dopamine receptors in the brain – that is, as body weight goes up, dopamine receptors go down.

This could suggest one of two things: people born with fewer dopamine receptors need to overeat to compensate for this reward deficit, or, as with other stimuli receptors, if chronically over-aroused, they simply switch off or diminish. The big question is whether this is cause or effect? The little answer, nobody knows. One thing that is known is that CRAP is a staple substance of abuse for very many people.

The road to addiction

The motivational drive to eat CRAP, to drink alcohol or to take drugs (the reinforcer) and the behaviours that follow are based upon our experiences and previous exposure to these substances, and our responses to them. In addicts, the response to the reinforcer, either immediately or gradually, but inevitably, is to assign supreme importance to the 'state' brought about by the drug. Consequently, the brain allocates all available resources towards attaining this state; acquisition of the reinforcer becomes paramount.

This reward region of the brain amplifies the value of the 'altered state' and places it central to functioning and decision-making. The reinforcer is then considered above all else as the chosen path; the addict shuns the mundane and boring existence that is life without the drug. It is the prospect of attaining the state (known as the predicting cue) which increases the likelihood and/or strength of the behavioural response towards indulging. Repeated consumption of the reinforcer strengthens the associations between the reinforcer, predicting cues and the binge. The addiction is building its doomsday machine.

The altered neural networks of initial addiction are accompanied by lower pleasure responses to other incentives, leading to loss of interest in things that used to be gratifying, and the social and creative world of the addict narrows. At the same time, a loss of conscious control and self-regulation causes impulsive and compulsive responses to the reinforcer. The addict is losing the ability to apply logical reasoning and reach rational conclusions. Collectively, these changes underpin addiction through reinforcement, changes to motivation and self-regulation, and habitual and inflexible responding[272]. The doomsday machine is being supercharged.

The vicious cycle escalates and, as dopamine receptors are downregulated, this counter-intuitively enhances responsivity to reinforcer and predicting cues (since CRAP promises a 'hit' that is big enough to overcome the blunted reward response). The result is a paradoxical pairing of increased 'wanting' and decreased 'liking', evident in all addictions. The doomsday machine is complete, and its clock is ticking.

What is the addict seeking?

In the most simplistic terms, the addict is seeking euphoria and or an escape from pain (emotional or physical). In the early stages of addiction, the fix provides this, but as addiction takes hold, the addict seeks merely to escape from the pain of withdrawal, the euphoria is gone, and the pain always returns. The brain of an addict must once again focus all its resources on obtaining the reinforcer to remove the pain. The outright fixation of the mind suppresses any resistance and reasoning offered by the pre-frontal cortex as it attempts to exert conscious control and resist impulses. Ultimately, diplomacy fails, and the addict succumbs.

Despite the devastation that binges cause, the addict ignores the downside of their behaviours and simultaneously pursues their addictions long after the obsession has ceased to bring pleasure. It is this loss of conscious control that is one of the most distressing aspects of addiction. The utter bleakness of repeatedly treading a progressively destructive path, over which the voyager has no apparent control.

Even during remission, the addicted brain works to lure the addict back to the 'preferred state'. One such mechanism deployed is known as euphoric recall. As the name suggests, the brain continually reminds the addict of the good times. Addicts also suffer obsessions of the mind, they rationalise the binges, upholding and justifying them through irrational thoughts and reflections. Mental blanks and a lack of any logical thinking that would normally prevent behaviours known to inflict pain, are a hallmark of addiction. Ignoring the pain and hurt, the immense damage to mental and physical health and the collective devastation wreaked by the drug is a cornerstone of the illness.

As this area of the brain is also responsible for other vital cerebral processes such as emotional response, anxiety and stress management, inevitably, the constituent psychological maladies of addiction involve negative behavioural and personality changes and a general decline in mental wellbeing. Comparisons between overweight people with similar BMIs show that those with eating addictions have significantly poorer psychosocial functioning in measures such as anxiety, depression and mental health.

Animal models of food addiction

There has been a lot of work done on laboratory animals to determine the effects of CRAP on brain-reward centres, and to compare these similarities with drug addictions. The examples below show that the consumption of CRAP triggers the same 'pleasure centres' and elicits the same chemical and structural changes that are seen in the brains of other substance addicts. A selection of the more memorable animal experiments is summarised below:

Example 1: A shocking study

One study divided a set of rats into two groups and fed one group foods such as sausage, bacon and cheesecake (the CRAP rats) while the other group (the chow rats) continued to eat chow, which is standard rat-pellet food. They then provided all the rats with CRAP but gave electric shocks to their feet when they accessed it. The chow rats quickly learned to avoid the unhealthy food, but the CRAP rats refused to let the shocks get in the way of their high-calorie binges. When the CRAP was removed and replaced by chow, the CRAP rats simply refused to eat, while the chow rats continued to chomp away[273].

Example(s) 2: Sugar

Many animal studies have asked the experimental question, 'Is sugar addictive?' and most found that it is. In these cases, sugary food altered the chemical balance of dopamine in the brain's reward circuits, mirroring changes in the brains of rats given cocaine or heroin. As these pleasure centres in the brain become less and less responsive, rats quickly develop compulsive overeating (to boost dopamine), consuming large quantities of high-calorie foods until they become obese. In some studies, the animals completely lost control over their eating behaviour – the primary hallmark of addiction.

Studies of the addictiveness of sugar frequently apply the four components of addiction to drugs of abuse: bingeing, withdrawal, craving and cross-sensitisation (substances or addictive behaviours) In these studies, sugar consumption is shown to be associated with long-lasting increases in reward values, cross sensitisation, reduced pleasure response in other normally pleasurable activities, and withdrawal symptoms. In other words, all signs that are present in classic drug addictions.

Such studies also note that sugar is noteworthy as a food substance in that it causes the release of opioids (as well as dopamine), and sugar ingestion and opioid production may exist in a reinforcing cycle. In rats, withdrawal from sugar causes symptoms such as anxiety, behavioural depression, tremor, teeth chattering and head shaking.

Repeated, excessive intake of sugar creates behavioural and neuro-chemical signs of withdrawal, just like withdrawal from morphine or nicotine. According to Professor Paul Kennedy from the Scripps Research Institute in Jupiter, Florida, "Junk food is as addictive as recreational drugs and tobacco". Collectively, these results support the argument for sugar dependency and addiction which likely translates to human eating disorders and obesity.

Example 3: a CRAP legacy

Numerous laboratories have reported changes in reward circuitry in the offspring of mothers fed a high-fat, high-sugar diet during pregnancy and lactation, which leads to an increased preference for CRAP in their children. These changes in the offspring are also seen as epigenetic markers that lead to long-term alterations in gene expression altering the release and response to dopamine and opioids, wiring a preference for CRAP foods. Further studies show that these changes last into adulthood for the offspring, creating a life-long risk for obesity and metabolic disease[274, 275].

Sugar addiction

Our brains are hungry for sugar. The human brain accounts for around 2% of body weight, but it uses about 20% of the total energy we consume (almost all as sugar). The brain consumes 5.6mg of glucose per 100g of brain tissue per minute, at a steady rate, irrespective of physical activity levels, cognitions or sleep. An average human brain weighs around 1.4kg resulting in a requirement of around 5g per hour, making its requirements for the day 120g, or 480kcal.

The brain really is something quite extraordinary, using just 0.0014g of sugar per second, it can fuel 86 billion neurons, each firing 200 times per second and each connecting to 1,000 other neurons, thus transmitting and receiving just under 20,000 trillion electrochemical signals in a second, all on 0.0056 of a calorie. To put it another way, one strand of cress would fuel fourteen such cycles of bioelectrical wizardry.

Thirty-five million years ago, a transilient layer of our distant ancestry, known collectively as the Old-World monkeys, are thought to have developed the sweetness receptor. A genetic adaptation that encouraged the consumption of ripe fruit and plants (naturally occurring sugars exist in thirty different classes of plants). Not only would this increase calorie intake, but it would help to avoid ingesting toxic substances, which are typically bitter. The sweet receptor mutation would have bestowed big advantages on the lucky recipient, providing not only abundant sugar resources for the brain, but increasing eating-derived pleasure, thus enhancing nutrient intake, greatly improving survival and reproduction prospects. Most recently, Homo sapiens have taken this evolutionary benefit to a whole new level, which, ironically, is now having the exact opposite effect that it had on the Old-World monkeys.

Blood-sugar disruption has a profound impact on humans, with glucose insufficiency posing a grave threat to the brain and its avatar. Therefore, the body is adept at breaking down carbohydrates (and fats or proteins if the need emerges) into glucose. As I have no doubt you are aware, careful blood glucose regulation is the key, and we ought to provide the body with foods that can enable gradual conversion and release of sugars rather than the substantial rush that accompanies sugary food and drink, which decouples eating behaviour from calorie needs and leaves the door open for unrestrained overeating.

The absolute pathways underlining addiction to CRAP (or, if you prefer, addiction to eating CRAP) are still under construction, but it is becoming ever more apparent that sugar will play a significant role in the final analysis. One laboratory study looked at the impact on the reward circuitry of 'intense sweet' against the reward effect of cocaine. For those researchers that relish a spot of suspense, there was a bit of a spoiler in the title of the paper: 'Intense sweetness surpasses cocaine reward'[276].

There is also the line of enquiry that suggests dependency on sugar may also be linked to the production of the brain's chemical serotonin. Serotonin synapses in the brain signal the alleviation of physical and emotional pain, and those deficient in serotonin are often quite anxious or depressed. When sugars are ingested, serotonin is released, subsequently, the default remedy for stress-management for many people is often to eat, especially sugary foods, and repetition and reinforcement of this cycle may result in dependency issues.

Although there are still the old die-hards (read 'captains of the food industry') that refuse to accept the deleterious effects of sugar on human health, evidence from epidemiological surveys and clinical studies has demonstrated that consumption of high-sugar foods and drinks result in increased risk for obesity, hypertension, insulin resistance, diabetes, harmful lipid disruptions, some cancers and, of course, cardiovascular disease[277].

Interestingly, one previous approach to treating alcoholics was to provide sugar and chocolates to satisfy the addicts' physical cravings. However, many sober alcoholics discovered that the sugary sweets were quite literally irresistible, and many recovering alcohol addicts who started with a modest consumption of chocolate eventually found themselves binge eating out of control. Rightly, the authors of the book *Eating Right to Live Sober*[278] show the benefits of avoiding sugar to help alcoholics to stay sober. They also found that sugar can lead some sober alcoholics to acute food dependency, even leading a significant number back to the bottle.

What are sugars?

Basically, sugars are soluble, sweet carbohydrates that can be single molecules (monosaccharides) including glucose, galactose and fructose, or dual molecules called di-saccharides, which are more stable and stick around longer like maltose (two glucose), lactose (one glucose one galactose), and the ubiquitous sucrose (one glucose one fructose). There are also long-chain, or complex, sugars known as starches, such as oligosaccharides and polysaccharides, which are more beneficial to human health due to their gradual breakdown into sugar.

Most of the sugar in a Western diet comes from either sucrose (50/50 glucose/fructose) or from high-fructose corn syrup (HFCS), which also contains roughly equal glucose to fructose (but there are variations to this ratio). Neither sucrose nor HFCS are natural products. While their constituents, glucose and fructose are both monosaccharides, fructose has been shown to be sweeter. It has a different chemical structure to glucose and follows a different metabolic pathway, leading to differences in how the body and brain respond. One difference occurs in the liver, which has to work hard to metabolise fructose, and, in doing so, succumbs to reduced glucose tolerance and an increase in the release of very low-density lipoproteins (bad cholesterol) and increased conversion of sugars to fats, which is one of the pathways linking fructose consumption to non-alcoholic fatty liver disease[279].

Fructose has come under much scrutiny lately and while it seems counterintuitive (because it is found in fruit), it may not be great for us. Typically, dietary carbohydrate is converted to glucose and the majority is taken up in muscle, fat and other peripheral tissues via the action of insulin; only a small amount is stored in the liver. However, fructose travels straight to the liver which converts the fructose to glucose before releasing it to the bloodstream where it can now be used to generate energy. These different metabolic pathways may lead to differences in how the body responds to each.

For example, compared to glucose, fructose produces smaller increases in circulating satiety hormones and a weak stimulation of insulin secretion. Since insulin increases satiety by blunting the reward value of food, it can be deduced that, taken together, fructose is less satiating than glucose allowing overconsumption of calories by failing to activate the body's signals to stop eating.

Glucose and fructose have different impacts on the brain. The main source of energy for the brain is glucose, and within the blood-brain barrier, are glucose transporters which shunt glucose from the bloodstream into the brain. However, these sugar shuttles don't work well with fructose, inhibiting the jump across blood-brain barrier. Subsequently, most fructose is left in the bloodstream.

Many people believe that fructose is healthy because it comes from fruit, but the vast volume of our fructose comes in the added fructose in our processed sugars (sucrose), which is implicated in a host of metabolic disease. In one study, the gram-for-gram replacement of fructose for glucose in the diet of children living with obesity reduced liver fat, blood pressure, circulating triglycerides, and harmful LDL cholesterol, while improving insulin sensitivity[280]. Furthermore, when it comes in fruit, fructose is accompanied by antioxidants, flavanols, potassium and vitamin C, all of which improve biological function. The fructose content of a peach is less than 10% by weight, whereas fructose accounts for half the weight of sucrose or high fructose corn syrup HFCS. A healthy diet should always include plenty of fruit. It is alternative sources of fructose (sucrose) that I believe are creating enormous health issues for millions of people.

Chocolate

Craving: 'to long for' or 'to desire intensely' (Collins English Dictionary). Chocolate is highly palatable, typically consumed between meals, and valued as a treat and a reward. It is cited as the most-craved edible item and its consumption is associated with ameliorating negative moods, including boredom, tension, anger, depression and fatigue. However, the common practice of eating to alter mood may be a source of inner conflict. A frequent psychological penalty for indulging in the hedonic pleasures of chocolate are feelings of guilt and remorse.

Many people consider themselves 'addicted' to chocolate. We could assert they are deluded or consider their notions fanciful, but I'm inclined to give credence to their self-assessments and subscribe fully to the concept of 'the expert patient'. Labelling oneself a 'chocoholic' is very revealing about your relationship with the key ingredient in 'the Devil's food cake'. In one study, self-diagnosed chocoholics were recruited into a study through a newspaper advertisement that began simply, "Are you a chocoholic?" Compared to a group of age and gender-matched controls, the chocoholics showed a greater desire to eat chocolate, but a smaller increase in salivation when exposed to chocolate[281] (greater craving, lesser liking)... sound familiar?

As flippant as it may seem to some, saying, "I am a chocoholic", in my view, is an important step; it acknowledges that eating chocolate is outside of your control (if you don't want to eat it but you do, then of course it is out of your control). Some argue that this shifts the locus of control to the food and places blame with the manufacturer, suggesting it contains dependence-forming substances. Such attributions, the detractors say, are a rational attempt to excuse personal behaviour and blame others. Well, I remind those people that, when people first started attributing addiction to cigarettes they were ridiculed and pilloried, and this went on for forty years and millions died.

This business of chocolate addiction being due to the presence of psychoactive or mood-altering compounds in the mystical cocoa bean is interesting. Published in the renowned journal Nature in 1996, this breakthrough study claimed to find "brain cannabinoids in chocolate"[282]. Since then, however, a series of studies have rained on their parade by concluding that such constituents play little or no role in chocolate addiction and craving.

Other substances present in chocolate raised as potentially pharmacologically significant, include phenylethylamine, theobromine, tyramine, serotonin, tryptophan and magnesium, but they are more abundant in other non-moreish foods, and anyway are neutralised in the intestinal mucosa, liver and kidneys. Anandamide (a cannabinoid relatively unique to cocoa) is present, but calculations by one researcher found that you would need to eat 25kg of chocolate in one sitting to achieve a noticeable high[283]. Caffeine is present in chocolate and regular caffeine consumers do become mildly dependent, but compared with coffee and tea, chocolate is an insignificant source of dietary caffeine.

Genetics and addictions

In the late 1980s, a single genetic marker for alcohol dependency was identified which was quickly confirmed as the same gene implicated in addictive drug use. Ten years later, Earnest Noble, M.D., published a paper in the *International Journal of Eating Disorders* resulting from his work with non-alcoholics who were obese 'food cravers and bingers'. Noble found that they had the same marker previously identified for alcoholism and other drug addictions. Noble made clear that the genetic marker was not a marker for obesity but rather for 'an internal chemical dependency on food'.

A little later, a survey of Overeaters Anonymous members in the US identified compulsive overeaters or food addicts and found that each had at least one blood relative also addicted to food or alcohol. Statistically, this was highly improbable and was explained as a genetic link to addiction (though some argued that this could be social conditioning with families following patterns displayed by parents and siblings).

According to Overeaters Anonymous, many food addicts are also 'users' of other substances. They wrote:

"It also is common knowledge that many members of Alcoholics Anonymous, while sober, use cigarettes, coffee, and sugar/flour/ fat products in abundance both in and out of meetings. What is not as well known is that there exists a large subset of members of Overeaters Anonymous and other food-related recovery programs made up of recovered alcoholics and drug addicts. Oftentimes after a few years of sobriety from drinking and using drugs, members of this group not only find themselves gaining weight (or using anorexic or bulimic methods to try to control their weight), but also eating in very similar ways to how they once used alcohol and drugs – by obsessing, bingeing, isolating and lying."[284]

Impulsivity and compulsivity

Impulsivity (acting without thinking) underpins addictive, compulsive and obsessive behaviours, and is ever-present in other problem behaviours such as gambling and thrill-seeking. The brain's cerebral cortex around the frontal lobes, where planning and complex cognitive behaviours like decision-making and the expression of personality and social behaviour occur, is thought to be the area responsible for impulsivity.

Food-related impulsivity is linked to weight gain via uncontrolled eating, but there are two components of food impulsivity: reward sensitivity (the hedonistic response to food), and rash-spontaneous behaviour (disinhibition with no regard for the consequences). While the distinction might be subtle, it appears that it is increased reward sensitivity that is the main problem for most people struggling with their weight, and this is the feature that generally leads to overconsumption. You can tackle increased reward sensitivity using mindful eating or the truncated Feel the breath, Find the calm, Use the strength technique. Impulsivity driven by rash, spontaneous behaviour looks to be the primary driver of binge-eating disorder (BED), and therefore therapies that focus on disinhibition would bear the most fruit.

If you identify with impulsivity or disinhibition, don't fall into the trap of accepting that this is who you are. Like many of our personality traits, these are modifiable characteristics that can be managed and curtailed with practice and perseverance. It may be true that this is who you have become, but that does not make it who you are. Be aware of feelings of impulsivity (feel them and explore them) and understand that you do not have to succumb to them, you are in control, and you can take a different path.

Compulsivity

Compulsivity differs from impulsivity in that it relates to feelings of limited control and an inability to rein-in unwanted thoughts and actions. The culmination of this is the need to repeat self-defeating behaviours despite a strong desire to avoid them. Therefore, compulsivity involves a mental tussle, where impulsivity encounters zero resistance. Known as behavioural inflexibility, compulsivity can lead to excessive habit-forming, and people can and do become defined by their compulsions. Compulsive behavioural addictions, as they are termed, include compulsive eating, gambling, computer use, sexual behaviour and compulsive buying.

Impulsive eating is a more benign and controllable state, but nonetheless should be considered the thin end of the wedge. If not acknowledged and managed, there is a danger that it could transition into full compulsive eating. This progression results in changes from positively reinforced food seeking, where heightened reward sensitivity (it tastes great – I eat it) is allowed to run amok, which can progress into the negatively reinforced substance-withdrawal stage (I don't want this, but I just can't stop myself).

Assessing eating compulsions

When general overeating problems spill over into full-blown compulsive eating, the situation becomes extremely bleak for the individual. Society sees people living with morbid obesity and says: "If I was that big, I'd do something about it". But that is a facile view; it is judgemental and prejudiced. Like all prejudices, such opinions are based upon a starting point of ignorance. I have learned the folly of disregarding the plight of compulsions and addictions, and in my work, it soon became apparent to me that, if I were to wear those shoes, I know I would struggle to cope. For this reason, I hold people living with obesity in high esteem, because I have an inkling of what they are dealing with. I admire their courage and fortitude.

Eating addiction or compulsive eating does not simply materialise one day as an all-or-nothing condition. Rather, it evolves over time, and typically, as time passes, the condition becomes more challenging and more immersive. Therefore, classifying someone as 'addicted' or not may be tricky, at least in the early stages. Perhaps more helpful would be to ask people to consider where they might presently reside across a range of progressive stages. I've termed this example the Eating Relationship Continuum (ERC). I suggest that the gradients may be summarised thus:

1. I have absolutely no eating or food issues. I can eat what I want when I want and don't ever feel guilty or lose control around foods.

2. Most of the time I'm fine but sometimes I do find myself eating too much of some of my favourite foods. I take practical steps such as managing shopping lists and not picking after a meal.

3. I am aware that I can overeat in specific situations and so I take steps such as keeping certain snack foods out of sight and trying to avoid shopping for my 'trigger' foods. I can impulse-buy foods that I know will be difficult for me to eat in moderation.

4. I have some weakness foods such as X, Y or Z, which feel more significant in my life than I think they should be. I have mixed emotions when I'm buying them. I can over-order when it comes to takeaways thinking I'll leave some for the next day, but I usually eat it all. Afterwards, I feel stuffed, but then find myself doing the same thing all over again the next time.

5. Food is on my mind more than it should be. Snacking is sometimes a problem for me particularly if I'm bored or feeling down. I reach for a biscuit and only mean to take a couple, but often I eat half the packet. I regularly buy snacks on a whim and regret it when I've eaten them. I am aware of trigger situations which invariably lead to eating and I try to plan to avoid them. I often overeat my favourite meals, particularly takeaways. Much to my shame, I sometimes eat in secret.

6. I have periods when things go fine but this can be disrupted by hectic events or emotional situations. I use food as a comforter and eating my favourite foods is one of the best feelings. I'm anxious about certain foods and constantly vow to cut down on those that I can binge on. When certain foods aren't available and I'm feeling vulnerable, I will go out of my way to obtain them. While I know at the time it's wrong, I can find myself planning for an eating session which will involve all my favourite things and far too much of them for my needs. Each time I tell myself this will be the last time and I'll change my ways tomorrow, but I find myself doing the same thing over and over.

7. I feel totally powerless around certain foods. I act normally when around others, but then I plan lone binges sometimes two or three times a week when I totally overeat to the point that I sometimes feel disgusted with myself. I plan ahead to ensure I can get the things that I want. I hide foods and I'm always eating in secret; I feel guilty about it all the time. A thought enters my head about a food, and I must have it. I wish I could stop; I feel guilt, remorse, and distress, but I just can't make the change.

If you feel you have an unhealthy relationship with food in general or just with certain foods, consider where you may be on the ERC scale. Reflecting upon this and accepting your situation if you do have an unhealthy relationship with food is a vital starting point on the journey of change. Anything below four and you are probably OK to keep managing things as you are and trying to apply perhaps some of the strategies in this book or those that have previously worked for you to manage your weight. Anything above four and I would recommend considering accessing support to help you to overcome what may be the development of a compulsive eating disorder.

Food sobriety

If your weight is a result of compulsive eating, food dependency or addiction to CRAP, then you will need to think long and hard about the notion of food sobriety. This requires the acceptance that CRAP is a substance which, when confronted with, you are rendered powerless, and that you will always succumb to it, and that it is the root cause of your weight, and any and all the corresponding health, social and psychological consequences that being overweight brings. You must accept that you will never be able to manage your relationship with CRAP and no amount of dieting, health drives, exercise programmes, weight-loss books (including this one) and medical weight-loss approaches will ever solve this intractable problem; they are futile distractions to the origin of your dilemma. Food sobriety is your only salvation.

The over-arching approach in traditional addiction therapy (and, ultimately, the only secure method) is absolute abstinence, and if you have an addiction or compulsion, then your only prospect of recovery is for you to treat your condition as an addiction and apply the principle of abstinence. But the notion of food sobriety for someone with a compulsion (which compels them to always have access to their controlling substance) is, to say the least, a daunting proposition. But it is important to see that people in remission from their addiction don't ask: "Can I keep this up forever?" Instead, they ask: "Can I manage this today?"

But people think that, where food is concerned, abstinence is not possible: "How can I stop eating?" However, recovering alcoholics do not stop drinking, they stop consuming ethanol in their fluids, and thus achieve sobriety. Recovering compulsive overeaters do not stop eating, they abstain from eating CRAP and so also attain (food) sobriety. If you suspect compulsive eating or addictions are implicated in your weight, now would be a good time to determine a list of high-risk items that you associate negatively with your eating behaviours – the causal CRAP, or substances.

Establishing CRAP as 'substances' in the context of food abuse represents the preparatory phase of change. It must be adequately considered and openly discussed with family and other significant people that will be involved in your recovery. Keeping this as a closely guarded secret will almost certainly lead to failure. The most important aspect of this preparatory stage involves coming to terms with your weight and its causality and being confident and sufficiently trusting to share this (either with a practitioner or trusted friend). This preparatory phase is more than simply a marker for readiness to change, it is an upholding principle upon which you will build your recovery.

In your diary, write something along the lines of:

> "My name is XXXX and I have an eating compulsion. I have no control over the CRAP that I have listed below. I accept that, unless I abstain completely from this CRAP, my life will be completely dominated by it."

As mentioned, truthful acknowledgement of your actual situation is the only starting point when contemplating change. If I were to attend Alcoholics Anonymous and as a client, stand up and say:

> "Hi, I'm Alan and I don't think I'm really addicted to alcohol; I just drink too much, particularly at weekends, and I've come along because I'd like to cut down a bit."

I suspect someone, rightly, will point out to me that I may be some way off starting my recovery. As any recovering addict will tell you, the first step of healing is the acknowledgement and acceptance that you are addicted to the substance. You must believe that you have no control over it and that it is a serious threat to you if you are to overcome your addiction. Without this mindset, recovery simply can't start.

It is accepted that alcoholics' or drug addicts' recovery cannot be effective while still drinking or using drugs. Similarly, a person with an addiction to food cannot recover while continually relapsing on CRAP. I learned early on in my career that applying the standard psychological behavioural-change techniques with which I had successfully treated many overeaters was simply ineffective with those people living with established compulsive eating or chronic food addiction. In these cases, the only course of action is complete abstinence from CRAP foods.

As with other addictions, for the food addict to have the clarity and truth in their lives that they will need, they must first be separated from the drug. If for no other reason, initially, this is to reduce the physical cravings to a manageable level so that they are no longer overpowered by CRAP each day. Detoxification is imperative to break the hold of the disease; without it, recovery cannot start. Becoming abstinent offers the addict a degree of functional normality to build upon. Until the distorted thinking of the addicted mind is remedied, with its manic lying, hiding foods, deceiving the self and others and its persistent upholding of the underlying lie that life without CRAP is not worth living, there will be no healing.

Even when someone has removed the CRAP from their lives, they will still suffer the legacy of the addicted mind. They will still need to overcome the inevitable denial of their food addiction and will need to grapple daily with the lurking self-destructive power of the addicted mind, which, without support, risks a relapse, and a full-scale return to addiction. If all of the above resonates with you and you believe that you are a food addict, a valuable resource that I would highly recommend is *Food Junkies*[285] written by a US physician and a recovered food addict – probably the most important work undertaken on food addiction and an invaluable tome for those dealing with food compulsions. The case studies and stories from recovering addicts are both uplifting and tragic, and reveal with shocking clarity the only salvation for the food addict. Philip Werdell concludes the book with a moving summary of his life as an addict. His final words sum up the prize: "Freedom from food obsession can taste better than anything you could possibly imagine".

As I'm sure you have gathered by this point, most cases of compulsive eating or food addiction are going to require considerably more support than that which can be provided by a traditional weight-management service, or a weight-management book for that matter. Food addicts require a high level of very specialised help and support and a framework that is designed from the bottom up to treat addiction and to attain food sobriety. Telling a person with compulsive eating to 'eat less' is about as effective as telling a person with clinical depression to 'cheer up'.

I am delighted to witness the emergence in the UK (and around the world) of a few outstanding organisations committed solely to food addiction. Their work goes way beyond anything that is offered in the conventional weight-loss setting and is centred around the reality of food addiction. While each has its own unique programme, the common theme is focused on enabling a chronic compulsive eater the possibility of finally seeing, telling and believing the truth.

Overeaters Anonymous (OA)

OA is a twelve-step programme that began in 1960 in the USA and offers around 6,500 meetings around the world in seventy-five countries. It is a fellowship of individuals who support each other to provide recovery from compulsive eating and food behaviours by sharing experience, strength and hope. OA is based on the twelve-step programme of Alcoholics Anonymous. Members recognise that they are powerless over food and help each other recover from unhealthy relationships with food. Compulsive eating in OA includes under-eating, dieting, starving, over-exercising, vomiting, laxative abuse and other symptoms related to eating and weight control.

Meetings are offered in many languages and are freely available due to members making voluntary financial donations and giving service. OA offers thousands of meetings online, in person or via telephone, making it easily accessible to those with barriers such as social stigma, mobility issues, and lack of diagnosis for disordered eating e.g., eating disorders and mental health issues.

OA is a self-supporting fellowship of individuals whose primary purpose is to stop eating compulsively and to carry the message of recovery to others. They freely share this experience to strengthen their own recovery from food obsession. Following the programme releases the need to eat compulsively while maintaining a healthy body weight.

The OA programme can work alongside mental health therapies such as counselling, cognitive behavioural therapy (CBT) etc, and dietary therapies such as commercial weight-loss groups, weight-management groups, dietetic support, and other multi-disciplinary treatment programs. It is helpful if the healthcare professional has basic knowledge of twelve-step programmes, but it is not essential. OA can be offered as an option with the suggestion that they attend meetings to learn about how the programme has worked for others.

Much evidence has been provided about twelve-step programmes. The most notable piece of evidence was a gold standard Cochrane systematic review in 2019, which demonstrated that they were more effective than CBT in chronic alcoholism.

To conclude, OA provides a promising option to those having difficulty with food and food behaviours. It is available free of charge, and when accessed online, support is available day and night. Healthcare professionals can signpost patients to OA without cost, making it a financially viable option for people dealing with eating disorders and disordered eating.

I'm delighted to say that more clinicians are now offering counselling and support for those with food addiction. In the UK, a charity called the Public Health Collaboration has researched a group intervention and published research on its promising outcomes[286], and is now expanding its efforts to provide these online courses internationally. These will be self-taught or coached. They are also developing courses for healthcare professionals to help them identify and support people with food addiction in their clinics. The website to follow for updates is www.phcuk.org.

Ellen's story

If anyone is still in any doubt about the reality of food addiction, then you need to read Ellen's story.

"I was obese from the age of nine years old. My factory worker and bus driver parents were told by doctors to give me plenty of low-fat, high-fibre foods. They dutifully obeyed. I was very happy to see the piles of pasta, potato, rice and bread on my plate every day. One of my favourite dishes was pasta bolognese with garlic bread. I had as much as I liked. Low-fat yoghurts or trifle – without the cream for desserts. I got bigger and bigger, and the professionals told them to reduce my portion sizes.

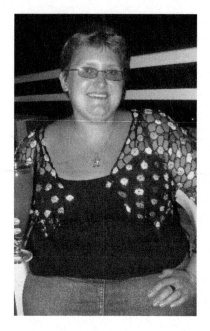

I remember one Sunday lunch of meat, vegetables, roast and mashed potatoes and stuffing (no oil or butter). My dad's portion was far bigger than mine. I asked Mom why I couldn't have a plate like Dad? I remember her saying, 'When you are an adult you can have as much as you want'. My mom probably said many wise things to me over the years, but my brain held on to this one. I thought, 'Right then, I will', and, as you will see from my story, I am quite a determined person – and I did.

By the time I left school, I was sixteen stone; unhappy, depressed and struggling to get work. The jobs I did get required a uniform that needed to be ordered in for my size and I struggled to get behind a till. Over time, I started dieting. One commercial weight-loss programme taught me that 'If you cook chips by part boiling them and using spray oil you can have as many as you like on green days'. But this advice was for normal people because I went home and made three full baking trays. The following week, having paid my £5 to be weighed, I had gained pounds – yet again.

Chocolate was the worst; I would buy two share bars and eat one before I got home and then offer some to my housemates. If they said no, I would never say 'Are you sure?' I used to pray they wouldn't say yes. Then two bars weren't enough and eating in my bedroom started. The first bite was chocolate, the second bite was salted crisps and then came the rapid alternating bites, I only came up for air for sugary drinks to wash it down. The day came when I could eat chocolate and lose weight – diet chocolate was launched. I went to Boots and bought all three flavours (they were always cheaper per item when you buy three), with the intention to have one per day. All three were gone before getting home and the rest of the time I spent on the toilet. The packet had warned me – it wasn't enough to stop me. I did it again and again. The weight continued to rise. Thinking back, it seems as ridiculous as someone hitting their head with a hammer to get rid of a headache.

I had one diet success – Atkins, as it was known then, low carb we now call it. I lost six stone and felt great. Still obese but in better physical and mental health than I had ever been before. The diet came to an end when professionals started telling me how dangerous it was to be eating as much fat as I did. I started introducing whole carbohydrates. This was fine until I had some bread and I soon escalated back to sweets, chocolate, crisps and biscuits. There was no hope, willpower or energy left in me to restart the diet. My weight went to twenty stone. At 5ft in height, that gave me a BMI of 55kg/m2 – a candidate for bariatric surgery. My determination came again: I WOULD NOT have surgery. I stopped weighing after that. What was the use? It only made me eat more. I never knew my heaviest. I got further depressed and suicidal.

The eating would not stop. I was stealing food and rearranging biscuit tins and cupboards to make it look like I hadn't stolen anything. I shopped daily, binged nightly, and before sleeping vowed the next day would not be the same. I searched desperately for pills to fix me. I found some capsules online – I still have no idea what was in them, but I had to stop as there was an immense pressure behind my eyes which disturbed my vision. I had fat-blocking pills from the doctors which made me have greasy diarrhoea; I didn't stay on them long as there was more than one time when I soiled myself at work.

I would wake up and, before opening my eyes, I would think of breakfast, and while eating breakfast I would daydream about what I'd have for lunch. One day, I thought, this can't be right, thinking about food like this. I asked my office colleagues what their first thought was in the morning, the answers were various. 'Oh no, got to sort the kids out.' 'Oh no, forgot to pay that bill yesterday.' 'I need a fag.' No one said anything about food. When it was my turn, I lied and said I thought about work. I concluded that I must not speak to anyone about this. It is only me that thinks this way about food. I am not normal, and I am alone. Eventually, in my isolation, I neglected myself, my job, and my family. I couldn't continue. I'd go to bed hoping that I wouldn't wake up the next day. I would wake up the next day disappointed that I hadn't died.

Then, I saw an advert in the paper that said, 'Do you have a problem with food?' My brain immediately went 'Yeah! I can't get enough'. I acted on it and joined a twelve-step fellowship programme for food. I found myself in a room full of people who were just like me. People talking about the insane things they did with food. Eating mouldy food, eating out of bins, eating salads when in company and making up for it when alone. Stealing food or money for food, lying to partners about needing to go out for vegetables for dinner, to get my binge foods, stealing the kid's advent calendars and having to replace them, and much more. I was not alone anymore. I got a sponsor and vowed to do what they said. I was so desperate, I'd have given them my credit cards – yet they never asked for a penny.

The first thing my sponsor asked me to do was to go home and have a shower and call her the next day. I was in a daze, and did as I was told as it occurred to me then that I couldn't remember the last time I showered. I made a daily call and shared all my food secrets to this stranger who didn't judge me in the slightest, in fact she nodded away as if to say 'yep' done that. I asked her for the diet sheet. She said we don't have any and we don't weigh people either. After my other weight-loss groups, this seemed a bit strange, but I felt like I'd found my tribe, so I went with it and went to meetings up to four times a week.

My food plan was developed with honesty and tears. Over time, she asked me what foods I felt like I could not live without. She wasn't daft as she knew it was highly processed foods. The first food I put down was chocolate. I remember the last time I had chocolate. Had I known it was to be the last time, my addicted self would have done better, as I had part of a Kit Kat. Someone had bought a four-finger bar and asked me and a friend if we wanted a finger. The other friend politely said no. I said yes. I put down chocolate that night and it was the hardest night of my life. I cried myself to sleep, convinced that if I did not eat chocolate I would surely die. My body ached from crying. Then the beautiful part of recovery started happening. I woke the next morning without thoughts of breakfast but with the knowledge that I will die if I keep eating chocolate. I decided that I had already consumed my lifetime's worth of chocolate and I could not have anymore. This was in 2009, and I haven't eaten any since.

Other foods went as I became more honest with myself. Chewy sweets, sugar in foods and drinks, crisps, popcorn, bread, cakes and biscuits. Still, the professionals say that I will become ill if I do not consume carbohydrates regularly. I remind them that I have been excluding them for over a decade and that I am eleven stone lighter because of it. What's more, I have maintained my weight for well over a decade. Professionals are kind and tell me that they wouldn't want me to feel deprived and to have cake on special occasions. When I have listened, I have fallen into a deep binge that is very difficult to get out of. Now I state firmly that you wouldn't ask an alcoholic to have a glass of wine on special occasions so why would you ask me to have cake? Their 'kind' advice is dangerous to someone like me.

It took two years to lose eleven stone. With excitement, I went to the doctors to see if I could set up a group in our local surgery to help other people like me take back control of their food. My kind doctor was stunned by my weight loss but said that he could only listen to dietitians. So, I went back to college, got my GCSEs and A levels in science, and applied to university. I was looking forward to learning about food addiction and perhaps finding out why I hadn't been told about food addiction or the twelve-step fellowship by healthcare professionals before; God knows, I saw enough of them. I learned for four years about how low-carb diets are bad, but, sadly,

nothing about food addiction. Luckily, views on low-carb eating have started to change. I qualified as a dietitian and started to practice clinically.

Now, as a research dietitian, I am determined to bring food addiction into the research arena, working with a charity called Public Health Collaboration, to help others with their food addiction and collating the masses of evidence on food addiction to provide to the World Health Organization (WHO) to include Food Addiction diagnosis to the ICD-11."

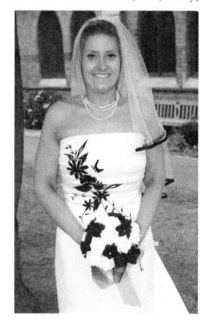

Ellen Calteau Registered Dietitian

(Edited by Deborah Spiers)

There really is only one way that I can end this chapter, and it would be reprehensible of me to conclude otherwise. I know that I have upheld my mantra of not telling people what to do throughout this book, but this is the one instance that am going to deviate from that path. If any of this chapter has resonated with you and you think that your weight is at least in part due to compulsive eating, then I implore you to contact Overeaters Anonymous and allow this wonderful organisation to welcome you home.

For those in the UK, visit www.oagb.org.uk. For those elsewhere, visit www.oa.org.

My final word on food and eating addictions: considering the weight of available evidence showing the addictiveness of eating CRAP, continuing to omit compulsive eating from the established spectrum of addictive disorders is, in my view, medically negligent.

Insight 3: Acknowledgement and acceptance

Revisit your notebook and read the words you wrote for Insight 2. Now it's time to acknowledge and embrace these as legitimate reasons that are underpinning your weight. By thinking clearly and by using logic and reasoning, you have determined these 'causes', and your challenge now is to accept them as the truth and never waiver from this.

You must also now think carefully about the consequences that your weight has imposed on your life, such as disadvantages, losses or restrictions that your weight has inflicted. Unwavering self-honesty and courage is required for this step. Don't leave any stone unturned, the further things are locked away, the deeper you must forage. Contemplating the consequences of your weight will not be easy and may lead to collateral emotional damage, but it is another important step on your journey.

Think about your physical and mental health and how the burden of your weight may have impacted each of these. Consider your family, friends and your relationships and the effects that your weight may have had on them as well as on yourself. Think about your quality of life and the opportunities for doing the things that you have wanted to do. Are there any future aspirations that may be stifled by your weight if nothing changes? How has your weight impacted you when you were younger (if you were overweight as a child)? Is there any leftover baggage from previous weight-related unhappiness or trauma? Try to consider everything and make a list of all that you consider relevant.

Take your pen, and write in your notebook:

"THESE ARE THE CONSEQUENCES THAT MY WEIGHT HAS HAD ON MY LIFE..."

The psychology of eating

"I'm not lost, but I don't know where I am"

Talking Heads, 1985

I remember Sandra, one of the first weight-management clients I had the pleasure of meeting over twenty-five years ago. One evening during her regular weekly group meeting, Sandra was aghast to see the scales tip 95kgs (209lbs), 1.5kg (3lbs) more than the previous week. After the meeting, Sandra sheepishly sidled over to me and asked: "Alan, avocados, are they fattening?"

Me:	"Well, they are more calorific than many other plant foods, but they are an excellent, nutritious food."
Sandra:	"Actually, this is all I can put it down to, I had an avocado in the week, and that's all I have done differently."
Me:	"Blimey Sandra, that avocado must have been the size of a beach-ball!"

An average avocado (150g) contains 240kcal, and Sandra had put on the equivalent of over 10,000kcals or forty-one avocados in one week. I worried about this for some time. How could one seemingly credible and rational person believe something that another person would deem utterly impossible?

Fifty years ago, physicians in the USA were confronted with the same problem: the sheer number of patients attending their practice, consistently gaining weight, while at the same time reporting low or moderate food intakes. They were puzzled as to what to do. It was an unfathomable nationwide explosion of weight gain with no apparent explanation. While the physicians wrestled with the phenomenon, their combined clinical data set off alarm bells upstream in the scientific community. The riddle of the inexplicably expanding US population spawned a plethora of research studies and epidemiological investigations aimed at shining a light on what was a nationwide medical mystery. Several highly funded research projects backed by the foremost scientific institutions set about designing experimental investigations to determine the truth.

To get to the bottom of matters, the scientific community set about a design that could accurately measure calories consumed against calories burned and relate this to an individual's body weight over time. The primary study involved people of varying BMIs keeping comprehensive food diaries for five days, while at the same time being measured accurately for energy expenditure. At the end of each study, food diaries were analysed for reported energy intake (calories in) and compared against how much energy each person had burned over the period (calories out). Precise body measurements were taken before and after, which provided energy storage information over the five days, enabling calorie intake to be calculated with a high degree of accuracy.

Actual calorie consumption was then plotted against self-reported eating (as estimated by the dietitians who were interpreting the food diaries), which revealed significant underreporting of calories consumed. This data was then plotted against BMI, to see if underreporting is weight specific, and it turns out that it is, with underreporting increasing in a linear fashion with BMI. For those with a healthy weight, food reporting is within 5% accuracy, but at the heaviest end of the spectrum, people underreport by up to 25%. Typically, this would equate to 750kcal/day of underreporting for heavier people.

There also emerged a selective reporting pattern for different food types, where snack-type foods are preferentially forgotten as BMI increases. This supports the existing body of evidence explaining that it is fatty and sugary (CRAP foods) that are underreported as BMI increases. One study carried the tongue-in-cheek sub-title: "Soda, chips and candy keep you lean", because these items were well represented in the food diaries of lean people but became increasingly absent from the diaries of people as their BMIs increased.

Research has proved (beyond doubt) that larger people are high-energy expenders, and greater body mass results in higher overall metabolic requirements[287]. To meet these higher energy needs and maintain the extra body mass, heavier people must consume more calories for the same levels of activity undertaken by smaller people. Despite many years of research, the mythical overweight person with a low metabolic rate (and subsequent frugal diet) has proved entirely elusive. The lowest free-living total daily energy expenditure ever accurately recorded over a lengthy period of time was a very lean woman at around 1,200kcals/day[288].

Secret Eaters

Aired on UK TV several years ago, a show called Secret Eaters was a documentary consisting of twenty-one episodes spanning three series. In each episode, the presenters met overweight people that were typically in a family situation or a relationship. The premise of the show was that their 'guests' are hoping to lose weight and become healthier, but presently they were somewhat mystified as to why they were overweight. With the use of discrete cameras, the families were then filmed in their homes for a few weeks (presumably when they were off their guard) and tracked by private investigators watching and recording everything that they bought and ate. At the end of a selected week, the hapless foodies were confronted by the presenter, who detailed exactly what they had all eaten that week. This aspect of the show was theatrically staged using incriminating footage of the secret eating and the widespread over-indulgence that each episode portrays. Their frequent visits to the local fast-food outlets to buy colossal portions of junk food were exposed for all to see, alongside the home binges where they devoured CRAP with great alacrity. When tackled with the evidence, the response from the foodies was always the same: shock, horror and embarrassment at how much they had actually eaten. If you have not seen Secret Eaters and you are interested in the psychology of overeating, then I suggest you go to YouTube and watch a few episodes.

This phenomenon (I'd no idea I was actually eating that much) has been termed the 'Eye Mouth Gap (EMG) – the eye did not see what the mouth took in, and is an accepted phenomenon of overeating for very many people. EMG is explained as a subliminal coping strategy to counter the damaging effects of continual self-blaming and remorse, which would otherwise lead to distress and anguish, following episodes of overeating. It appears that the brain has an in-built mechanism to protect us from the pain and potential mental health consequences of 'repeat offending', by learning to blank out such events as though they never happened. This calorie warp avoids the internal conflicts and psychological trauma from constantly worrying and stressing about what has been eaten. If you omit to register it in the frontal lobes (where we make sense of the world), then it simply doesn't count!

When submitting food diaries, those concerned about their weight tend not to report the 'naughty foods', because they didn't think they had eaten them, and this is because they 'don't register' (in the frontal lobes). Therefore, EMG is not a deliberate ploy to deceive doctors, dieticians, researchers or themselves, and they are not in denial so much as subconsciously parking the pain. While it is unlikely that EMG represents a complete elimination of a memory of the event, it is thought to be buried so deep as to avoid consideration, thus averting the psychological pain and discomfort that would surely accompany such transgressions.

The same happens when parents complete diaries for their overweight children – the calorie values are always significantly lower in the diaries than what the children have actually consumed, with the 'naughty' foods most underreported (EMG by proxy). The same thing also happens when you ask people about their exercise and activity levels, only in reverse (they report more activity than they have actually performed). G. H. Beaton summarised matters in the opening sentence of his paper on diet reporting, with the words, "Dietary intake cannot be estimated without error and probably never will be"[289]. Food and activity diaries should be renamed food and activity liaries!

Therefore, both Sandra and the thousands of overweight people attending their physicians in the US with reports of meagre diets were purely a result of underreporting of food intake. EMG is identified as a considerable barrier to changing behaviour in many people, particularly those with substantial weight to lose, or those where their weight leads to significant distress or low self-esteem.

To help my clients understand the ramifications of EMG, I would discuss with them such experiences at one of our group meetings. In my opinion, these discussions are best held during such meetings, where people feel secure alongside peers who understand and relate to their problems (which has probably got a lot to do with the reason that group meetings are more effective for weight loss than one-to-one sessions). In such circumstances, openness and candour flourish, and acceptance and problem-solving opportunities are optimised. "So, what do we think is going on here?" I would muse. What typically emerged is that people would agree that it is easier to 'forget' the naughty foods and the snacks, 'the ones that don't count!' People also regularly said that, if no one saw them eating, then that didn't count either!

Those in the groups that I discussed this with generally acknowledged EMG as a coping strategy for those living with obesity. As one of my clients said to me: "It means that you don't have to face up to what you are doing to yourself." I cannot overstate the importance of thinking deeply about EMG for anyone considering embarking upon the momentous journey of permanent weight loss. The eyes must see what the mouth takes in, and the mind must acknowledge and accept it – or there can be no self-credibility and no healing.

Weight-loss support groups

I am a big fan of weight-loss groups, and it is my experience that they are extremely helpful for very many people. However, they can only work if people are ready to change, and therein lies the rub. Another anomaly of human behaviour was unearthed when a recent study looked at how people would respond if they were offered weight-loss support that was either free or paid for. One study [290], found that, when doctors offered a referral to people living with obesity onto a free weight-loss programme provided by the NHS, the take up was quite good (40%). However, if doctors offered a referral onto a service that the patient must fund themselves, then take up was virtually zero, well, actually 2%, even though the outcomes on both programmes were comparable (the free one did not outperform the paid for one).

The psychology behind this is interesting, and it's worth giving it some thought. For instance, I don't think that the results of this experiment were a reflection on how much people value weight loss or weight-loss services, but instead, I think it tells us more about people's expectations for such programmes:

> "It will no doubt be someone telling me to eat less and exercise more, eat more fruit and veg and less ice cream etc. It probably won't work, but as it's free, I'll give it a go – I might lose a few pounds through herd conformity or osmosis or something."

They know what I know – telling people what to do diminishes the prospect of change (which is particularly true if you are telling people what they already know). If this is the mindset of someone attending such a programme, then I can guarantee that it won't work, so of course they would be correct, and they will have done well to save their money. If you go to a popular commercial slimming club that involves 'Watching your Weight', then you will know that, providing you follow your points, you will lose weight. Therefore, you are not paying for someone to tell you what to do, or to provide you with information that you either did or did not have previously, you are paying for a system, and as long as you stick to it, then it will work, but only while you stay on the programme (actually, it's a brilliant business model).

People know that, to lose weight, they should eat more healthy food, cut out the CRAP and do more exercise, and so if this is your primary message, why would people pay for it? Do the doctors promoting the programmes imagine that the course leaders have some secret knowledge or dietary revelation up their sleeve that until now has been kept away from the general public. "People will be amazed to hear what we have to say, and weight loss is virtually inevitable." I don't think so, and nor do the people that took part in this study. However, I imagine if I advertised a 'hypnotic cure' for obesity with a 90% success rate, then I could charge whatever I wanted, and people would form a queue around the block. People desperately want to lose weight, but it is all about expectations, and the mundane (yet correct) messages of eat less CRAP and take more exercise are no longer news to anyone. But teaching people how to think differently transcends the futile dissemination of banal information.

On a somewhat related theme, numerous trials that involved paying people to lose weight have taken place, and what is always found is that, in the short-term, financial incentives do improve weight-loss outcomes. This is because the theory of behavioural economics suggests that we want to maximise benefits and minimise costs, and increasing the benefits of weight loss (by also getting paid) therefore helps to outweigh the considerable challenges of making the necessary lifestyle changes and enduring the perceived denial of overeating.

In a 2020 US study, men were randomised onto an online twenty-four-week weight-loss programme called Gutbusters! Some were offered a cash incentive, some weren't. The cash incentive meant that, if they were successful each week for the duration, they would earn a grand total of $1,200. The incentive group's average weight loss was 4.5kg at twelve weeks and 3.8kg at twenty-four weeks. The Gutbusters alone weight loss was less than half, at 1.7kg and 1.5kg respectively [291]. A previous UK programme for both men and women called Pounds for Pounds was evaluated with much the same result – a 4kg average weight loss at twelve months for those incentivised using cash (no control group was used)[292].

There are advantages and drawbacks to this incentive approach, and in support, it obviously helps to shift the pounds by temporarily increasing motivation. But the drawbacks are clear, as some of the incentive for change is based upon the cash prize, once this enticement is removed, motivation will evaporate proportionately. Moreover, if you place more value on the cash than your health, this may skew your judgement of choices for the future. The other important point, of course, is that anything that is based around a diet programme (with a start and an end) won't work, because diets don't deliver permanent weight loss, since you always have one eye on the target weight or completion date, and after that, it's business as usual.

To assume we are fully in control of what we eat is naive. How many times did you ask yourself, why did I eat that? What made me reach for the biscuit tin at home, or grab the sugary/salty snack in the queue at the petrol station when I wasn't even hungry? Why do I often go back for seconds when my initial portion was fine? Why do I crave particular foods at certain times and why do I sometimes totally lose control around these foods? Why is it that there are some things that I simply can't resist if they are there? What is it that means I can't make the food choices that I planned for when I'm confronted with other options? What is this potent, omnipresent force that appears to be in charge where food choices are concerned? Why do I feel so powerless when it happens?

If I had a Jammie Dodger for every time someone asked themselves one of the above questions, I'd no doubt bump Jon Brower Minnoch out of the *Guinness Book of Records*. The multitude of contributing factors leading to our food choices means that there is no easy answer to these difficult questions. If you have asked yourself such questions from time to time, then you may wish to think about re-framing the question. Rather than asking: why did I just eat that? You could ask: why do I feel unhappy about eating that? The first question may be impossible to answer, but the second should be within your grasp, and you should aim to answer it, if and when it arises in the future (the opportunity is probably in close proximity). This will help you to understand better how your brain works and how you can start to reach the decisions about food choices that are compatible with your long-term goals. These thought processes are important to revealing the answers that are the critical insights needed for change.

Another thing that has puzzled me in the past, is why people on a weight-loss diet that have a temporary slip, can react by tearing up the rule book.

"That's it, I've strayed from my eating plan today by overeating at lunch, so I'm going to push the boat out tonight and have a real binge." People pursuing other lifestyle changes don't react the same way to lapses. If someone trying to follow a plant-based diet was careless enough to eat a pork pie, would they respond by going to the kebab house that evening to order the full elephant's leg kebab with chicken wings on the side? Or would they think, hey, what happened there? I'll make sure in that situation next time I don't make the same mistake.

Peddlers and pushers

If someone has a problem, it makes it easier to share this with someone else, which is a very reasonable thing to do. However, some people interpret this to mean that if they behave in a damaging way to themselves, then getting others to do the same will normalise their behaviour and make it more tolerable, and therefore make them feel better about it and about themselves. These are the peddlers and pushers. When someone tries this on with you (plying you with CRAP that you are trying to avoid, which they know you are, because you have told them), then you need to respond accordingly. Normally, you might think, "I don't want to upset them because they are always so generous and kind with their gifts of food, or they baked it especially for me (peddlers and pushers know every trick in the book), and I know how happy it makes them when I eat it. I suppose on this occasion I'll eat it because I don't like upsetting people." What you are really saying is: "I'm prepared to break my promise to myself and ruin my own self-credibility and risk going back to being miserable and depressed, so that they can feel better about eating their CRAP".

What is food?

On meeting my clients for the first time, one thing that I might say to them, much to their bewilderment, is that it would be my hope that together we can figure out a way for them to eat more food. As a starting point for this, I will often use a group workshop imaginatively entitled: What is food? And it works like this. Two tables are placed either side of the meeting room. On one table are vegetables, fruit, rice, eggs, fish etc. The second table contains chocolate, sweets, cola, ice cream, crisps and so on. Everyone together is given a simple instruction to go and 'stand or sit by the table of food', nothing further is said. After various shenanigans, the group, to a person, invariably ends up next to the 'healthy' table. They are asked why they have chosen to stand by this table when asked to stand by the food? They say:

Group: "It's healthy, natural – it has not been processed or modified."

Me: "Yes, all of that is right, but it's too vague. Try again."

Group: "These are fresh, with nothing added. These are good for you."

Me: "Getting warmer!"

But I won't let them off the hook until they hit the nail on the head. Sometimes we are there for quite some time. Finally, someone will say it:

Group: "These foods have grown!"

Bingo!

'These foods have grown.' It is clear that the cauliflower, the beetroot, the fish, and the eggs have all been living things, and it is plain for all to see that they have grown. Thanks to truly miraculous cells in plants known as chloroplasts, they have captured the energy of the sun, combined this with carbon dioxide and water and created edible carbohydrate, that we can eat, or the fish or the chickens can eat, and then we can eat the fish, or the chickens or their eggs, thus releasing the energy locked in by the sun for use in our bodies. Only plants can do this (photosynthesis), and it enables the power source of our solar system to become a usable form of energy for our bodies. We then expire the waste CO^2 and the plants oblige once again by soaking it up and combining it with water to create more glucose and releasing oxygen for us to breathe. This marvel of plant respiration is represented by the equation: $6CO_2 + 6H_2O \rightarrow C_6H_{12}O_6 + 6O_2$. Every now and then, I stop and think about this miracle of creation, and I wonder to myself, could this all really have happened by chance?

Back to my group: "So, if this is food, what are those things on the other table?" The group quickly conclude that these are the treats, the feel-good gulps, uppers, stimulants, or comforters. They are what we turn to for a lift, a boost, or simply to indulge and wallow in serotonin and dopamine-induced pleasure for a few fleeting moments. They are the fix, and until you can stop thinking about CRAP as food and recognise it as a recreational drug, then it is my guess that you will always struggle with your weight. They are the fix, but they are not food. Don't ever confuse the two, and don't allow yourself to think of them as food. They are edible substances that we use and abuse. The purpose of this workshop, of course, is to help people to see things in a different way, to consider these deleterious edible products as substances (and, like all substances, they can be, and often are, abused). If you can disassociate these ultra-processed materials from food, you can in fact think differently about them and in turn behave differently around them. People have in the past accused me of demonising food, but my answer is always the same. "I never demonise food, I love food!" My final message to my clients: try to eat more food. I hope this has given you food for thought.

Cage the Pig

In his book *Never Binge Again*[293] Glenn Livingston PhD. adopts a novel approach to overcoming your 'fat thinking alter ego', enabling a return to control from overeating. At first, it seems a little crazy and the book does require an open mind. However, as you read on, this entertaining and empowering book makes it plain to see how such an approach (which is logical) will work if people adopt and embrace the way of thinking that he proposes.

Dr Livingston considers that the negative thought process of 'fat thinkers' is underpinning destructive feeding behaviour, and that the accompanying doubt and low self-esteem are the drivers of such overeating behaviours. He suggests that identifying and caging your fat-thinking self is the start of recovery and of reprogramming how we think about food and nourishment. He refers to this alter ego as 'the Pig', and the first thing you must know is that the Pig is not you. You have dreams and aspirations, but the Pig lives only to binge; it will say whatever it can to get you to feed it!

Thankfully, says Dr Livingston, "You are the only one that can feed it!" If you learn to ignore its squeals, you are well on your way to overcoming your eating difficulties. By reframing the urges to binge as the clamours of the demanding Pig and not yourself, this conceptual framework allows you to separate your own real thoughts from the cravings. You are in control; the Pig exists because you say it does, and you give credence to its thoughts and wants.

Never Binge Again insists upon strict food and eating rules that you create. Dr Livingston is crystal clear that you must own these rules 100%, and you must stick to them. They must be clear and unambiguous (the Pig loves ambiguity). Livingston puts it like this: "The question isn't whether you will have freedom of choice vs becoming enslaved to a food plan. The question is, will you choose to live your life as a slave to the Pig's impulses and demands, or put the animal in its cage so you can exercise your human freedom?"

I agree with Dr Livingston 100%. For people with serious binge-eating disorders, if they think that the latest new diet or a few minor modifications to their existing diet will help, or hope that perhaps simply the passage of time will put their weight into decline, then sadly they are wishing on a star. For most people with this type of disordered eating, over time, things will only get worse, unless they can find something that works for them.

Personally, I'm very inclined to pay credence to a man that was formerly obese and has self-overcome his own eating failures, and someone that, with hindsight, has the confidence and integrity to admit that his own earlier work was wrong, in the light of his enhanced understanding. This book is worth a try for anyone that eats compulsively.

Emotional eating

Stress and other negative emotions, such as depression and anxiety, can lead to increased food intake through emotional eating (EE), which is particularly associated with weight gain in women[294]. EE is a maladaptive coping strategy to ease negative emotions or to fill an emotional void, rather than to satisfy hunger. It involves changing normal or appetite-based eating by altering food choices, typically substituting healthy foods for unhealthy options, and increasing the volume or frequency of consumption. The purpose is to regulate emotions and to make oneself feel better or to meet emotional needs by regularly activating the dopamine and serotonin release that 'treat' foods elicit. Clearly, EE doesn't fix emotional problems, moreover it often leads to its own considerable psychological and physical dilemmas. A feature of EE is that it leads to poorer dietary choices and an expanded waist circumference.

A 2022 study found that people classified as an 'emotional or very-emotional eater' were significantly less likely to be categorised in the 'healthy dietary pattern' of eating, which included regular consumption of fruits, vegetables, olive oil, oilseeds, legumes, fish and seafood. Instead, their diet was of the 'snacks and fast food' kind, which favoured sweet bread, breakfast cereal, corn, potato, desserts, sweets, sugar and fast food. Consequently, emotional eaters have significantly lower fibre intake, folic acid, magnesium, potassium, vitamin B1, and vitamin C, and higher sodium, lipids, and saturated fats[295]. Could it be that this malnourishment is contributing to, or even causing, the mental health and emotional difficulties associated with EE?

Life is often upsetting, but if, each time we become upset (which is inevitable unless you've had a frontal lobotomy), you turn to drink, or CRAP, or stimulants, or relaxants, or become angry or violent, then you will only make matters worse. EE is a problem for many people, and the addictive aspect of CRAP makes it very difficult to disengage from once the pattern of stress → negative emotions → self-medication, emerges. It is not news to anyone that this way of handling emotions does not solve matters, instead, over time, it deepens the relationship between the stressed state and the maladaptive behaviour of using CRAP to self-medicate. But, as you are aware, knowing what to do only loosely correlates with behaviour change. Assuming you don't want things to deteriorate when you are already dealing with a challenging situation, then learning to manage upsetting emotions without using substances to soothe the self is an important part of the tricky balancing act of life.

In an emotionally charged situation, the best thing to do is to stay calm (easier said than done), and, as you know this to be true, you just need figure out how best to go about it in a way that will be effective for your own personality and psychological characteristics. When challenged by acutely stressful events, I remind myself that if I can find thirty seconds, I've got a reasonable chance of successfully traversing the pass without saying or doing something I'll later regret. If feasible, I close my eyes, feel the breath (ten seconds), find the calm (ten seconds), use the strength (ten seconds). Now I feel I've wrestled the control back from my delinquent emotions and I'm better placed to make rational decisions and avoid impulsive actions. If successful, after the event, I give myself credit for staying in control, and acknowledge what is a considerable act of personal growth and development. It doesn't always work and sometimes I respond angrily, which, by way of a solution, I guess is the verbal equivalent of guzzling a bag of doughnuts and a bottle of cola.

Mindfulness

During weight loss, hunger is never far from the door. As you start to lose weight, the natural response of the body will be to increase your appetite. If you are not expecting this, you will be caught off guard and typically start to blame yourself for being weak, greedy etc. Therefore, strategies should be in place to ensure you can deal effectively with this. Delay and distraction tactics are good ways to combat cravings, which, like all feelings, come and go (as you will be aware). When cravings start to arise, the best thing to do is to keep a daily log. Keep a note of what it is you are craving, rating the crave on a scale of 1-10, and noting your distraction action (be sure to have a few different plans for this).

Simply knowing that cravings are transient and will in time pass is important, but probably not enough in isolation. Exploring and understanding such feelings when they land, and gaining greater insight into how they make you feel, is an important first step in taking control over the previously automatic response of satisfying your craving. Our stress-fuelled, time-challenged, information-overloaded lives are not conducive to mindfulness, rather they are more aligned to that of mindlessness. Using strategies that can help us to unleash the power of our minds and learn to channel our energy into our positive plans and aspirations, can only add value to our lives. Mindfulness and meditation-based exercises are potent tools in helping us to achieve our goals.

'Surfing the urge' is a mindfulness technique allowing us to observe cravings and develop mindful control. Urge surfing is helpful against damaging, spontaneous actions that occur resulting from a crave or an urge. This could include snacking, impulse purchases or even flying off the handle with someone. Mindfulness techniques are often linked to breathing, because breath is the life force – inhalation brings oxygen and exhalation removes waste. By focusing on breathing, we can bring the power of the mind and body to bear, calm ourselves and resolve internal conflict, by bringing the mind back to the breath.

Urges (cravings) behave like waves, rising, cresting, and petering out; they will almost always pass (usually within twenty or thirty minutes). When urges crest, it can feel like they are overwhelming and that they will never go away, but this is wrong. The idea is not to 'feed' the urge by fighting it, being afraid of it, dwelling on it, trying to suppress it, or, of course, by giving in to it. Positive distraction may work and that may be the first thing to try, but if that does not work, urge surfing may be the answer.

Mindfulness posits that you can't forcefully rid your mind of an urge, but you can 'embrace' it and ride it out. Cravings and urges are uncomfortable and distracting, but by centring on them, you can experience them in a different way, so their discomfort and power can be controlled. For this, we must adopt an enquiring and curious mindset towards the urge, observe it with interest, and resist the temptation of going into battle with it.

Here is one technique for urge surfing (but there are others). I hope that you will find this effective, and if so, I would suggest you consider learning more about mindfulness to help you achieve your weight loss and other life ambitions. Before you have a go at this, please be aware that many people find this a crazy notion, or even a little bit silly. I would just say to that, mindfulness is one of the most helpful thinking tools I have come across for aiding us to overcome the idiosyncrasies of the mind. So, if you are experiencing an urge:

1. When you first notice it, focus on the physical feeling of the urge. Where is it in your body? How would you describe it? Is it in more than one place? What does it feel like? Really delve deep into your resources to answer these questions.

2. On a scale of 1-10, how strong is it? Try to periodically evaluate this and note it.

3. Now clear your mind and bring your attention to your breathing. Don't alter your breathing but concentrate on the gentle inhalations and exhalations. Allow your shoulders and neck to relax, and empty your mind. Now, think about everything that you can feel (your feet on the floor, legs on the chair, clothes on your body and so on). Be in the present and simply be aware of your breathing from moment to moment. Be aware of thoughts and emotions, try to think about them without trying to change them. Do this for a couple of minutes.

4. Slowly move your attention back to the urge and think in as much detail as you can about the sensation. Can you add anything to your initial description? Is it any clearer? What is the current strength rating (1-10)? Has it crested yet?

5. Use your curiosity to examine any changes to the sensations over time and don't be afraid that the urge won't pass or that your focus on it will make it stronger – it won't. Your attention is on the examination and understanding of what it is, this is the exploration of an urge.

6. If the urge starts to become overwhelming, then turn all your attention back to your breathing. Focus on the calm that this brings and the energy it gives. Continue until you feel more strength and control.

7. After a couple of minutes, revert to the urge. Rate its strength and note any changes in sensation. If it is still rising or cresting, you can use the 'surf' metaphor to Ride the Wave. Your breathing is the surfboard, and your ability to apply mindfulness is your skill as the surfer. No wave is infinite and even the mightiest waves must eventually kneel before the master surfer.

Rather than waiting for an urge to come along (and then start scrabbling for this book), you can practice urge surfing based upon your memory of and understanding of past craves using this technique. Think about an urge that you recently experienced and imagine the sensations that occurred at the time. Can you remember how these sensations altered over the brief time the urge was with you? Try to recreate it and use your breathing to help to centre yourself, to be calm and to ride out the wave. Practice this a few times before a real crave ambushes you while you are defenceless.

If you are caught off guard, close your eyes and resort to the control summary: **Feel the breath, find the calm, use the strength.**

Mindful eating (ME) has also been shown to reduce body image dissatisfaction, abnormal eating patterns and emotional eating among people with weight difficulties. ME stems from the philosophy of mindfulness, and like mindfulness in general, ME brings into focus thoughts and physical sensations in the now, thereby bringing enjoyment and enhanced awareness to foods through emotional and sensational experiences. ME builds gratitude and appreciation of food, which is a core belief required to move to a higher nutritional level, thus respecting the food and the body simultaneously.

ME has been described[495] as non-judgemental awareness of internal and external cues influencing the desire to eat, our food choices, the quantity we consume, and the manner in which we consume it. Mindful eaters make food choices that bring maximum benefits to oneself, while minimising harm to others and the environment, and, through awareness, mindful eaters can not only improve their own health, but also contribute towards planetary sustainability. ME, if used regularly, will reduce consumption of CRAP, total energy and fat intake[296]. To learn more about mindful eating, visit www.thecenterformindfuleating.org

Planning for dietary emergencies

It is inevitable that, sooner or later, you'll end up in an overwhelming situation where your coping strategies don't work, at which point you will need an emergency action plan, which can be a simple matter of contacting a trusted friend. Being aware of the risks and alive to the warning signs such as:

1. Recognising familiar trigger patterns (people, places or things) – stop and evaluate.

2. Emotions are running low – act early, think differently.

3. Thoughts turning to lapse or relapse – feel the breath, find the calm, use the strength.

4. Cajoling or pressure from others to partake (in a binge) – use 'No' responses.

5. Thoughts and plans flicker towards buying or eating CRAP – very high risk, try to share this burden with someone and remember, you can choose never to go down that path.

Emergency action plan

1. Someone to call, close friend or relative ("Hi, I just need some motivational support…)

2. Getting out – if possible, leave the situation and walk for ten or twenty minutes. Breathe and give yourself time to make a plan.

3. Do both – walk and talk.

The skill of saying no

The ability to refuse an offer of CRAP may be the single most important interpersonal skill in relapse prevention. You should practice this, going over in your mind a variety of different situations – you will always encounter pushers and peddlers. Vague or apologetic answers are ineffective, and you should imagine what you would say to family and friends in similar circumstances:

Bill: "Hi, Bob, how about joining me, Frank, and the boys from the rugby club for the all-you-can-eat Korean BBQ on Wednesday?"

You:	*ineffective:*	"Oh, I'd love to, but I think I will be working late on Wednesday."
You:	*effective:*	"No, thanks, I don't need an all-you-can-eat, but you boys enjoy it."
Sheila:		Hi, Grace, we are having cream tea on Thursday afternoon. Can you join us?
You:	*ineffective:*	"Sorry, Sheila, I'm trying to be really good. Maybe next time."
You:	*effective:*	"No thanks, Sheila, but would you like to meet for a dog walk later in the week?"

By using a strong and concise response you will hear yourself rejecting these foods, which is very empowering. Note how the effective statements start with the word 'No'.

Expanding social support

Loneliness and boredom can be relieved by the social aspects of eating (and drinking), and this is a big risk that can lead to relapse. Therefore, the development of a wide social network that centres around activities and interests that don't involve eating can reduce the chance of relapse. Regular contact with friends and family and the informal support of social connections are important to avoid loneliness and boredom and to maintain a positive outlook. Being aware of the value of avoiding social situations where there is a focus on CRAP, or inappropriate food consumption, goes without saying.

Delay discounting

There is an interesting phenomenon known as delay discounting (DD), which states that, given the choice, we normally favour smaller rewards now, compared to larger ones down the line. I'll take £20 now rather than £60 in a year's time. I'd prefer two biscuits now instead of four tomorrow. In other words, we discount the value of delayed rewards against things we can get our hands on right now.

DD postulates that it is our proximity to the benefit or consequence that determines the value we assign to it. Also known as 'Time Preference' (immediate rewards are preferred to delayed rewards), it shares a significant relationship with being overweight. A study has shown that individuals with a low weight also have low time preferences (that is, they are willing to wait for delayed rewards), and are therefore more likely to invest in activities in a bid to reap future health benefits. This contrasts with people with higher BMIs, who, the study says, are more inclined to seek immediate rewards and discount any benefits further down the line[297]. The big problem is, delay discounting skews lifestyle judgements and scuppers our best intentions to make healthy choices, leading to actions that do not align with our plans.

Because food loaded with fats and sugars have such a powerful hedonic impact, setting out to swerve them invariably involves delaying gratification, the naughty but nice foods offer pleasure now at the expense of long-term costs or harm down the line ("I know that is not good for me, but the consequences are so far away I've discounted the risk"). DD also works on discounting the value of beneficial effects. "I know a healthy diet now can help me to avoid cancer in years to come, but it just seems so far away, and anyway it probably won't happen to me." This notion, that because it is a long way away, its value is less, is the central but false principle of delay discounting. We ought to consider healthy lifestyles as the equivalent of an instant-access, high-interest bank account. The benefits accrue instantly (you feel better straight away) and compound over the years to build the best defence against disease and decay over a lifetime.

Delay discounting is commonly associated with risky behaviours and is most evident in younger people. The problem is that repeatedly applying the DD rule (taking gratification now and discounting future health consequences) becomes habitual. Therefore, it is important to consider and value the concept of 'compounded health interest', which is the theoretical opposite of delay discounting. Nothing can guarantee health, but continually banking good choices gives us the best possible chance.

The boffins of behavioural economics are hoping to identify behavioural profiles such as those inclined to delay discount, and they suggest that this will help to predict unhealthy activities in some people, so that they can be intercepted before any damage is done. However, while I can see the theory behind this, I'm not sure of the practical application. I can picture the scene though:

Therapist:	"Mr Jones, our questionnaire has identified that you have a risky behavioural phenotype and have difficulty in making choices that support future health, instead, favouring immediate rewards. I think a course of cognitive behavioural therapy would help?"
Mr Jones:	"How long will that take?"
Therapist:	"There's a nine-month waiting list, and then, if you are invited, it involves a three-month course of treatment, once each week for one hour."
Mr Jones:	"Leave that with me!"

The Stockdale paradox

The Stockdale paradox emerged from Jim Collin's book *Good to Great,* a corporate success and leadership book[298]. It is based upon James Stockdale, a high-ranking naval officer who was captured and held as a Vietnamese prisoner of war for more than seven years. Stockdale was repeatedly tortured, and many of his fellow prisoners died. He had little reason to believe he would survive, but somehow he managed to find a balance between the grim reality of his situation and a cast-iron optimism for a good outcome. This formula, it transpires, proved to be his salvation. Stockdale's ordeal epitomises both the importance and the difficulty of striking a balance between realism and optimism, hence the paradox. It describes how to achieve success and overcome difficult obstacles in a way that transcends mere unbridled optimism.

What Stockdale learned is that you need unwavering faith to prevail, while simultaneously having the discipline to confront the most brutal facts of your current reality. Stockdale describes how optimism alone fails. He tells how, many of his fallen comrades expected to get out each year, and when they didn't, it broke their hearts and they died. Stockdale's tricky balancing act involved positive visualisation and absolute faith in achieving success, offset against the notion that, to realise this, he must prevail over the most difficult of circumstances every single day. Stockdale said: "It's not about choosing which side to take, but instead learning to embrace both opposing feelings and realise they're necessary and interconnected".

For those not facing death in a Vietnamese POW camp, what does this tell us? Well, for a start, blind optimism in isolation is futile, but if, at the same time, you don't have absolute faith in reaching your destination, you probably won't make it. You must reconcile this faith and determination against the practical hurdles that you know you must overcome each and every day. Keep your eye firmly fixed on the goal but be brutally realistic about the daily hurdles that you must overcome if you are to succeed. Make sure you know exactly what these hurdles are (refer to Insight 2). However, unlike Stockdale, when you escape the shackles of your weight, your journey and your labour will continue.

Freud

It would be remiss of me to speak of behaviour without referring to the work of Sigmund Freud and his development of the field of psychoanalysis. Aside from his astonishing revelations, his greatest achievement was that he taught us to think about thinking. If you are hoping to make changes to your choices, decisions and behaviours, then thinking about how you think, and understanding how your mind works, will be central to your success, because only through thought can we change our behavioural trajectory.

Freud's ideas have evolved into a collection of theories and therapeutic methods that seek healthy development and growth in troubled people. The principle of his work, which he termed psychoanalysis, is that our early experiences contribute to the formation of our current sense of self, and that we all harbour unconscious thoughts, feelings, desires and memories (especially painful or traumatic memories and unwanted thoughts) from our past. Freud taught us that the mind works hard to keep these difficult memories out of our awareness to avoid the pain and trauma that they evoke. The aim of treatment is to 'release' repressed emotions and experiences so that they can be dealt with, rendering the person free to move on in whatever direction they choose.

Perhaps Freud's most enduring and important idea was that the human mind has two competing combatants and one mediator. Freud's personality theory, written in his famous book in 1923, The ego and the Id[299], set out that the psyche is made up of three distinct elements: the id, ego and superego, each developing at a different life stage. According to Freud, the id represents the primitive instinct of the mind that seeks only things that feel good. The superego operates as a moral conscience, seeking to steer the ship in accordance with socially acceptable rules. And the ego is the umpire. They each have unique features but interact to form a whole, and together they determine an individual's personality and behaviour.

The id

The id is part of the unconscious mind that contains urges, desires and impulses, its processes are illogical and irrational. It is chaotic, selfish and unreasonable, and considers that all of its needs must be met immediately, regardless of the consequences – if it feels good, do it above all else. Freud called this the pleasure principle. A new-born child's personality is all id (the id makes sure we get what we need), the ego and superego are not formed until the child is much older. The id is thus infantile, it is not affected by reality or logic and does not learn or change, it will always be this way because it is detached from the external world and cannot develop through learned experiences. The id is what we must learn to manage if we are to grow and develop and have a balanced and healthy life.

The ego

The ego resides in the conscious mind, and it is probably the closest thing to what you think of when you think of 'yourself'. The ego forms the decision-making part of our personality, and unlike the id, it is rational and logical. The ego's role is to help control the needs and urges of the id by avoiding impulsivity (grabbing food off someone else's plate because the id demands to eat). The ego applies the reality aspect of reasoning, it knows that the desires of the id must be satisfied and aims to find a way to do this that is both socially appropriate and within the 'rules'. Using rationality, compromise, or delaying gratification, the ego seeks a solution. It is the mediator between the selfish uncompromising id and the moral requirements of society and the demands of the real world. The ego is conscious and weak, whereas the id is deep in the subconscious and very strong. Freud said that the ego is "like a man on horseback, who has to hold in check the superior strength of the horse."

When the ego fails to control the id, this creates anxiety and engenders the classic feeling of loss of control. At this, the conscious ego responds with problem-solving cognitions, if the first plan does not work, it is re-computed until a solution is found. This is known in psychology as reality testing, to exert conscious control over the id. An important feature of behaviour-change approaches is to enhance ego functioning by developing insight and learning to explore options. If the ego cannot control the id, chaos will prevail.

The superego

According to Freud, the superego develops around the age of four, through learning about rules and acceptable ways of behaving. Portrayed as the guardian of morality, it uses 'codes of conduct', prohibitions and 'don't' statements to guide us by trying to convince the ego to do the right thing. The superego can oversee feelings of pride and satisfaction following virtuous actions, but also administers punishments by way of feelings of shame and guilt when the id takes over and our behaviour errs. The superego strives to pursue perfection using the conscience and the ideal self. The conscience, or our 'inner voice', notifies us that we have transgressed and punishes us through feelings of guilt, theoretically guiding us to avoid repeat offences. The ideal self is the person that you feel you ought to be and how you should behave, based upon everything that you have experienced up to this point. If this were a cartoon, the id would be the devil on one shoulder, and the superego would be the angel on the other.

Psychoanalytic therapy

Guilt and shame are central to superego. But it is not healthy to wallow in guilt, and we therefore have defence mechanisms to protect ourselves. These are unconscious psychological strategies used to avoid excessive anxiety arising from guilt and shame. One defence is for our subconscious to distort reality so that our conscious mind is better able to cope with a situation (remember the Eye Mouth Gap). Freud's approach was to resolve unconscious conflict from the past between the id and the superego, by bringing these distortions into the conscious mind for resolution. Thus, make the unconscious conscious, whereupon internal conflicts can be resolved. To Freud, the unconscious is a vault where difficulties that we'd rather not face are locked away. But as we all know, ignoring emotional problems seldom resolves them; they tend to fester and, rather than go away, they gnaw away, resulting in lasting conflict and turmoil. Freud knew that awareness is the first step in the cycle of change, and without it there can be no liberation from the struggle within.

The pain-pleasure principle

Freud proposed the pain-pleasure principle, which states that people make choices to avoid pain and increase pleasure, and this is at the core of all the decisions we make. The id rules exclusively by applying the pleasure principle, but seeking pleasure (instant gratification) may conflict with our ultimate goals. Take eating comfort foods, watching hours of Netflix or expensive bouts of retail therapy. Part of development is that the ego learns to wait and to endure the pain of deferred gratification, and thus, over time, Freud argued that "an ego thus educated has become 'reasonable'". The ego now obeys the reality principle, which also seeks pleasure and avoids pain, but takes account of the consequences of our actions in a real situation.

Strengthening the ego

Practising techniques that build and strengthen the ego helps the conscious mind to overcome the demanding id, but ego strength requires ongoing effort and dedication. Anything that develops insight, increases the power of the ego, and learning and self-reflection are important aspects of ego-strengthening. Think about the things that you do every day that require praise and self-recognition. Give yourself credit and acknowledge your achievements for routine good choices. Save your best praise for when you overcome lapses, even if you didn't get back on track immediately, the fact that you got back on track is the main thing.

Accept that you have unhelpful thoughts and behaviours just like everyone does. It's about working to change these thoughts, which can be done, and one way to practice this is to develop the use of affirmations and positive self-talk. These are confidence statements that challenge and aim to overcome self-defeating or negative thoughts. A positive mindset is a key ally when losing weight, as negative mood regularly triggers overeating in those trying to eat well. Now would be a good time to write down some of your own affirmations in your book, and practice saying them to yourself. You must truly believe them and believe in the power they will bring to your ego. Here are some examples to help you to get started:

- Today I will make a positive difference to my wellbeing.
- I am worthy of health, wellness and happiness.
- I believe in myself.
- I know I have power, and with this anything is possible.

- I am so grateful for all the good things that I have in my life.

- Today I choose success.

We can also strengthen the ego by challenging or testing our thoughts and beliefs. One way of doing this is by inviting opposing points of view and new experiences into your mind and openly considering their validity. This develops mental flexibility and resilience that fosters rational logical thinking, conversely, rigid, closed minds encourage irrational and illogical reasoning. Think of something that may clash with your current beliefs and bring it into the court of personal opinion. Imagine you are the judge; you must remain entirely impartial and keep an open mind to all opinions expressed. Here are a couple of opinion-dividing scenarios that you could use to practice on:

- People that leave our shores and are convicted of terrorism charges overseas should have their citizenship removed, irrespective of how old they were at the time they went.

- Elon Musk should focus his billions on fixing Earth rather than trying to set up a human colony on Mars.

Stuck in a rut?

Cognitive neuroscience (the study of how we think) has recently shown that we are much more motivated to avoid threats than to seek pleasure – the brain's main goal is survival. Why is it, then, that we take the pleasure of the cream cake over the threat of furred-up arteries? Doubtless, delay discounting is involved, because if a cream cake instantaneously furred up our arteries, leaving us clutching our chests and grappling for our mobiles, then we wouldn't eat them. And of course, this wouldn't happen from eating one cream cake, and so we also apply the drop in the ocean concept.

The answer to why we get stuck in decisional ruts, in part appears to be that, without intervention, our subconscious brains draw upon the same 'fixed' data from our memories and experiences to draw its conclusions: "the last cream cake didn't kill me, but it did make me feel good!" Where the data remains the same, and the computer is the same, the results will always be the same – "Could I have jam with that cream cake today, please?"

Only now do I understand something that totally mystified me thirty-five years ago while providing phase 4 cardiac rehabilitation for clients from St George's hospital, which was on the doorstep of Tooting Leisure Centre where I was working. Many of our clients were recovering from heart attacks, caused in many cases by a lifetime of smoking. Regularly, I'd look out of the window following a group-exercise programme and observe one of my hapless clients lighting up a Benson & Hedges the minute they walked out of the door. Why on Earth do they do that? I would think.

Putting the addictive element of nicotine to one side, I'm guessing my clients had no idea that their id was still demanding the pleasure of nicotine while their superego was trying to convince the ego of the folly of such actions. Their ego was drawing upon all previous data and experiences, and, despite the new data (the recent myocardial infarction), was reaching the same conclusion – the id wins, and the cigarette will be lit. I don't think for a moment the rational mind concluded: "I value the pleasure of a cigarette over the risk of a further (probably fatal) heart attack". But I now realise that my clients probably knew nothing of Freud and his theories about how the mind works, and subsequently I can only imagine they probably thought something along the lines of:

> "I know, I know, I shouldn't be smoking but I've always been poor at making choices. I don't know why I never seem to be able to do the right thing."

From all of this, we can see that a person's behaviour is primarily driven by their unconscious urges balanced in part by the view of the self, as the conscious mind tries to steer the bus down a route that is both socially acceptable, avoids pain and adheres to the principle of self-preservation. In the middle is the referee (the ego) that makes the call. Freud states that our personalities ultimately are shaped because of these struggles between the id and the superego, and emotional and psychological problems such as depression and anxiety are often rooted in conflicts between the conscious and unconscious mind.

Self-evaluation

You may never have considered 'locus of evaluation' as a concept central to how you think about yourself. Basically, it refers to where you draw your reference points from when making judgements about yourself, and for that matter, for assessing what is right and what is wrong. The two primary options being mainly internal or mainly external signals, to get your cues from. Those with internal locus judge the world and themselves based on their feelings, emotions, instincts and personal beliefs, this is the self-anchor that represents who you believe you are. People with an external locus of evaluation too often judge themselves according to the views of others – in this case, the onslaught of judgemental experts, eager to exert their (irrelevant) points of view upon us. Accepting these external signals diminishes any value we have in our own self-evaluation and will quickly erode or override any positive self-values that we may hold.

We all like to receive praise and recognition; it makes us feel good. All our efforts to conform and to be accepted are rewarded, the respect shown to us increases, and our stock worth in society elevates. Intoxicated by this heady mix of praise and our perception of social attitude, it is forgivable to see why some people believe that courting the approval of others is a worthwhile activity. If, however, we give praise and positive endorsements from others excessive importance and authority, we risk moving the needle too far away from making our own internal evaluations of our worth. All very well when the external feedback is positive, however, this only renders the unavoidable negative comments more crushing when they finally land. The accompanying sense of worthlessness brought on by external rejection and disapproval is internalised and reinforced, leading in time to an alignment with the destructive views of others. Focusing on external praise or criticism leads to false beliefs about ourselves, distorting the reality of who we really are.

Because our behaviour reflects how we feel and think about ourselves, any negative self-beliefs that we hold will inevitably lead to behaviours that validate these views (I'm hopeless, I can never get things right, I'm a lost cause!), which in turn authenticates the external disapproval, and so things go from bad to worse. "I told you he was a basket case, just look at him now!" This acceptance of others' opinions about us often starts at an early age and is evident in adolescents and young people who constantly meet with the condemnation of surrounding adults: "Everyone thinks I'm useless, and so I must be. Well, if they think I'm delinquent, then let me show them how right they are!" Furthermore, the ubiquitous presence of social media, with its integral skulking trolls and keyboard warriors, ensures an endless panel of judgemental experts, ever-present to criticise and demean our efforts and intentions. For those trapped in the toxic web of external validation, now more than ever is a time for re-evaluation and reorientation.

Carl Rogers[300], founder of this theory, believed that much unhappiness and inner conflict is a result of abandoning our own perceptions and judging ourselves by the standards of others. His work made it clear that your prospects for happiness and contentment are significantly greater if you can find your values from within. Understanding what we believe about ourselves and why, and where these beliefs come from, will also give a sense of rationale for our actions, and thus provide a platform for change.

On a similar theme, be mindful of the theory of suggestibility. Some of what you consider true is based upon make-believe, fabricated by another person to suit their own ends. The principle of suggestibility holds true in us all, to a greater or lesser degree. That is, we are all inclined at some level to accept and base our behaviours on the suggestions or ideas of others, without fully researching or verifying the authenticity of such propositions. "That's not me!" I hear you say, but it is, it's all of us! If a new idea is forcefully or repeatedly imposed upon us, it can stick and distort our views and alter our memories, or fill in missing sections of our recollections, leaving us with an overall impression that can be a long way from the truth. People with heightened emotional states are thought to be more receptive to suggestibility, as, of course, are children. Suggestibility does have a purpose and must have contributed to our success, probably social cohesion, or something along those lines.

For people at the higher end of the suggestibility scale, it is problematic, as navigating complex mazes (such as maintaining a healthy weight in a world that promotes weight gain) can be tricky if your head is full of ideas that suit other people's agendas. This could be disingenuous advertising from a company eager to sell their food, or online influencers and health gurus clamouring for more followers, or simply some whacko down the street peddling their bonkers idea. But I remember fifty years ago at school, in the early stages of the computer, we had a presentation: 'Garbage in, garbage out'. The central message of this was that sloppily programmed inputs inevitably lead to incorrect outputs. To be successful in your quest for a healthy and balanced life, you must have credible information and clarity of thought. Test information thoroughly (check your inputs) and consider your own level of suggestibility.

Free will and conscious control

Do you believe in free will? How would you feel if I told you that free will is an illusion invented to comfort ourselves? Also, if you're upset about this idea, well, that's just too bad, as being upset is not for you to choose either! It may well be that we don't make free choices at all, we just respond to our feelings and desires, which, as I've just stated, we can't choose either. As our actions (responses) are based upon how we feel, and we can't choose how we feel, then it is illogical to believe that we can choose our actions.

So, what does determine our actions? Well, it seems that our actions are the result of our individual genetic makeup (shaped by evolution and chance mutations), alongside a lifetime of entirely individual environmental, social and emotional interactions and intelligent learning. Therefore, if an entity knew all that there was to know about you, it could predict your actions in any situation. If actions are therefore predictable, how can they be at the whim of our will?

This is the theory of determinism, which is the philosophical doctrine that all events, including human actions, are causally inevitable, meaning that, when a person decides or performs an action, it is impossible that he or she could have made any other decision or performed any other action. A deterministic model will thus always produce the same output (event, thought or action) from a given starting condition or initial state, making determinism incompatible with free will.

Consider the most powerful quantum computer in the world, running the most advanced and complex algorithm ever written. Its function, to determine the weather. It sucks in all the vast amounts of data available to it and runs its sequence. The outcome: the computer urges us to dash out and invest in an umbrella. How is this any different to your own onboard computer and the algorithms that it runs, computing all the data available to it, on all the decisions that you face each day? For instance, consider the impact of animal farming on climate change. Let's say your computer gathers all the data available to it, crunches the numbers and translates this into inner feelings of despair and sorrow, that your conscious mind interprets as a desire to want to eat less meat. You would say that you chose by your own free will to eat less meat, but did you? Did the weather computer choose by its own free will to tell us to buy umbrellas?

If that is determinism, what's fatalism?

Fatalists believe that we have only one true and inevitable 'fate'; a destiny that we cannot escape. We may take whatever twists and turns along the journey that we want, we can make whichever decisions and choices that we care to, but we cannot avoid our eventual fate, which is out of our control. What decides this fate depends upon the brand of fatalism that you subscribe to, for instance many religions require you to believe that your fate resides only in the hands of your God.

Fatalism tends to focus on final events rather than the steps that lead to them. "I was never going to get that job, no matter what I did." "It was always the case that I would get diabetes." It is clear to see how a belief in fatalism can lead to feelings of hopelessness and resignation, as fatalists believe they can't do anything to change their situation or 'fate'. However, fatalism tells us that we can choose our own path (even if we don't know our final destiny) and it is important to distinguish between fatalistic beliefs and things that are genuinely within, or out of your control. Consider the question:

> "I know the planet is heating up, and during my children's lifetime, I worry that the world will become an inhospitable furnace. Is this our fate and are we powerless to stop it?"

We can never know our fate until death is almost upon us (and even then, it's guesswork as to what happens next), but how you view fatalism will decide how you answer this question. You may believe that all the ingenuity and resourcefulness of mankind could be enough to avert disaster if only we applied ourselves. In this case, you are likely to modify your behaviour such as adopting a better diet, less consumerism, conserving energy and being better at recycling. If, however, you believe it doesn't matter what we do, as our fate is sealed, you could use this as a reason to continue over-consuming the resources of the planet with gay abandon.

Because our ultimate fate is unknown (and determinists will say already determined), it is far from certain that any efforts to avert disaster can affect the outcome, so you could say, why bother? But the key point here is that you will probably already have made a choice, conscious or otherwise (to recycle or not) and you can continue to make new choices. These choices will undeniably have an impact on the outcome (albeit small) even though we don't know what that outcome will be. In this way, I guess I'm a little fatalistic myself, as I accept what will be, will be. But I include a tiny caveat – depending upon how all of humanity reacts!

It's kind of chicken and egg stuff, but I suppose it all comes down to taking the decisions that you think will give you the best chance of a favourable outcome (which you may decide is enjoying life to the max because – que sera). But I prefer to look to the wisdom of the East, and as they say: "Have faith in Allah, but always tether your camel!"

To take control or to not, that is the question

So why am I blithering on about all of this and what on Earth does it have to do with your weight? Well, in short, this could very well be the elephant in the pantry. In terms of life choices, if you want to do something (let's say, lose weight or change your eating habits) and you know what to do, and how to do it, and you have the necessary resources to achieve it, but all of this is insufficient for you to realise your wants, then something else must be controlling your actions and preventing you from doing what you want to do. As I see it, this is the essence of the behavioural sciences.

If this is the case, then you have no option other than to figure out what it is that is forcing you down route 'A' when you would prefer to go down route 'B'. If you can successfully think this through to its logical conclusion, then you will have taken the first and most important step towards taking the control that you desire, and only once you have done this, can you start to investigate your options for change. With respect to the theories of fatalism and determinism, theoretically, they both allow you to set and achieve your own goals, in fact you were always meant to. I was always meant to write this book, and you were always going to read it.

Visualise a situation where you could use the unimaginable power of your own mind to learn something new and to find a way to accomplish all your goals. Now imagine that the entity that knew all about you assessed you both before and after this 'enlightenment'. Surely it would conclude that your prior course (for example, weight gain) would be route 'A', but following your enhanced knowledge and understanding, you will now go down route 'B' (weight loss). The learning experience predicted your change of course, not any decision that you made. The entity would also say that, following this enlightenment, you could take no other possible course other than route 'B', the path to a healthier future. Therefore, it is learning and enlightenment that changes outcomes, not decisions.

What if I still can't change?

If, however, you find that, following considerable thinking, soul-searching and deep contemplation, you still have no idea why you find it impossible to take control of your actions, then you have only a few limited options available. It's worth mentioning at this point that some people will reach the conclusion that, "I'd like to change, but I'm too weak!" This is inadequate as an answer. It's rather like taking your car to the garage with a fault, and after a thorough diagnostic, the mechanic says to you, I'm sorry but your car is broken, and that's all I know. I doubt you would accept this from him, and, in the same way, you mustn't accept that you are too weak, as that is not true, you just haven't given it sufficient contemplation.

If you are still oblivious as to why you can't control your own actions, you could engage with a psychotherapist who would help you to make this link, and together you could explore new ways of thinking. This could help you to break free from your dilemma, or at the very least could help you to find ways to cope and feel better about your situation.

Alternatively, you could choose to buy fully into the idea of fatalism and determinism and alter your psyche accordingly. Forgive yourself for any previous torment you may have inflicted upon yourself regarding perceived transgressions, choices and beliefs, and live in contentment knowing that this is your chosen life course (albeit chosen by a force other than yourself). Embrace your life and rejoice in the beauty and meaning of your life and all that is around you. Banish the worry and anguish that your weight (or whatever) has previously caused you, and seek to find balance and happiness in the way of life that has been bestowed upon you, and that you have 'chosen' to accept.

It may or may not be true, nonetheless it comforts me to believe that we do have control over our lives, although each of us will command a unique level of control. Choosing our preferred path will be considerably more attainable if we have been fortunate enough to have acquired the necessary fundamentals during childhood. Specifically, a loving, supportive upbringing that has nourished us physically, educationally, emotionally, spiritually, and, of course, nutritionally. Without these foundations, things will be much harder (but never impossible). In fact, it is worth noting that, even for those gifted with these reserves, things still do go awry, and so there can be no guarantees of success, irrespective of privileges. But if there are shortcomings in this formative nourishment, then optimum growth and development will be elusive, and so any insufficiencies in these areas must first be rectified. Take a little time to review your own circumstances with respect to the five pillars of nourishment mentioned and run an inventory of how these rudimentary aspects of your life feature in the person that you are today. Are these foundations strong and sturdy or are they in need of structural reform?

To be in control, we must know and understand ourselves. This means not only recognising and accepting our weaknesses, but also working to improve such limitations, because this is fundamental to personal progress and development. We should also appreciate the treasures that are our individual strengths and learn to call upon them for the power and confidence needed to overcome the challenges we face. Such a transition also involves discovering truthful and relevant information, and taking sufficient care to assimilate and to understand this new evidence so that it can become part of a tangible and personalised roadmap of what must be done. This is the premise of *Weight Wisdom*. Learning (primarily about yourself) will change your life course more effectively than mere decision-making, which is fragile and subject to amendment at some point in the future. Learning and development lead to permanent change, whereas decisions are ephemeral.

In the context of exploring change, it is also necessary to thoroughly examine and test our wants, to be sure they are what we actually want, and that they are realistically achievable. Assuming, since you are reading this book, that weight loss is one of your wants, then it will be important to qualify this. Why do you want it? How much do you want it? And what impact on your life do you anticipate it will have when you achieve it? When you are clear on these emotions and beliefs, they need to be reconciled against the practical aspects of your life that will need to change. So here we are at the nub of the matter: if this is what you want, this is what must change.

It is probably naive to assume that, if most adults were offered happiness and health, this would be more than enough to satisfy our wants. But while this may suffice for those that are unhappy and unhealthy, what about those that are already healthy and happy? You can't have more of it, and so presumably they would want for something else. If you asked all the great thinkers of the world, with respect to health and happiness, they would probably tell you, other than enlightenment and self-realisation, there really is nothing else. The point, I'm hoping to make, is that if your wants (for weight loss) are based upon a desire for health and happiness then your weight-loss goals are probably on a sure footing. Hopefully, the process of change and the growth and development that this will lead to, will also involve enlightenment, and perhaps even allow glimpses of the self-realisation to which the great thinkers refer.

Finally, I can't tell you if events are random or determined. I believe that our lives are in flux, and our paths reflect the growth, learning and development that we achieve throughout our individual and unique journeys, which changes over time as we remodel ourselves with every thought, choice, action and interaction that we encounter. These imperceptible nudges accumulate to shape and reshape our futures, setting new trajectories and forming longer-term designs for our future selves.

Insight 4: Forgiveness

Blame, guilt, anger, resentment, shame and bitterness are the antithesis of growth. The events, decisions and happenings of the past that have led to your current weight, occurred for reasons that you will have now come to terms with. Accept that the past is passed. We are where we are, and we are who we are. Harbour no ill will towards yourself or others that you may have concluded had a hand in your weight. Instead, accept that no one (including yourself) had any ill feelings towards you and there was never any malice in their actions, only love and caring in their intentions. If there is any blame, erase this from your mind and forgive yourself and others. Only by loving yourself and those around you can you truly find your path. Acknowledging and accepting our circumstances is the only route to emotional balance and peace of mind, this frees us, and allows us to grow and to flourish.

I FORGIVE MYSELF FOR:

I FORGIVE OTHERS FOR:

Change

"Obstacles are what you see when you take your eyes off the goal!"

Helen Keller (1880–1968)

Life is change

If you do what you've always done, you get what you've always got. And if you are not happy with what you've got, then change is all you have. Life is change, and so learning to embrace and develop 'change skills' is the foundation for a successful and happy future. Breaking out of a comfortable cycle feels threatening and can be frightening, which is why we often turn away from change. But most psychological approaches are about rationalising your fears and facing up to them, in order not to become stuck in an irrational pattern of behaviour. You are not a hostage to your mind; you *are* your mind.

However, you couldn't simply read a book about learning to play golf and claim to be able to play golf. You must get the clubs in your hand and get on the driving range, putting green and, finally, on the course. To play golf, you'll need repetition, consistency, staying power and other people around you who also like to drive for show and putt for dough. You need to practise. In the same way, you can't read this book and immediately start to think differently, you must practise thinking differently and developing positive self-talk in your head. You need to approach it like you would learning a challenging new skill like golf.

An important principle in approaching change is first finding the space and time to achieve the clarity of thought needed to enable your brain to figure out the right route. If you work in a cluttered workshop, you won't get much done, and sooner or later you will trip. Techniques that keep you thinking rationally and in line with your objectives, and those that teach you to recognise unhelpful, disorganised or chaotic thinking, will prove invaluable. I am willing to bet that your weight loss or healthy-eating plans have been undone in the past because you encountered challenging circumstances that you were unable to think your way around. Some of the techniques in this section will help you to avoid the entrenched thought patterns that may have thwarted you in the past.

Change starts by learning to think differently. I'm always surprised that people work so hard to change their waist circumference and their focus is on the material things around them and the physical aspects of their body. But by changing the psychological landscape, the physical form will follow. The principle of neuroplasticity ('things that fire together, wire together') posits that the brain can and does rewire itself and change as our experiences change. Therefore, removing neural connections in your brain (through abstaining from one behaviour) and establishing new ones through new behaviours, teaches the brain to recognise and reinforce different, more healthy patterns of behaviour. Even though you may not feel it now, this is within your power, and this power is within you, and only you can access it.

The contradiction of human behaviour that is wanting to do something but not feeling able to do it has always intrigued me. The multitude of competing emotions, stimuli, triggers and barriers that define health-related behaviour are complex, to say the least. For many of us, there is a dispute between what we want to eat and drink and how much we want to move, and our desire to be healthy and slim. While most of us know that eating CRAP is bad for us, and taking exercise is generally beneficial, we want to eat what we find tasty, and we'll swerve the gym if there is a better option or an excuse not to go. This is part of the slippery slope of negative behaviours becoming the norm. But the more frequently we do something, the more normalised the behaviour becomes, and therefore the less reason there is to question or challenge it – it's just what we do!

My interest in behavioural-change was first aroused by my experiences as a young (irreverent) personal trainer. I recollect one conversation with a woman, let's call her Val, that I had met at a social event. On hearing that I worked in the wellness business, she introduced herself and mentioned her concerns about osteoporosis due to family history. She wanted to know if she would be better off eating more yoghurt or cheese or drinking more milk to increase her calcium intake. In response, I recollect saying something along the lines of:

Me:	"Actually, from what I know, while dairy products have a lot of calcium, they don't have the best balance of other minerals such as magnesium, phosphorous and potassium required for good bone health, which is why you may be better augmenting your diet with lots of green leafy vegetables which have a good balance of all of the nutrients required for strong bones."
Val:	"I don't like those, I mean sprouts, cabbage, broccoli... yuk, I can't eat them."
Me:	"Oh, OK, well, actually then, I think you would benefit from regularly loading your bones by doing some resistance and impacting exercises. Any gym will be able to do you a programme that will help. This is because you can eat all the calcium in the world, but if your bones are not sensitised to absorbing it, then you will just end up with calcium-rich stools. Loading bones helps them to absorb minerals."
Val:	"Actually, I've thought about joining a gym, but I really don't have time."
Me:	"Ah, I see. Well, I hope you don't mind me mentioning, but a little earlier did I see that you were smoking?
Val:	"Yes, it's my one vice, well, other than the wine!"
Me:	"Well, has your doctor not mentioned to you that smoking is a big risk factor for poor bone health, because it impacts vitamin D levels and subsequent calcium absorption?"
Val:	"He might have done, and I've tried stopping in the past, but I always end up coming back to smoking."
Me	(with a cheery smile): "Ah, well, good luck with the osteoporosis then!"

Thankfully, I think my behaviour-change techniques may have undergone subtle improvements since then.

Don't be afraid to fail

The fear of failure often keeps many people in a state of perpetual inertia. But ask yourself, if you try and it doesn't work out, what is the most awful thing that can happen? Will you perish? Will people think worse of you for trying? Will you have lost something, or will you have gained from the experience? Will you learn anything? Will you feel pride in the fact that you tried? Because it did not work out this time, does it mean you can never try again? Have you burned your bridges?

Imagine you wanted to learn to play the piano, which for someone new to music would be a considerable challenge. But what does learning to play the piano mean? Do you want to become competent at 'Do-Re-Mi', or is your target to become a concert pianist? The mistake many people make when contemplating doing something new, is that they look at it like a project, rather like they would building a house, it has a start and an end – you lay the first brick, you lay the last brick. But developmental life skills are not building projects, they are open-ended journeys that help to characterise who we are. Viewing weight management (which, after all, is just a healthier way of living) in the same way as learning to play the piano, will bring about a much better chance of success.

Learning the piano means that you are committing to embracing a new skill into your life that will bring enrichment and satisfaction. To achieve this prize, you realise that you will have to work diligently each day, patience and perseverance will be needed in pursuit of continual improvement (success is a journey not a destination). As Bernard Barton reminds us in his classic poem Bruce and the Spider: "Perseverance gains its meed, and patience wins the race". The goal? An enriched life with the trappings of heightened pride and confidence – but only for as long as you engage in continual improvement.

Another important thing to do when contemplating weight loss is to reflect upon how you would normally approach a new challenge. For example, some people would describe themselves as an all-or-nothing type – I will throw myself in at the deep end, and either sink or swim. I'll be a success or a failure at this mindfulness programme; it's either my perfect diet today or it's Armageddon. While this personality type is innate in many people, if you identify with it, be aware that rigid dogmatic approaches to change can sometimes work, but often this way of trying to control yourself does not lend itself well to dealing with inevitable lapses.

You may, on the other hand, describe yourself as someone inclined to take a more cautious approach to change, preferring instead to take things one step at a time and trying to build upon each success. This is a logical, reasoned approach to change, but can run the risk of running out of steam if the road is long and the sequential changes don't immediately fulfil your aspirations.

The point is, neither of these two differing approaches is right or wrong, but you need to consider your own tactic for change and think about what is more likely to work for you, based upon your experience. Remember that life is not either black or white, it's mainly shades of grey.

Before tackling a new challenge, each of us will have an idea about the prospects of making our new habit stick. For instance, some people would rather start a task that they know they can easily achieve, perhaps something they have done many times before (I'm going back to my home yoga course). While others would be more motivated to start something much more challenging (I'm going to run a marathon). However, think about what I have said about not starting something that you realistically cannot keep doing forever. Are you really going to keep running marathons as a way of controlling your weight? Perhaps…

Decision-making

Mark Manson, in his impressive article '3 Reasons Why You Make Terrible Decisions (And How to Stop)[301], reminds us that everything we do in life is a trade-off between cost and benefit. These are not always immediately apparent and often they are subtle, but either way the cost/benefit algorithm is always reckoning. As Manson says: "Gain and loss are simultaneous. For everything you say or do, there is an infinite number of alternative choices you must forgo to say or do them."

Therefore, from our starting allocation of 'fortune chips', when we think we gain one way, we lose elsewhere. I like to think that our bequeathed cache of prosperity is like the energy in the universe – it's finite, you can't have more, and you can't lose any, but through our choices, the benefits or the drawbacks simply re-occupy different time zones (you win now, you lose later).

The trick, as Manson sees it, is to properly see what we're giving up and what we're gaining. Because, of course, it comes down to what you value. If you value hedonistic pleasure over longevity, you may see an early death from a self-indulgent lifestyle as an even result. Similarly, if you are one of the 'Health Saints' that values life above all else, you may decide that living an abstemious life justifies the 120 years that you hope to enjoy.

But good decisions are tough; you must suffer short-term loss now, while waiting for the long-term gain, which is likely to be a long way away. In contrast, bad decisions seem easy because we get the benefit right now.

Perhaps this is why, as you get older, making the right decisions appears to get easier because of your closer proximity to your final destiny. This may also explain why affluent people with a good life value the future more than someone struggling, with poorer people reporting being less motivated by health when making food selections. We are back in the realms of delay discounting, but this is how we make our choices. As Manson asks: "What are you willing to give up in each moment for something else? What is worth giving up? What is the 'something else' worth pursuing?" These questions are at the core of what we all struggle with daily. If everything is a trade-off, then a good life means making good trades. It means getting a lot of benefits for whatever costs we incur.

We are also poor at compounding the interest on our behaviours. Doing something frequently accrues the benefits or drawbacks, and over time, this is what really counts – it's not what you eat all the time that matters, it's what you eat most of the time. When we make a poor choice, we think, well it's only the once, it won't matter! If it is a good choice, we say the same – how much value will it add? We don't consider the long game, but life is a long-distance run, not a short dash. The economics of compound interest apply to lifestyle choices, but when we over-value the now and under-value the future, we don't contribute sufficiently to the health nest egg that we desire for our retirement.

It is our values that determine what we perceive as the significant benefits in our lives, and Manson suggests that if we are not clear on our values, then we can't make decisions that will benefit us. He says: "Find your cause, find your values, discover the costs and benefits of your actions, and taking action becomes infinitely simpler".

Motivation

It goes without saying that, to change, you must first want to change. However, wanting to change is not on its own sufficient, as most people want to change something but can't. Motivation is the drive needed to achieve your goals and is influenced in part by your desire for that goal and what your personal expectations are if you achieve your goal. Contrary to popular belief, motivation is not something that we either have or do not have. We all have motivation, which exists along a continuum, from a little to a lot. At any given time, it is situation-specific and is continually affected by external influences and personal circumstances. For instance, someone currently might not be too motivated to eat healthily, but they are super-motivated to achieve a very challenging task at work.

Motivation can result from external rewards such as more money, trophies, social recognition and praise, or internal forces such as self-gratification and a desire to achieve a challenging task. Engaging on a weight-loss programme may be the result of external forces such as pressure from a spouse or a healthcare professional. But external motivators in isolation are fleeting, and as soon as the authority of the referring medic is removed, or the pressure from a spouse subsides, so too does the motivation. Combining extrinsic and intrinsic motivators can be powerful (ask any elite sportsperson). They keep their eyes on the prize while figuring out how to delve deep into their internal pool of motivation and keep going back to the well, time after time.

If you feel that your motivation to achieve or start something is low, then keep in mind the idea of behavioural experiments. Sometimes, starting something big can be overwhelming, and so there are plenty of reasons to be ambivalent about such undertakings. For instance, if you have not exercised for many years, then starting can be daunting or even intimidating for some. However, if instead of thinking about making the 100% commitment to a regular exercise programme, you could instead think, "I'll just see what it feels like to do one session and I can see how I am after that. I don't have to make any commitments, I just want to know how I would get on and I can then take things from there." This will allow you to have a go without the massive commitment that is all-or-nothing thinking, which is not good when contemplating change.

You may want to think about rewards for when you achieve your goals (I've been keeping active now for three months, I'm going to book a weekend away as a treat). However, be mindful that, if you are enjoying being active, then a reward might act as a demotivator. Psychologists have found that rewarding enjoyable behaviour decreases motivation and they refer to this phenomenon as the over-justification effect[302]. If you are finding the activity enjoyable, then this should be reward enough. Perhaps reserve the rewards for things that you find more challenging.

Even the most determined person will struggle to achieve their goals if they allow low self-esteem, doubt and self-criticism to creep into their mind. Self-esteem is generally linked to our perceived competence in areas we consider to be important, and we are most vulnerable to low self-esteem when these self-imposed measures of proficiency fall short of our ideal. Be proud of yourself and celebrate the progress that you have made so far. A lack of trust will perpetuate a feeling of failure before you even start. Remind yourself of your greatest achievements – you are still that same person, in fact you are better – you are now older and wiser, and with that comes power.

Many people use visualisation (seeing yourself in your new lifestyle) to motivate themselves and help them achieve change, and, if it gives you power, I'm all for it. However, it is important that, when you visualise success, you visualise the steps towards becoming the person that you want to be rather than just on the end outcome. This is because research has shown that fantasising about the future endgame, predicts poor achievement by sapping available change motivation and energy; in essence, seeing yourself as a slim athletic person without visualising yourself doing the doing, keeps it a fantasy. Therefore, visualisation will be more effective if it encompasses the steps towards the goal.

It is OK, to take a favourite photograph of yourself or an image that you like and put it somewhere you can look at it each day. Imagine how you will become this person, build a clear picture in your mind of the lifestyle required and how life would be if it were to happen. Visualise what you will wear, where you will go, and what activities you will do. If you cannot 'see' yourself doing something, then how do you expect it to become reality? Visualise eating the healthy food and being the active person, rather than visualising yourself as thinner. Don't focus on the destination, concentrate on the journey.

Be sure to talk about your goals with family and friends and enlist their support. Ask them: "How can you help keep me motivated?" You might be pleasantly surprised by their creativity and support. Try not to make too many changes to routines all at once, and celebrate each small change, as small changes will compound to make a significant difference over time. Take things gradually and never underestimate the importance of the goals that you have set – keep them close to you and refer to them regularly. If health goals are tied to your future thinking, this can assist in positive behaviour changes, so consider your health alongside future plans.

If you are looking to unleash your motivation to change, then it is important to start by identifying negative or counterproductive behaviours or beliefs, with a view to testing their authenticity, as these will suppress any motivation to change. These ought to have been identified when you completed Insight 2, and be sure to remind yourself of the strategies that you have in place to ensure these old habits don't reappear. Praising yourself for trying, even if you don't have success the first time, will help you to stay motivated to continue working toward your goal. Also, you could consider opportunities to form social networks and meet and discuss your ideas with others facing similar challenges. You could try a weight-loss forum, such as that to be found at www.weightwisdom.co.uk, where you can chat to others and I try to answer as many questions as I can.

Willpower

Willpower is a battle between logic and emotions. Emotions are strong, and logic requires continual reinforcement and recognition to compete with its overwhelming power. When the brain is tired, emotions will always triumph over logic (because logic requires more resources to reach conclusions). Stress also depletes willpower and gives emotions the edge, which is why you might grab a drink if you have had a stressful time, even though you are trying not to drink during the week. A lack of willpower is a big problem, as many mental health difficulties can be a result of conflict between an immediate impulse to do something that is not in your long-term interests and the physical or psychological consequences of your actions if you go ahead and do it.

Willpower is related to our earlier subject of delay discounting, in that it is described as the ability to resist short-term temptations for long-term gain. Resisting temptation is therefore considered to be willpower. When people consider that they lack the willpower to exercise, for example, what this actually means is that they lack the willpower to resist the short-term lure of the comfort of being sedentary. It is not the exercise that is the problem, it's the relationship with the couch that needs attention! Reframe your mind to put the sedentary behaviour at the centre of your change strategy.

Willpower is also heavily influenced by our upbringing, which plays a significant role. For instance, the famous marshmallow experiment in which five-year-olds are given the option of having one treat immediately, or, if they are prepared to wait a short while (seven minutes), then they will get two marshmallows. This is a measure of someone's ability to delay gratification, and the experiment, which has been replicated many times, shows there is a socio-economic aspect to the outcome. It has been postulated that people growing up in poorer households may be inclined to take the smaller, short-term benefit now, rather than wait for the bigger prize later, because the long option may never arrive. In childhood, this was probably self-preservation at work, but, if it has persisted into adulthood, it is no longer rational and requires a change of thinking.

Willpower is also closely linked to incentive, and the difference between non-exercisers and super-fit people is not necessarily the willpower required to get up and put in the extraordinary workouts, but the incentive to do so. If, for instance, you excel in sport, then you may be able to win something, either money, recognition or even fame, and subsequently you will have a strong motivation to work very hard. If, on the other hand, there is no chance that you will ever receive any material gain from exercising, then there is no incentive and thus little motivation. Professional footballers have a big incentive to train hard, but the average person (including many recreational footballers) does not rely on super fitness to be successful.

Our beliefs inform our motivation and this in turn impacts our willpower, and so motivation and willpower are reliant on each other. As they are both situation-specific, they may hold firm for one activity but crumble for another. Consider someone that is very motivated to get fit because they want to go skiing. They may well be able to resist the lure of the sofa on Saturday morning when it's time for a run, but on Saturday evening when their friend offers them a cigarette, their willpower crumbles and they succumb.

You can be motivated by the prospect of both positive outcomes (if I keep practising, I will pass my driving test) or by negative ones (if I don't get this tax return done, it's a £100 fine). We only keep doing things that we are not motivated to do when we feel compelled to do them (going to work or going to the dentist), but this doesn't apply to optional activities such as healthy eating and exercise. Therefore, if you are not motivated to do something that is optional, the reality is, whether you like it or not, if it has little priority in your life, then you won't do it. Sooner or later, you must face up to this. If that optional something is instrumental in achieving your most important goals, then rationality in your life has broken down and your brain is short-circuiting the indisputable logic that is: goals need priorities, and priorities need priority.

The reason that you are not motivated to do something that is intrinsically linked to one of your life goals, is that you simply haven't joined all the dots together in your mind. There are logic gaps that are not allowing the circuits to connect, obstructing the information from flowing. By thoroughly working through the Five Insights, you will bridge these gaps and mobilise your motivation and bolster your willpower.

Another important consideration when you are contemplating willpower and the motivation to change, is that viewing a task as an obstacle or a problem rather than as an integral part of the solution, will create conflict and stifle progress. If you are aware that you need to exercise to manage your weight, but you don't want to exercise, then what you are effectively saying is that you don't want to manage your weight, because exercise is an integral part of weight control, and therefore you are not approaching it realistically. To put it another way, "I want to be an astronaut, but I don't want to bother with all the work of getting my PhD. in Astrophysics or whatever it takes". In other words, I don't want to be an astronaut (or I do want to be an astronaut, but I realise that it's a fantasy).

If you find yourself in such a conundrum, you could internalise the discussion and feel ashamed or conflicted and turn to despair to help you out. Or you could open up and discuss it with someone that you trust and see if they can help you to understand the situation better (which is why the talking therapies are so helpful). What you will almost certainly find is that any self-criticism you harbour about your ambivalence is unjustified and probably helping to keep you stuck in your behaviours. Further to that, you will probably learn that there is a solution to be had, and by discussing it, you can explore your options. You don't need to go to a therapist necessarily, speak to a trusted friend or family member, or join a self-help group or online forum.

If you accept the finite energy analogy (you either win now and lose later, or vice versa) then to move you closer to your goals, you need to bolster the rationality argument to allow the conscious part of your brain to overcome the emotional control centre (ego over id). Because the rational position is irrefutable. If there is no clear connection between your goals and your priorities, the incentives and motivations which are essential to generate willpower will not be present. In this case, you need to take a step back and re-establish your goals and the behavioural priorities that will achieve them. By writing them down you can see where the process is breaking down. Only by accepting and regularly reinforcing the link between your behaviours (priorities) and your goals will we find the motivation and incentive needed to overcome the low willpower that is currently pinning you to the sofa or not allowing you to make the right food choices.

When contemplating change, you also need to give thought to time, which is a frequent reason cited for failing to realise a goal. Time management is priority management, because time is just a device to stop everything happening at once. The most productive person in the world has the same amount of time available as everyone else, and if you set out the priorities in your life as the things that are most central to your goals, then you will always find (make) time for them. "I don't have time" simply means that it is not as important to you as what you're doing right now or what you intend to do next. Make sure your priorities are your priorities and that they represent your most important goals.

A practical scenario

Let's imagine that your one life goal is to lose a substantial amount of weight. Imagine that you described the motivators for your goal as:

> "I fear for my health, I think I'm heading for diabetes and my mobility is really suffering. My quality of life is deteriorating, and I am afraid."

Weight Wisdom acknowledges the complexity of behaviour change, but the facts in this scenario boil down to this:

1. Without change, there is a very serious threat on the near horizon.

2. Weight loss will involve:

   a. Abstinence from the consumption of CRAP and the adoption of a healthier diet.

   b. More movement (exercise and physical activity).

   c. The adoption of a) & b) as a new way of life.

The *goal* is substantial weight loss. The *motivator* is the fear of a catastrophic loss of health and dramatically reduced quality of life. The *priorities* are a), b), and c), and the *incentive* is the prospect of a healthy and normal life. In the face of all of this, you must ask the question: "What does *willpower* have to do with it?" And the answer is, sooner or later (probably sooner), you will be faced with the prospect of going for a brisk walk or staying at home to watch your favourite TV show. You will have to forgo CRAP temptations multiple times every day, and you will have to be disciplined enough to not succumb to frequent snacking that has been customary for probably most of your life. Boredom will come knocking and the lure of just one last binge for old times' sake will loom large. Friends, family, pushers and peddlers, and historical triggers will be hammering the door down to encourage you to engage in old habits, to justify their own compulsions. This is the reality for many people, and this is when willpower is needed.

Recent work suggests that willpower may be a finite resource and trying to exert too much all at once (fighting on too many fronts) can cause willpower fatigue. The good news, though, is that the utilities of willpower and self-control are modifiable and not immutable. With practice and process, they can be developed and strengthened. Here are some of the ways that you can strengthen your willpower:

- Recognise, reward and praise yourself for your achievements, no matter how small they may be. Make this a life habit.

- Regularly reinforce the link between your goals and your priorities, and always be aware of your incentives and motivations, make sure they are crystal clear and always at the forefront of your mind – they are your salvation!

- Believe in yourself and draw on your strengths, credit yourself when you do well.

- Use affirmations – "Today I will overcome!"

- Give time and energy to planning and scheduling – chaos is your worst enemy.

- Feel the breath, find the calm, use the strength (to make the right choices).

- Practise, practise, practise (all the above).

- Don't try and go it alone, join a group – feel the love.

- Oscar Wilde could resist anything except temptation. Be prepared, it will surely come!

Popular change strategies

The challenges that people encounter when faced with the need to change is what led me into the field of behaviour change. Over many years, I researched and trialled the populist ideas and practices and introduced these highly theoretical models into everyday wellness and weight-management services, deploying them alongside my colleagues to help people to solve their behaviour-related problems. In the context of weight loss, I found that some work better than others. In particular, the techniques used in cognitive behavioural therapy (CBT) and the Trans Theoretical Model (TTM) I found to be very helpful.

A central pillar of CBT is to help people to see things in different ways, and hopefully benefit from an alternative and more appropriate perspective. When people can see things differently, they can also think differently, and this is a prerequisite for change. But most people seeking to lose weight don't undertake a course of cognitive behavioural therapy, or indeed engage in other specialist behavioural programmes, they simply set out on a path that they consider will be the most successful. This might be joining a weight-loss group, buying a book, or simply making their own plans based upon what they know and what has worked previously.

But, as you will know, changing course is not easy, particularly where eating and moving is concerned. Mark Twain astutely observed, "You can't just take bad habits and toss them out of the bedroom window; you have to coax them down the staircase one by one". To give yourself the best possible chance of success, it will be helpful to examine the main behaviour-change models and understand how they operate to elicit change, and to help coax each one down the stairs.

First, let's look at how we typically get others closest to us, such as our family, to make the changes that we want from them. I would normally workshop this in a group situation, as this is where the best ideas and contributions are always to be found, and I'd like to share with you the results of many such meetings. I also want you to think of your own personal examples and experiences, particularly where you have tackled conduct at home that has gotten on your nerves to the point that you need it to change. Those I've discussed this with, typically cite the following family behaviours as the 'most annoying':

- The kids won't tidy their rooms.
- S/he leaves their dishes in the sink when I'm constantly loading the dishwasher.
- Everyone in this house (except me) always leave the lights on when they exit a room.
- I'm always pushing the kids to do their homework.

- Who needs to take a twenty-minute shower?
- Why am I the only one that can put the bins out?
- I can't get them off their phones.
- Why are bedtimes always such a battle with the kids?
- S/he watches too much TV.

So, the question is: "How do we get other family members to change their behaviour (presumably so that the house can be more harmonious, and we can all be more productive, happy and successful)? I would expect many of the following common responses as strategies for domestic change:

1. I ask nicely a few times and then I normally end up screaming!
2. I threaten to remove their pocket money.
3. I get my own back by doing something that really annoys them – how do you like it?
4. I just leave the dishes until someone else has to load the dishwasher.
5. I break down and cry, and hope and pray that they will change.
6. I apply sanctions such as the removal of privileges (no Xbox, phones etc).
7. I use bargaining tools such as if you do this for me, I'll do this for you.
8. I just keep going on and on, drip, drip, drip, (Chinese torture) and try to wear them down.
9. I have a tantrum and don't speak to anyone for days.
10. I bribe them with money and treats to do their homework.
11. I try and reason with them and explain why it is important to change.
12. I just leave them all to it and take the dog for a walk.
13. I down tools – make your own dinner, wash your own clothes, get yourself to football!
14. I make jokes or use sarcasm about their behaviour to get them to change.

There are other methods not mentioned here that people use which they think will lead to changing the behaviour of others. However, some of these are offensive, unacceptable and against the law, and include controlling coercion, psychological bullying and violence. I won't give this any credence other than to state that they are all utterly pointless as change strategies, and this is probably not the underlying reason for such behaviours in any case.

So, let's look at our list of fourteen family behavioural-change strategies. I'd like you to add to these your own methods, and then, when you have a complete list, in your notebook, put them into one of the following six broad approaches:

- Threatening and coercive: using my authority and status, I'll force my will upon them.
- Pleading: I'll beg them to change and hope they take pity on me.
- Bargaining: Making it beneficial for them to change.
- Ignoring: Just let them get on with it – see if I care!
- Trivialising: Make a joke out of it.
- Rationalising: Explaining why change would be positive.

Now we need to consider which of these categories has any prospect of modifying behaviour over the long term. It may be that you think that some of these fall into the category of 'unlikely to facilitate change', or perhaps 'will make a short-term difference' (to assuage you and disarm the situation). But we are not interested in temporary change, we get that every day from the weather.

Threatening and coercive: Unlikely to engender long-term change. Once the threat or intimidation is removed, the prevailing behaviour is likely to return. Furthermore, as threats and punitive sanctions become commonplace, so you must continually up the ante to get the required result. A raised voice becomes a shout, which becomes a scream, which becomes hysteria. This is why smacking children to control their behaviour is a very bad idea.

Pleading: Unlikely to work, as you can only play this card once or twice until it becomes emotionally passé. Also, it's a position of weakness that relies on a benevolent and compassionate response from those you are appealing to. It might work as a temporary measure if people feel sorry for you, but that won't last.

Bargaining: May work for a while but there is a danger that it may teach people that you only change if there is something material in it for you. You must keep incentivising people to maintain the change. Once the incentive is gone, the behaviour is likely to return. Also, you always have to be prepared to 'buy' change from people by conceding something that they might want.

Ignoring: Probably little chance of working over the long term (but may make you feel better). Could make people reflect on things and may make them feel bad about the situation, but that is not a great starting point for long-term change. People might interpret your stance as sanctioning their behaviour (on the basis that you don't seem to mind), or they might find a workaround that could even make matters worse.

Trivialising: Making a joke of matters or being sarcastic is one way of raising the issue while trying to avoid any conflict. It may work by keeping the behaviour in the mind of the perpetrator, but trivialising things is unlikely to result in change, and being humorous about a behaviour may just encourage it.

Rationalising: This is the only method with any real prospect of a long-term change. Enabling people to think about why a change is important and allowing them to explore all outcomes, hopefully they reach their own decision that change is right and will bring long-term, tangible benefits for themselves and others.

Here is how I grouped the fourteen change strategies (you may have grouped them differently, and that's fine):

- Threatening and coercive: Using my authority and status (1, 2, 3, 6)
- Pleading: I'll beg them to change and hope they take pity on me (5, 8, 9)
- Bargaining: Making it beneficial for them to change (7, 10)
- Ignoring: Just let them get on with it – see if I care! (4, 12, 13)
- Trivialising: Make a joke or be sarcastic (14)
- Rationalising: Explaining why change would be positive (11)

Therefore, it appears that from our list of fourteen common strategies used at home to try to elicit change, only one has any real prospect of long-term success (number 11). Yet, we plug away with these other hopeless strategies in the belief that, in time, they may work. Perhaps more correctly they have just become habitual knee-jerks to when something annoys us. Consequently, if we draw on our own family traditions for change, is it any wonder that when we want to change our own behaviour, our successes are limited? The purpose of considering all of this is to help you to think more clearly about behaviour change and how it works.

To deepen your understanding of how the human mind works when faced with the prospect of change, I believe an examination of the established theoretical models of change will be most helpful. Of course, by their very nature, talking therapies don't lend themselves too well to a book, but the plan here is not to expect you to read these theories, have a Eureka moment, and run down the street shouting, I'm cured! Rather, to introduce you to the ideas and techniques that have assisted millions of people to overcome some very serious and entrenched psychological and behavioural problems, in the belief that you too can learn to think in ways that will enable you to make lasting change in your life.

I hope this introduction to these ideas will enable you to think differently to solve your weight problems and may also inspire you to learn more about techniques that you feel may be helpful to you for now or in the future. This may lead to you seeking support from one of the many available options, such as one of the excellent online interactive programmes, joining a self-help group or perhaps engaging with a change therapist, any of which I would consider a hugely positive step on your journey towards your weight-management goals.

An examination of habits

Habits are behaviours that are automatically repeated and can be difficult to control as they are triggered by environmental cues and decoupled from the original reason for the behaviour. Quite simply, habits enable us to do things automatically without having to think about the action, they are useful and time-saving devices. Habits allow us to perform lots of everyday mundane routines without distracting us from other tasks, allowing our brains to focus on processing more important information, thereby rendering us more productive.

All habits that we form will originally have served a useful purpose, otherwise we would not have done it in the first place and kept doing it for the fifteen or so repetitions that it is estimated are needed to form a habit. However, we often forget to switch these instructions off once they have served their useful purpose. It is important that you realise that habits are just fragments of behaviour that once had a purpose, and no longer do ("When in the school staff room for morning break, we had chocolate biscuits with tea every day. It was a ritual that was seen as an important bonding session. I don't work there anymore, but still do it"). Habits are not part of you and they can be changed, they can be turned back off. Someone once said to me, "I'm not a fat person, I'm a thin person with a lot of fat habits!"

Habits get in the way of change by suppressing the modifications to beliefs and attitudes required for change. Habits get us stuck in 'ruts' and lower our motivation to learn and engage with new information. This is particularly the case if new ideas or ways of thinking are at odds with our habitual behaviour. To overcome long-standing habits, sometimes behavioural experiments can help.

Case study: Geraldine, movie aficionado

Geraldine likes the movies very much and goes once a week without fail. Worried about the effect on her weight, she raised it as one of her 'risky behaviours'. The reason for the risk rating, Geraldine explains, is that, from an early age, the family movie was always accompanied by a big bag of sweets and ice cream. "And now, I habitually buy sweets when I go to a movie; always!" This 'pairing' intrinsically links the sweets to the movie and becomes an integral part of the enjoyment of the movie.

I ask Geraldine, "So, why do you do this if you are worried about your weight?" She explains that she knows she would not enjoy the movie the same without the sweets and ice cream. (This is what is known as the 'maintaining mechanism', the central belief that the movie will not have the same enjoyment without the pairing with the sweets.) It is important that, if Geraldine is to break this habit, then we need to remove the maintaining mechanism and debunk this dysfunctional belief about her inability to enjoy a movie in the absence of sweets and ice cream. This is where the experiment starts.

Geraldine's normal routine is to meet her boyfriend after work midweek and aim for a 7pm screening. Sweets are duly acquired and eaten (mainly by herself). After the movie, either a drink on the way home or a bottle of wine shared back at home.

As I may have mentioned previously, I'm not in the habit of telling people what to do. However, for purposes of behavioural experiments, I ask that people indulge me and try to do things differently, just to test the outcomes. Together, we agree that this week the couple will book a slightly later viewing and meet at home beforehand. Geraldine agrees to prepare a preferred meal at home before they go, and she settles to take just a bottle of water into the cinema for each of them. I bid her farewell and wish her luck with the experiment. The following week we meet, and here is how the conversation went:

Me	"Hi, Geraldine, how did the movie go, what did you watch?"
G	"Oh, wow, we watched Titanic, amazing! Leonardo DiCaprio etc. etc..."
Me	"Did you stick to the plan?"
G	"Yes, just as agreed."
Me	"What did you cook, before you went?"
G	"Spag Bol, lovely!"
Me	"How did it feel, not getting the sweets?"
G	"It was fine. I'd given it a lot of thought since last week and I sort of knew I'd be OK. I felt prepared."
Me	"How did you feel when others around you had sweets?"
G	"Absolutely fine, I felt a little bit smug actually, I was not at all envious."
Me	"Geraldine, do you need sweets to enjoy a movie?"
G	"No, it's all in my head."
Me	"And so are all the answers."

Theories of learning

To better understand the principles of behaviour change, it is first worthwhile taking a brief look at some of the theories of how we learn. If we understand how we learn, surely this will help us to figure out how to change what we have learned (and un-learn some things) and subsequently change how we think and behave.

The theory of learned behaviour

The theory of learned behaviour states that the things we experience and our environment are the drivers of how we act. Psychologists J.B. Watson and B.F. Skinner believed that, if they were given a group of infants and could control their environments and the way they were raised, this alone would ultimately determine their behaviours and actions, not their parents or their genetics.

Stimulus response and positive reinforcement are key in the behavioural learning theory. If a child receives praise for solving a puzzle, they are much more likely to try other challenging tasks as they see a direct correlation between problem-solving and praise. If they don't receive praise, they experience negative reinforcement (you did well, so what?), and they get bored and give up. Motivation and positive reinforcement play an important role in behavioural learning. Good behaviour → praise and recognition → a learned preference.

An extension to behavioural learning is Social Learning Theory[303], which argues that behaviour is much more complicated than simple stimulus and response. Instead, we learn through observation, and then consciously decide to imitate behaviour based upon the attitudes and emotional reactions of others. We are further influenced by peer pressure and a desire to fit in.

Classical conditioning

Russian physiologist and Nobel Prize winner Ivan Pavlov discovered classical conditioning, which is learning through association. This is where two stimuli are linked together to create a new learned response. In his most famous experiment (Pavlov's Dogs) he repeatedly rang a bell to his dogs, and the dogs became used to the bell and did nothing (neutral stimuli). However, he then rang the bell just before he fed them (pairing), and, after a few repetitions, the dogs salivated when they heard the bell. The bell had become the conditioned stimulus and salivation had become the conditioned response.

Therefore, in classical conditioning, when a neutral stimulus (phoning a friend, for example) is paired with an unconditioned stimulus (we snack when we chat) it creates a conditioned stimulus which, if repeated often enough, develops the conditional stimulus – use the phone and respond by snacking. If done often enough this could create a desire to phone in order to snack. Pavlov called this a conditional reflex.

Based on Pavlov's observations, John Watson was convinced that this classical conditioning was able to explain all aspects of human psychology. In his infamous experiment 'Little Albert', Watson and his accomplice Rosalie Rayner encountered a remarkably fearless child known as Little Albert, who was scared only by loud noises. In an ethically and morally bankrupt experiment, they somehow convinced Albert's mother to allow them to prove their theory of associated conditioning by inducing a phobia (an irrational fear disproportional to the danger) in the child, using his fear of loud noises!

Albert was shown a white rat, a rabbit, a monkey, and various masks, and showed no fear of any. He would reach out to touch and play with the rat. However, predictably, what did frighten him was when a hammer was struck against a large steel bar being held behind his head, at which Albert would burst into tears. When the white rat was presented to Albert, seconds later the hammer was struck against the steel bar. After several 'pairings', Albert cried and avoided the rat and became ever more fearful as the episodes of rat/loud noise pairings continued.

After only a few weeks of this, he would cry and attempt to crawl away from the rat even in the absence of the loud noise. This fear would fade as time went on, however the association could be renewed (cruelly) by repeating the original procedure a few times! The egregious Watson and Rayner also found that their actions made Albert develop phobias of objects which shared characteristics with the rat, including the family dog, a fur coat, and a Father Christmas mask (this is known as generalisation). The relevance of this is how the associations and responses of others to eating (pairings) can have a profound influence on our learning about food and dietary habits[304]. While this is strongest in childhood, it continues throughout life.

Operant conditioning

Operant conditioning[305] adds the idea that the consequences of a response to our actions determines whether it will be repeated. Behaviours that result in pleasant outcomes are 'reinforced' and will likely be repeated, but those which result in unpleasant outcomes or punishment will be avoided. This valid explanation, at least in part, accounts for how children learn about the consequences of their actions. However, punishment as an influencer on behaviour is only short-term. Punishment has also been linked to increased aggression, and it can create fear that can generalise. That is, a child punished at school for stealing could become fearful of school in general, rather than simply abstaining from the behaviour that led to the punishment while at school. Furthermore, punishment does not encourage desired behaviour – whereas reinforcement tells you what to do, punishment only tells you what not to do.

When was the last time you thought about how you learn? What was the last thing that you learned? How did you learn it? You may think that you have learned a few things from this book, but hearing or reading and retaining information is merely building your encyclopaedia, which normally involves learning facts or remembering stories (most of which will be forgotten over time). True learning involves teaching the brain how to use the information held in the encyclopaedia. What will the CPU do with all the digital data on the hard drive? How will I respond in a given environment or under particular circumstances based upon the data I hold? Learning how to think is learning.

Evidenced change strategies

"To improve is to change; to be perfect is to change often."

Winston Churchill (1874-1965)

Are you frightened of being hungry, or afraid of the sensation of vigorous exercise, or anxious at the prospect of never eating CRAP again? Perhaps you are not afraid, but these scenarios make you feel uncomfortable or worried. Are these fears or concerns rational? You must learn to test your beliefs, because it is your beliefs that lead to how you feel, and how you feel dictates how you behave.

Consider the following questions and, **out loud**, answer yes or no to each. Think carefully and only answer truthfully:

- Does the short-term discomfort of exercise outweigh the long-term discomfort of my weight?
- Is my relationship with CRAP more valuable to me than my health?
- Is my fear of hunger more powerful than my fear of chronic illness and unhappiness?
- Are my cravings for CRAP more rational than my cravings for health and happiness?

If you answered yes to one or more of these questions, then your beliefs about eating and exercise are dysfunctional. While this remains the case, your behaviours will always remain incongruent with your wants and desires. You must un-learn the flawed programming of the past and re-teach your brain how to learn and respond in a way that will enable you to reach your life goals. And this you can do by using the techniques shown in the strategies for change outlined in this chapter.

If you answered no to all of the above, then these need to become central pillars of your change strategy. Write them out in bold in your notebook and use them daily as powerful affirmations of your intentions to change:

- **The short-term discomfort of exercise does not outweigh the long-term discomfort of my weight.**

- **My relationship with CRAP is not as valuable as my relationship with my health.**

- **I fear chronic illness and unhappiness more than I fear hunger.**

- **I crave health and happiness infinitely more than I crave CRAP.**

When considering change, some of my clients would say things like, "I want to lose weight but avoiding CRAP and committing to exercise most days seem really drastic, and I don't think I'll be able to do it". This is known as ambivalence (I want to lose weight, but I'm not sure I want to commit to changing the things that are causing my difficulties). Such thoughts and beliefs require exploration, because unless this ambivalence is resolved, change will continue to be elusive.

Where ambivalence exists, it is important to explore and resolve this psychological conflict. This is normally achieved by talking this through using the framework of motivational interviewing (which guides the client to find the answer). In most cases, people invariably conclude that the reason they are afraid of eliminating CRAP from their diet is because they have a compulsion to eat it. Therefore, a strategy for managing this compulsion is required, rather than facing the only other option which is to deal with the angst of ongoing ambivalence and the accompanying life dissatisfaction.

People may also be afraid of committing to daily exercise because they know that in the past they have always lapsed when trying to maintain exercise. In this case, the approach is to discuss this and lead the conversation to its logical conclusion, where the client deduces that their options are binary: to continue as they are, or to learn to expect and anticipate lapses as a normal part of life, and not see them in the terminal way that they previously have, thus increasing the prospect of re-engagement.

The idea is that the discussion helps the client to see that it is these thoughts that are holding them back, and until they can resolve them, they have little prospect of change. Thankfully, when people are taught how to adopt 'rational change talk', more positive and helpful thoughts emerge:

Irrational talk:

> "I don't think I can give up the CRAP in my life and I know that if I try to exercise, I'll just give it up sooner or later."

Rational change talk:

> "At the moment, I'm still somewhat fearful of eliminating CRAP, because I can see how central it has been in my life. However, the fear of ill-health is a far more powerful force in my life. I am also aware that, if I take up exercise, I may lapse, particularly if I don't find a physical-activity programme that is suited to my lifestyle and time available. I now also know that lapses are a normal part of change."

Changing damaging and defeatist thoughts (and internal talk) are the start of the change process, but people make the mistake of trying to change their behaviour before they change their thoughts. But, of course, our thoughts and beliefs control our behaviour, so in this case you are putting the cart before the horse and that won't work. By allowing your mind to think dysfunctional thoughts, you are maintaining the illusion that you can't change, and you will forever remain trapped in your existing 'safe' behaviour. But, as you are aware, this behaviour is not safe, in fact, it is quite the opposite, and you must continually remind yourself of this.

Despite how you may feel right now, it is absolutely within your power to eliminate dysfunctional and sabotaging thoughts and change how you think. But as with anything that you want to change, you must first want to change. You must *want* to change how you think. Facing up to the fact that it is the way that you think above all else that is holding you back from change, is the first stage in the process of change. If I could give you a tablet that would cure the madness of thinking that eliminating CRAP and exercising is more drastic than vascular disease, diabetes and chronic mental health issues, I guess you would take the tablet.

What follows is a short overview of some of the more effective talking therapies (tablets) and how they help people to move away from dysfunctional thinking and embrace self-change talk to escape the damaging behaviours that are controlling their weight.

Kubler-Ross Change Curve (KRCC)

Psychologist Elizabeth Kubler-Ross was interested in helping people deal with grief. She developed a theoretical model now famously known as the Kubler-Ross Change Curve (KRCC). Kubler-Ross intended this for people facing death or bereavement and their relatives. The theory has subsequently been applied to a multitude of situations where change is desired, and is now a popular and flexible change tool, used in scenarios as diverse as dealing with chronic disease, to culture change in the workplace. Personally, I have always found it very helpful for supporting people to manage the changes required to lose weight. There are several stages, which she described as performance points, set out in her memorable visual (shown overleaf).

Performance points

- Shock and denial: The first reaction to the change is usually a shock, sometimes resulting from the lack of information and fear of the unknown. This is often followed by denial – this can't be happening to me; the news/diagnosis must be wrong.

- Anger and depression: A realisation that the news/diagnosis is correct brings anger. As time passes and the condition worsens, depression, apathy and isolation can take their toll.

- Blame: Looking to unload the burden onto someone else. Eventually, though, blaming oneself.

- Bargaining: Seeking to change the situation through good behaviour.

- Acceptance and integration: A more optimistic and positive mindset emerges – acceptance that change is inevitable. The last part of the process is the integration of feelings of hope and trust.

For someone facing a terminal illness, the journey involves exploring a series of self-knowledge processes that aim to bring realisation, acceptance and peace towards the end. Ross described them as defence or coping mechanisms for all concerned (today, experts in this field have expanded the stages to include 'yearning' and, finally, 'meaning').

From here on, I would like you to think about the KRCC in the context of lifestyle change relating to health. Take a moment to study the change curve, before reading on.

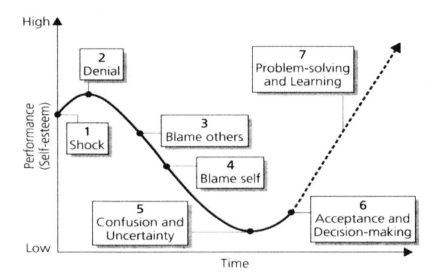

Normally, I would introduce the change curve in a group situation which allows for a full exploration of ideas and enables people to hear other views and exchange their thoughts. We would start by asking the question: "With respect to your weight, where are you on the change curve? Are you still shocked about your weight or perhaps there are some that are still in denial about their weight?" These are important questions that are difficult to answer without extensive consideration, and the group dynamic is a potent catalyst for open and meaningful discussion. We would discuss all seven of the stages of the curve, but, in my experience, discussion seems to disproportionately centre around the stages of blame. Once the corporate world and the government and schools and supermarkets had been blamed, it always saddened me to hear people blaming themselves for their size. Correcting this is a key milestone in anyone's weight-management journey.

One of the important conclusions that I hoped the group would reach (and that you, too, will reach), is that, where your weight is concerned, if you are trapped on the left-hand side of the curve (stage 5 and below), a successful outcome is very unlikely, and weight-loss attempts will probably end this time as they always have before. Furthermore, my hope is always that the KRCC workshop results in the realisation that significant life changes unavoidably set in motion profound transformations in our thoughts and beliefs. The critical aspect of this is that this is a bi-directional effect and, crucially, profound transformations in our thoughts and beliefs set in motion significant lifestyle changes. These paradigm changes to thoughts and beliefs will only arise from considerable inward searching, reflection and an exploration of the self, if you are to achieve the self-realisation needed for lasting change.

Now would be a good time to revisit your notes regarding the reasons that you think you are overweight (Insight 2) and your acceptance of these reasons (Insight 3). This, if done with absolute candour, represents stage 6 on the curve. You are now preparing for the journey that is stage 7 on the KRCC, which is problem-solving and learning. In terms of *Weight Wisdom*, this represents Insight 5 – The roadmap.

Dealing with trauma or grief

Trying to manage personal foibles while dealing with trauma or grief is very difficult, and at times impossible. A constant yearning to deal with this pain offers a rationale for wayward behaviour, and impedes healing, growth and development. Ignoring or suppressing feelings relating to trauma or grief is not advisable, and so seeking help to overcome such emotions is highly recommended. If you suspect your weight is connected to personal difficulties in the past or emotional pain and suffering over years, then this must be the focus of your recovery before trying to concentrate on matters of body weight. A trusted friend may be a starting point, or you may wish to consider professional counselling as an option. Your doctor may be able to arrange for you to attend a grief-counselling service or other talking therapies.

Readiness to change

Goals, priorities, incentives, motivation and willpower (summarised as 'need') are all required for change, but there is another ingredient required, which is that you must believe in your ability to change. This is called self-efficacy. A simple formula to express this idea is need + self-efficacy = readiness to change. We touched on this earlier when I asked the question:

■ How important is it for you to change? (need)

■ How confident are you that you could change if you decided to? (self-efficacy)

One of the most frequent grievances I would hear from people attending a programme, would relate to their motivation and self-efficacy: "Why am

I just so rubbish at sticking with anything?" This is perhaps the biggest challenge facing anyone intent on significant change. Resistance to change is often a sign of low self-efficacy and this can result from looking too far into the future or expanding the task way beyond the brief. For someone that would benefit from being less sedentary, they may well think: "I can't possibly see myself becoming a fitness freak!" Sometimes, people with low self-efficacy make negative and possibly unrealistic predictions about the future ("I'll probably do it once or twice and then give up"). They often focus on the memory of prior relapses without considering periods of adherence to exercise when things were going well.

But we all know of (ordinary) people that have achieved amazing things, and we think of them as awesome individuals who are in total control with high self-efficacy and huge dollops of motivational drive. But they don't think of themselves in that way, and they will often say: "If I can do it, anyone can!" And they really mean it, and they are 100% correct to say so, because they have no more motivation or drive than you or me, it's just that they have managed to engage their brains in a way that follows the logic of getting what they want.

One of the goals of therapy is to elicit 'change talk', as it is important for the client to hear themselves talking about change, which can be the first step towards making change. It's tricky when you are reading a book, but you should still have these discussions, but instead of having them with a practitioner, you will be having them with yourself. Stay neutral, avoid confrontation and argumentation, and always have empathy with the other opinion. It might seem odd at first but try it and see how it works out (obviously, try to do this in a place where people are not going to see you and think that you are going off your rocker). To help you to understand how reasoning and probing can and does help clients to think differently, here is a typical motivational interviewing exchange in just such a situation:

Practitioner:	"So, tell me, what part of becoming more active seems most impossible?"
Betty:	"I just don't think I'll be able to keep it up if I start. I'll just relapse again. It happens every time."
Practitioner:	"Would it be OK if we examined that statement a bit more closely?"
Betty:	"Sure. It's just that I've always relapsed, every time I start, I always stop."

Practitioner:	"So, you've had many relapses before, I understand… but when you say: 'It happens every time', this means that you have been active quite often. What if we were to add up all the good exercise days that you have had, I would think that this would be quite a total?"
Betty:	"Well, quite some time ago I was in good shape, and then periodically here and there I've done OK. I went on a walking holiday in my forties once, and while I was worried about it beforehand, actually it was OK."
Practitioner:	"So, some good successes over the years – is that right?"
Betty:	"Yeah, I just wish I could stick with it."
Practitioner:	"So, when you did get it to stick previously, how did you do it?"
Betty:	"I suppose back then I was fitter and had more energy so it wasn't as hard, so I could keep up with it."
Practitioner	"I see, so I'm wondering if it is just a matter of getting the right programme that is right for you at the moment."
Betty:	"Yes, if I felt it was manageable, then that would be a big help. I think if I could keep it up, then I would be happier to give it a go."

At this point, I should remind you that lapses and relapses are to be expected and are a normal part of the process of change. Lapses are to be embraced and considered opportunities for learning. Why did I lapse? What led to it? What was the trigger? What can I do to avoid this in the future, and when it does happen, how can I get back on track quicker? Each setback therefore contributes to the solid platform upon which to build sustainable change for the future.

A further goal of relapse prevention is to not only reduce the incidence of lapses, but to decrease the likelihood that brief lapses will become relapses, and that relapses will become collapses. The core of relapse management is to have a detailed exploration of the chain of events leading up to the episode, and this must be very specific to be useful. This is often uncomfortable to do, but if you do lapse or relapse, I can't tell you how important it is to think very carefully and to document all the preceding events that lead to it, so that you have a better understanding of what led you there. This will help you the next time lapses threaten.

Also, bear in mind that the all-or-nothing thinking of ambivalence is not conducive to change. Remember the use of experiments to test beliefs and attitudes which avoid the sink-or-swim dilemma. Rather than taking something on where there is huge pressure to make it work, you can instead take part in a 'trial' in which the outcome is unknown (that is what experiments are). The purpose is not to see if you can continue forever, but instead to see what will happen and how you will feel if you go just once or twice. This approach is less threatening and will allow you to put yourself in new situations with an open mind as to the outcome.

In Betty's case, she may have been apprehensive about joining a walking group because of how it would make her feel. She may also be harbouring thoughts that others in the group would reject her or that she would not fit in, and that she would feel awkward. The experiment could be to attend a walking group to see how this made Betty and others in the group feel. This may seem challenging for Betty, but what is almost certain to happen, is that if she does turn up, she won't feel awkward, nor will any of the other people in the group. No amount of reassuring Betty – "No one will feel awkward" – will make any difference, she must experience it, and this is the power of behavioural experiments. This is worth thinking about if you have reservations about doing something that you are harbouring negative thoughts about. Rather than think, "I really must start swimming again" (big call, I could swim, or I could sink), why not think, "I'll go to the pool just once and see how I feel after that" (no pressure).

Be prepared for the bad days

Having a bad day can send us off track and this is far more likely if we have not prepared for the predictable faltering day or two. When this does happen, we feel bad because we have not performed how we wanted to. This feeling down is a prompt from the superego to remedy the situation, but people often interpret this to mean they have failed, and it can lead to feelings of 'totally losing the plot' and letting all our plans for progress turn to dust. We need to realise that 'feeling bad' about not performing well is a rational emotional response. The uncomfortable emotions of guilt and shame conjured by the conscience part of the superego are urging us to respond appropriately. In this scenario, you could either:

A. Go on a binge to make yourself feel better (the id wins and pleasure-seeking to soothe the self is chosen). The dire consequences are, for now, kicked into the long grass and the principle of delay discounting bolsters the demands of the id to convince the conscious mind that bingeing is the answer to your problems.

B. Recognise the destructive thoughts of the pleasure-seeking, chaotic id proposing that bingeing is the answer. Accept your mistakes and try to salvage the day by making any remaining choices good choices, thus finishing the day feeling back in control. Tomorrow, be proud that you turned things around and are still piloting the ship in the direction of your choice.

The id will push forceful suggestions by creating powerful urges, while the superego will try to counter by making you feel bad. But your conscious mind (ego) must always make the final call. In this way, if you are organised, determined and regularly practice and strengthen your conscious control, you can ensure the selfish and childish id doesn't get its way (cage the Pig!)

The Trans Theoretical Model (TTM)

TTM[306] is the most popular stage model in health psychology, and has been an important theoretical advance in understanding health behaviour. Initially developed for use in substance abuse (drugs, smoking and alcohol), in recent years it has been applied to the adherence to positive behaviours such as exercise. TTM describes an individual's movement through stages (in relation to behaviour) from pre-contemplation to relapse. Strictly speaking, it is not a model for change but more a framework for determining if you are ready for change. The stages are:

1. Pre-contemplation – not yet acknowledging that a problem exists.

2. Contemplation – acknowledging the problem but not yet ready to make changes.

3. Preparation – getting ready to change.

4. Action – currently changing behaviour.

5. Maintenance – maintained behaviour change for more than six months.

6. Relapse – which can occur at any time during any stage of change.

The way I have found TTM most helpful is to simply ask my clients where they are on the six-item list with respect to their weight management (or exercise, or diabetes plan, or whatever). It is important to explain the practicalities of such theoretical models in order that the person at the centre of the service can make sense of them. The main points that I would make about TTM are as follows:

- You may remember the lifestyle continuum. TTM is a similar tool, and we don't find ourselves fixed forever on one of the six points. We are merely passing through one stage to another in a continual state of flux for all the activities in our lives.

- Moving between stages is normal and to be expected, and finding yourself in relapse or pre-contemplation about something that you think is important is OK, it happens to everyone, all the time.

- Being aware that laziness, apathy or intransigence has nothing to do with not moving through the stages, these are not reasons for inertia. What normally pushes us off course are other priorities, and for whatever reason, our target behaviour isn't sufficiently important now, compared to the myriad of other competing priorities to warrant a move up the scale. This is also OK.

- Most importantly, recognise that going straight to action is not required. If you have gone from stage one to two over the last couple of weeks (or months), that's fantastic (success is a journey etc...)

TTM is flexible and can be applied to the multiple changes to behaviour that would typically be associated with pursuing a new goal. For instance, if I took the fanciful notion of becoming a Tibetan yak herder, then if I really wanted to do it, I'd have to commit to learning a lot of new skills, such as: building dung fires, butchery, yak eating, embracing Buddhism, mastering difficult equestrian skills, learning the Tibetic language, nomadic camp building... in fact, I'd have to become a 'yak of all trades!' – sorry about that one!

Now while I'd be quite motivated to do some of these things because they appealed to me, others (butchery and yak eating), I imagine, would be pretty challenging, and so straight away I can feel my motivation waning for these tasks. I'm drifting into pre-contemplation over the yak slaughtering, while I focus on the more engaging aspects of Tibetan hill life such as Buddhism and horse riding. But I can't do the job without the other skills, so I need to figure out how I can move from pre-contemplation to, at the very least, contemplation for the things that don't appeal to me.

At this point, I would suggest that the best course of action would be to set out a strategy to tackle the behaviours to which I know I have an aversion. I need to have a plan to move me from pre-contemplation to contemplation, then to preparation, and finally to action. I'm simply not going to pick up a knife and kill the poor yak – I would think that this would almost certainly put an end to my potential new career. Fortunately (though not for the yak), I have a method for helping me to move through the stages of change on page 211. There is no need to visit that now, suffice to say you can practise using this when tackling your own challenges, and planning your personal strategies for change. For now, the message is: don't just jump into changes without ensuring you have fully thought everything through.

Another important lesson you can take from TTM is that you must be sure to consider each of the multiple behaviours in isolation, rather than thinking where you are in relation to starting your weight-loss programme. Where am I in relation to removing CRAP from my life? Where am I in relation to preparing more of my own food? Where am I in relation to my plan for weekly intermittent fasting? Where am I in relation to my exercise programme? This is vital in that it allows you to think individually about each behaviour, some of which you will find easier than others. It is also very important that you plan to implement them gradually and not all at once. There is no pressure to start everything immediately, in fact this may be too overwhelming.

To understand TTM better, it is easier to apply it to a real-life situation. Take a moment to think where you are with respect to a few different aspects of your many life ambitions. These could be anything: managing finances, using less energy round the house, exercising, recycling, healthy eating or reading more. In fact, anything that you have thought to do that might improve your life (or the lives of others) in some way. Think of a few behaviours that you feel need to be involved in your weight-loss strategy and make a note of where you are on the TTM for each. Notice how you will be at different stages for each and remember that this probably will change as time goes by.

Now pick just one of your aims and consider whether you are ready to move along to the next stage, from, say, contemplation to preparation, and if so, ask yourself, what would it take to make that move? What would have to be in place and what other things may have to give way? What adjustments in my life would I have to make, and what can I expect if I do move along? What is holding me up? Are there any barriers that I need to overcome first? Over the next few days, you can continue to think about this and hopefully you will start to put in place some of the adjustments that will facilitate your move to the next stage of change, but only when you are ready. TTM is just another way of helping you think about all the things that are going on in your life, and how you can best manage them all.

Decisional balance

Decisional balance (same as cost-benefit analysis) is the assessment of the perceived advantages weighed against the disadvantages of a behaviour. It compares the anticipated benefits and drawbacks of change against those of not changing. Someone in the pre-contemplation or contemplation stages of readiness to change, probably perceives that the negatives far outweigh the positives. At the preparation stage, perceptions of the positives and negatives are roughly equal, and, at the action or maintenance stages, the perceived positives probably outweigh the negatives. From this, we can conclude that there is a shift in perception as a person moves through the stages (the benefits seem greater, or the barriers seem lower).

If you are thinking of a behaviour (contemplation stage), you may find the decisional balance matrix helpful. Simply put in the boxes the pros and cons of either change or no change, to help you decide if change will be worthwhile. This can be helpful, as most people don't consider the drawbacks or the costs of not changing, which are often very high.

Decisional Balance Sheet

	Disadvantages	Advantages
No Change		
Change		

The Health Belief Model (HBM)

The Health Belief Model is worth considering when a health condition is driving the need for change. HBM examines core beliefs to determine if change is likely. The theoretical requirements are that the client must have a certain level of knowledge about their condition, as well as an acceptance of the impact that it has upon their life. A further important requisite belief is that the client feels vulnerable or threatened by the condition. To better understand HBM, think about a health condition (or you can use your weight as a 'condition') and then work through the questions below, and try to work out why HBM states that it is necessary to satisfy yourself that you agree with each belief.

If you don't agree with one of the indicators, try to get to the bottom of why you disagree. Test your beliefs through research and learning and by discussing them with other people that you trust. Remember, the answers to all of this are within you, and while others can help to bring them into focus, ultimately you must find the answers.

According to HBM, if you can answer yes to all the following, you are in a good place to progress your change plans with respect to your condition:

- Do I possess sufficient knowledge about my condition – do I understand it properly?
- Do I view the condition as threatening and see myself as vulnerable?
- Do I have confidence that I can perform the required 'change actions' adequately?
- Do I believe that it will be beneficial for me if I can make these changes?
- Do I have time to do what's required?
- Do I believe that I can overcome the barriers facing me?

Working through these six points should provide you with another indicator of your proximity to change, and help to answer the question: "Are my current beliefs compatible with my desire for change, and is it likely I will be able to change?"

Cognitive Behavioural Therapy (CBT)

Certain ways of thinking can be destructive, and CBT aims to modify these patterns under the premise that our thoughts (or cognitions) are malleable, so we can control their sequence and substance. This enables us to change our judgements and reach more helpful decisions and conclusions, which in turn enables us to act differently. Thus, CBT helps people to think less negatively, which helps to overcome problems such as anxiety, depression, panic, phobias and stress, supporting them to change behavioural course.

CBT aims to modify the dysfunctional or unhelpful thoughts that uphold the unwanted behaviour. For instance, depression is maintained by characteristic depressive thoughts and assumptions about oneself, the world and the future. In bulimia nervosa, the 'dysfunctional' maintaining mechanism is the judgement of self-worth in terms of shape or weight: "Everyone is judging me by my weight, and unless I become super skinny, my life will have no value". People can become trapped in these negative and damaging beliefs, which feed the harmful behaviours leading to illness and undermining mental health.

Part of learning about ourselves involves questioning our beliefs and the ideas that are in our heads. When dysfunctional thoughts come along, as they always will (generated by feelings from the selfish id), you must forensically examine them. Is this a logical thought? Is it true, or are there other forces at work here? Is there an alternative angle on this? What other thinking routes are open to me and what are the consequences of taking each route?

CBT is orientated to short-term problematic situations and is focused on the present and the future rather than the past. It involves the systematic identification and evaluation of dysfunctional thoughts and assumptions, with the participant active in the change process. The central theme of CBT is that we can choose how to react to a situation. Topics central to CBT are addressing negative thinking, relapse prevention and problem-solving. The diagram of the classic CBT model is an example of how the way someone 'chooses' to think about a situation affects how they feel.

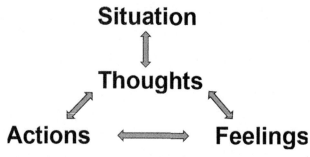

Classic CBT model

	Unhelpful	Helpful
Thoughts	S/he ignored me – they don't like me. I must have really upset them.	S/he looks a bit wrapped up in themselves – I wonder if there's something wrong?
Emotions	Depressed, sad and rejected.	Concerned for the other person – want to help.
Physical feelings	Stomach cramps, low energy, feel sick.	Feel optimistic – I can act positively and help the situation.
Action	Go home and avoid them, stay out of sight for a while.	Get in touch to make sure they're OK, ask if you can help.
Outcome	Isolation for both people.	Build friendship, strengthen support network, feel empowered.

Situation. You're feeling down and so you go for a walk in the park. As you are strolling, someone you know walks by and apparently ignores you. Which way do you choose to think about this?

CBT can help to make sense of overwhelming problems by breaking them down into smaller parts and identifying the connections between the problem and its effects. How a person thinks about a situation can affect how they feel physically and emotionally, and therefore can determine the actions they may take, thus impacting the final outcome. There are helpful and unhelpful ways of reacting to most situations, depending on how someone thinks about them.

For example, negative thoughts (the unhelpful column on the left) can set in motion a vicious cycle: negative thoughts → negative emotions → feel physically bad → harmful actions → negative thoughts, and so on. This leads to self-deprecation, and, when distressed, we are more likely to jump to the wrong conclusions and interpret things in extreme and unhelpful ways. In contrast, the outcome of the helpful column on the right is likely to be a sense of wellbeing and positivity.

CBT teaches people that they have a choice about how they think about things through 'thought chaperoning', and that, by practising positive thinking, they can avoid the negative path that can lead to the dark places that people find themselves in. If you recognise your thoughts taking you in a negative direction, stop and challenge the thought process and then change the way you consider the situation.

CATCH IT → CHECK IT → CHANGE IT

Here are some examples of self-defeating and destructive thoughts, alongside more productive options, should you choose to take them:

☹ I feel silly praising myself when I have achieved something.

☺ I'm learning how my brain works and I see how praise and recognition will strengthen my resolve and help me in the future.

☹ I ate something I didn't want to, so the rest of the day is cancelled in terms of being healthy.

☺ That didn't go well back there. Ah well, I'll try to do things differently next time and I'll make sure the rest of the day goes better.

☹ I can't inconvenience other people in the family by not having CRAP in the house.

☺ How inconvenient to everyone will it be if I'm a physical and emotional wreck because of my weight?

☹ I just can't resist sometimes.

☺ I know I don't get it right every time, but every time I will try.

☹ I have the right to eat whatever I want.

☺ I deserve to eat the foods that will make me happy and healthy.

☹ I hate wasting food, so I must eat it all.

☺ I need better plans to recycle food so it does not get wasted, and so that I don't have the excuse to eat more than I need.

☹ I don't think I can keep making all the sacrifices.

☺ I'm not thrilled about giving up some of the things I like, but it sure beats the alternative.

Rational Emotive Behavioural Therapy

REBT is really an extension of CBT. According to the theory of REBT, humans are happiest when we have life goals and purposes, and we actively strive to attain them. Therefore, 'being rational', in REBT, means things that help people achieve their goals, and 'irrational' means actions that prevent this. REBT reminds us that putting oneself first (to achieve our goals) sometimes requires putting others a close second, and this is OK (unlike the philosophy of selfishness, where the desires of others are neither regarded nor respected)[307].

REBT posits that there are no higher powers (such as those involved in religion), stating that devout belief in higher beings can foster dependency and increase emotional disturbance. The focus of REBT is on free will and personal choice. REBT borrows ideas from the teachings of some of the ancient philosophers (Confucious, Loa-Tsu and Gautama Buddha), who state that people are disturbed not by things or events around them, but by their view of those events and the way they think about them. Therefore, it is *how* we think about or interpret external incidents that brings emotional distress.

Getting what we want brings positive feelings and emotions, and this is both rational and pragmatic, but when we don't get what we want, the opposite is true. These are healthy responses that don't interfere with the pursuit of our goals. Irrational beliefs differ and tend to be absolute or dogmatic, expressed as rigid 'musts', 'shoulds', 'oughts' etc., and interfere with normal, flexible thinking, derailing our goals through negative emotions such as anger, anxiety and guilt. Ultimately, this leads to emotional disturbance and self-defeatism. However, like CBT, REBT holds that humans have the power of choice to change their dysfunctional thinking through realising the disturbance caused by their irrational beliefs. In many cases, dysfunctional beliefs are reflected as absolutes, as in "I must", "I should" or "I can't".

- I need to be perfect to be valued by others and achieve self-acceptance.

- The challenges and conflicts in my life prove that I don't deserve happiness.

- I have no control over my own contentment, others will determine this.

Unyielding beliefs of this nature leave little room for healthy responses to problems and can only result in disappointment and emotional distress. During therapy, these rigid patterns of thinking are challenged to help people respond rationally to situations that would typically cause emotional upset. Some of the key concepts are:

- You are worthy of self-acceptance no matter what, even when you struggle or make mistakes; there is no need for shame or guilt.

- Others are also worthy of acceptance, even when their behaviour in your eyes is poor.

- Negative things happen in life – it's not positive all the time. There's no rational reason to expect it to be.

REBT, like CBT, helps you to: identify the activating event → figure out beliefs that led to your negative feelings → change those beliefs → thereby changing the emotional response[308].

A: Activating event – something external in the environment around you.

B: Belief – your thoughts about the event or situation.

C: Consequence – your emotional response to your belief.

Motivational Interviewing (MI)

Motivational interviewing evolved from experience in the treatment of alcohol abuse and was first described in an article published in *Behavioural Psychotherapy* in 1983[309]. It is a technique that, by definition, requires two parties, but an understanding of MI helps us to think more clearly about how we reach our own conclusions. I believe MI is the only realistic approach to supporting change in someone else (you, in this case). It wraps comfortably around all the previous techniques we have covered.

Most people are ambivalent about changing their behaviour, and say, "Yes, but…" Their approach (to avoid conflict) is common, such as, "I want to do more exercise, but I feel embarrassed that everyone will be looking at me". The classic dilemma for everyone facing behavioural challenges is ambivalence; they want to change, and at the same time they don't want to change. Ambivalence (which is normal and to be expected) is one of the things that keep people stuck and unable to make lifestyle changes, even when they want to.

The theory of MI assumes that all clients are ambivalent and says that, if you fail to explore your own ambivalence, then your resistance to change will be predictable. To oversimplify a little, if you were not ambivalent, it would be easy for you to change. The reality is that people have powerful reasons for continuing their current behaviour. Here are the common one's people have told me about why they keep eating CRAP foods:

- It feels and tastes good, so why should I give it up?
- It improves my mood and helps me when I'm down.
- It helps me to escape my problems and takes away the pain.
- It's convenient and suits my busy life.
- It has become a way of life and I don't think I can change now.

Ambivalence is normal, and those embarking upon change who don't adequately address their ambivalence will run into trouble. People I have met that have enrolled on a programme will tell me they are 'underway' with change, and they are already well on the way to their promised land. They avidly pronounce that they will never eat CRAP again! But if, when you probe about what they see as the benefits of eating CRAP, they tell you, "Nothing, it's awful and killing me", then I would wonder why they were here!

But, of course, they have not fully explored their ambivalence. Instead, they are just brushing it under the carpet, which frees them from the pain of considering the problem fully. They fear that, if they 'admit' that CRAP foods have had an important role in their lives (and still have a significant charge over them), this may somehow compel them to return to that relationship. Their flawed strategy is to imagine that none of it ever happened and that CRAP will lose its potency just because they want it to – but this naive approach is just wishful thinking. You must confront your ambivalence and thoroughly test all your beliefs that are holding you in a state of inertia.

Motivation for change occurs when there is a perceived discrepancy between behaviour and goals. The spirit of MI requires that motivation to change must come from the client, but the practitioner supports the client's self-efficacy through guidance and affirmations. It is for the client to articulate and resolve their own ambivalence (the practitioner merely guides them to consider each side of the case). It is the practitioner's task to help to reveal both sides of the ambivalence and develop the discrepancy between what the client wants and how they are acting, and to keep returning to this until the client can see with clarity the conflict between their wants and their actions.

If current behaviours are acting as barriers to goals, MI gently and gradually guides people to the realisation that this incompatibility must be addressed. In MI, the practitioner does not fight client resistance, but 'rolls with it' and fosters a belief that the solutions to the defined problems are entirely within the grasp of the client. Practitioners invite clients to examine new perspectives, but do not impose new ways of thinking. The practitioner maintains an absolute belief that the client will succeed and uses this to build their confidence. There is no right or wrong way to change, only the client's way.

In contrast some health practitioners habitually try to change patient behaviour through 'expert-driven direct persuasion', which seldom works and which has the potential to progress into destructive disagreement, resulting in increased resistance to change. Direct persuasion, confrontation and coercive approaches, are the theoretical opposite of MI. The principle of MI is a strong therapeutic alliance, where the practitioner and the client share equal authority in helping to resolve ambivalence to change. The practitioner above all else values client autonomy regarding their own destiny, and the central idea behind MI is that the practitioner guides the client to find the answers that are within them.

Many years ago, while working as a guest lecturer at the University of Chester on their MSc programme, I had the great pleasure and privilege of sharing a platform with the esteemed psychologist Everard Thornton. His profound understanding of MI and its application afforded him the status of 'legend' in my eyes. Everard's eloquent summary of MI and behaviour change ought to be enshrined in its teaching. He recounted to those fortunate enough to be present:

> "I would say to my patients, imagine I am holding in front of you a huge bunch of keys. One of these keys certainly will unlock the difficulties that you are having. But you must find that key, because only you can."

Case study – Harry

Harry was a lovely man. I often wonder how he is getting on. He was part of a men-only weight-management programme that I was managing on behalf of Portsmouth Primary Care Trust many years ago. Harry was an older gentleman, and sadly he had recently been bereaved from his wife of forty-five years. Harry had relied more or less entirely on his wife for meals, and now that he was on his own, he was struggling. From memory, here is an excerpt from our initial consultation:

Me: "Hi, Harry, lovely to meet you. So, tell me a little about what brings you here."

Harry: "My doctor suggested I come. Since my wife passed, I go to the café most days for breakfast and sometimes lunch. Also, I find I'm having lots of takeaways. I've always been a big lad, but over the last twelve months, I'd say I've put on two or three stones."

Me: "Tell me, Harry, why do you think that you are spending so much time eating out?"

Harry: "I'm bored, I think, and I'm not very good at cooking myself – I've never done it much. Anyway, I don't think it's worthwhile just cooking for myself."

Me: "I see, are there any other reasons that you think that your weight has increased so much recently?"

Harry "Well, I've always liked a beer. Since my wife passed, the only thing I really look forward to each day is going to the Derby Tavern for a few jars with the boys. I go most nights."

Me: "And what's your favourite tipple, Harry?"

Harry: "Normally, I have four or five bottles of Newcastle Brown Ale."

Me: "Newkie Brown, lovely!"

Harry "When my wife was alive, she would always tell me to drink less and blamed my weight on the beer. When I saw the doctor, he would also try to get me to cut down on the beer. More recently, I went to see the surgeon about my knee which is getting worse. He told me the beer was not helping with my weight either and that with the inflammation and the extra weight, this was putting more pressure on my knee."

Me:	"I see, Harry. Is there anything else that you think is important about your weight and anything that you think could help you to lose some weight."
Harry:	"Well, since my knee has got worse, I can't really walk that far. In fact, I'm so worried that if it gets any worse, I won't be able to make it down to the Derby, at which point I may as well pack up, as that's all I've got left these days. It already takes me fifteen minutes each way, and I've got to sit on a wall halfway. I'm sure if I could be more active I could shift some of this weight and things would be a lot better."
Me:	"OK, Harry, thanks for talking that through with me. In that case, why don't we get a plan together to get you more active?"
Harry:	"OK."
Me:	"I've got an idea that I'd like to share with you. I have a couple of home exercise bikes that I lend out. We could set one up at your house in front of the telly, and you could have a little peddle every day while you watch Countdown? Did you know that exercise bikes are good for knees in that they don't have any impact or loading on the knee, and you can just go at your own pace. How does that sound?"
Harry:	"Sounds champion."
Me:	"Well, that's great, one of our instructors will bring the bike round this week and he will show you how to use it and give you a programme that you can follow. Just start very gently and slowly build up. If you have any pain in your knee, then I would use a bag of ice after each session to calm it down. If it persists, you could ask your pharmacist for something for the pain and swelling. All OK?"
Harry:	"Yes, that's all OK."
Me:	"Great, Harry. Well, it's been lovely meeting you today, and I'm really looking forward to seeing you again on Wednesday at the group meeting. I'm sure you are really going to fit in well with the other chaps, they are a great bunch and we have lots of laughs. I'll see you Wednesday night."

And so Harry started the programme and came along faithfully each week. A popular member of the group, Harry would keep our spirits up and entertain us with his stories and jokes. I kept an eye on Harry's progress, and sure enough, each week, half-a-kilo here, quarter-of-a-kilo there, he was progressing nicely. After about twelve weeks (and three to four kilos of weight loss), Harry called me over:

Harry:	"Alan, can I have a word?"
Me:	"Sure, Harry, what can I help with?"
Harry:	"Well, something's been bothering me. I can't stop wondering why you haven't asked me to stop drinking yet?"
Me:	"Tell me, Harry, when your wife asked you to stop, did you?"
Harry:	"No."
Me:	"What about when your doctor asked?"
Harry:	"No."
Me:	"What about when the knee surgeon asked?"
Harry:	"No."
Me:	"Then why would I ask you? The point is, Harry, you know what is best for you, because no one knows you like you do. You figured out what was right for you, and of course you were right. You have lost loads of weight and, as you say, your knee is so much better from the cycling. That was your idea to get more active, it just happened that I had a spare bike."

Several more weeks went by, and Harry told me that he had made a few changes to his pub routine and was now enjoying just two or three brown ales each night. I was delighted to hear that he was also having breakfast at home and cooking himself a couple of meals each week. Harry had found his path, and he was surely walking it.

Insight 5: The roadmap

The answers to Insight 5 are to be found in Insights 1 and 2. Visit your notes and think about what will have to change in your life to become the person that you want to be. Be truthful and write down what you think are the most important differences between your life now and the one that will be permanently free from the weight difficulties that you currently endure. Be specific about the choices and behaviours that will need to change. For now, don't think about how easy or difficult or how likely these changes may be, simply put down the facts of what needs to change. These are the causalities.

THE CAUSALITIES (things) THAT WILL HAVE TO (PERMANENTLY) CHANGE IN MY LIFE TO ACHIEVE MY GOALS ARE...

A strategy for change

Throughout the book, we have examined weight gain and the thoughts that surround it in considerable detail, and I hope that you have learned a lot about your own weight and your relationship with it. It would be wrong of me to conclude that you have now taken the decision to lose weight, and even if you have, it might be that you are minded that now is not the right time to start. Nonetheless, you may have decided that the time is right to start your weight-loss journey, and I hope that this is the case; if so, *Weight Wisdom* has achieved the first part of its objective. But remember what we learned earlier: decisions are ephemeral and don't always lead to lasting change. It is learning and development that changes our behaviours, and subsequently alters the life course. For this reason, your approach must always be one of enquiry and curiosity, constantly seeking to learn more about yourself as your journey unfolds, because I can guarantee that this will not be a straightforward or predictable route you are about to tread.

If you wish to change, first we must make a strategy for change, because up until now, throughout the entire book, we have merely contemplated whether you believe you need to change, want to change, or are ready for change. If you have now reached the conclusions that you need to, want to and are ready to change, then you must set out your plans in detail. Changing behaviour, especially modifying ingrained long-term habits, is not easy and requires practise and a strategic approach. The important qualities of resolve and fortitude can only flourish in a supportive framework for change that has been carefully and thoroughly thought through. You have all the critical insight and knowledge about your weight; now you must weave this into a strategy for change.

Through the Five Insights, you now understand why you are overweight, and this you know is the truth. Insights 2 and 5 detail the causalities and the changes that you must make if you are to achieve your goals, and permanently escape the weight difficulties that are currently yours to endure. You are aware that these changes hold the key to the future that you are seeking, and that without change, in all these behaviours, you will always be overweight, and perhaps increasingly overweight as each year passes. Now is the time to accept that this is the binary choice that it all boils down to. Do I change, or do I stay the same?

Close your eyes, gently breathe, and feel how your breath gives you life. Look inward and find the calmness that is everywhere within. Now seek the inner strength that is building and use it to empower your mind. Concentrate on your breathing, feel the tranquillity and simplicity that it brings, think about your journey and what it means to you, feel the strength that lies within. Practise this every day. Use this when you feel tempted to stray, use it when you feel stressed, apply it when you need direction – feel the breath, find the calm, use the strength.

Below is a simple framework to remind you of some of the important steps when planning change. You may be happier with your own methodologies but look at some of the ideas in the framework and see if you think they would be useful to give you more structure and support. The insight work that you have already done forms the foundations for this summary exercise. This is a final reminder of some of the key points, and, as you are now aware, you cannot make changes to established behaviours unless you fully understand them. The deeper that this understanding develops, the more the power moves away from the behaviour and moves closer to you. You cannot revisit these thoughts and beliefs too many times.

Some of this may seem repetitive, and that's the idea. Each time you cover a point from a slightly different angle, you will observe it with a little more clarity, and your perspective may just move a little, perhaps sufficiently to help you see things somewhat differently than you did previously. When confusion and uncertainty are holding you back, then the process of thinking things over and over until certainty emerges is the only option available. Remember, change is not about saying, "I won't do that again" and imagining that this will be the case. Change is about learning and developing. Write out a framework of exactly how you will achieve change, be prepared to modify it, and let it evolve as you learn and grow alongside your plans. Change is ongoing: "Tomorrow, once again, I'll walk down the path I have chosen".

Keep in mind that changing behavioural habits (going to bed late) is different to tackling dietary changes (no more sugary fizzy drinks), and this is because eating and appetite are controlled in a far more complex way than other adopted behavioural habits. Therefore, practising changing more straightforward habits first is a great way of preparing yourself for the more challenging dietary changes that will no doubt be required. For this reason, you may feel happier starting with what you see as the more manageable changes at first and you should think carefully about this. Most importantly, before you consider any change, be sure that you can answer yes to the following question: "If I make this change, is it realistic, and am I committing to it becoming a lifelong change?"

A framework for change

Step 1: Write down the habit you would like to change.

Step 2: Why did it start? Revisit Insight 2, Part 1. Write it down to remind yourself.

Step 3: Now, draw the following table and complete the decisional balance matrix. This will establish the incentive and develop motivation.

Current Behaviour		Changed Behaviour	
Benefits	Drawbacks/ costs	Benefits	Drawbacks/ costs

Step 4: What is maintaining the behaviour? Insight 2, Part 2 – revisit and remind yourself.

Step 5: On a scale of 1-10, how important is it that you make this change? (Consider this alongside the big picture of everything that is going on in your life.)

Step 6: On a scale of 1-10, how confident are you that you can make this change? (A measure of your self-efficacy for this task currently.)

Step 7: Revisit the Trans Theoretical Model and consider if you need to move from one stage to another before attempting change. Are you at the preparation stage?

Step 8: What are the barriers to making this change? (List as many as you can and be completely honest. Think creatively and don't brush over this one. Consider each carefully.)

> **Step 9:** Can you think of any ideas that may help you overcome these barriers? (These need to be realistic and achievable; they will need resourcing.)
>
> **Step 10:** What will the personal cost be of failing to make this change? (Perhaps the most important question of the exercise. Most people never consider the cost of inaction.)
>
> **Step 11:** How will I deal with the inevitable lapses? Make sure you have plans and expect lapses to occur.

Available to download at www.weightwisdom.co.uk

Now make a plan

You know the drill – if you fail to plan, you plan to fail! Take your list of causalities from Insights 2 and 5 and plan how you will tackle each required change. Don't lump them all together, but have clear proposals for how you will go about each change. Perhaps rank them in order of priority and start with the more manageable changes first. Don't attempt them all at once, this journey does not need you to be fired from a cannon to start. Tackling everything at once could be overwhelming – you have all the time in the world; take small steps and target one each week and focus totally on the one change until you feel you are able to tackle the next.

By way of example, some of the things you should be considering in the development of your plans (let's say the example to tackle the CRAP in your diet):

- Identify it – what is your interpretation of CRAP – what needs to go?
- How much will go? All of it? Some of it?
- Why is it in your life and house? Who else is it for? Do they need it? Have you discussed it with them?
- What will replace it?
- Is there a time cost? Is there a financial cost? Is there an emotional cost? How will you fund each? What resources do you need?
- What is your buying, shopping, storing, cooking strategy?
- How will you plan for others around you and how might they be impacted?

- Have you planned for lapses and relapses? Relapse is part of the process of change.

- Do you have your emergency action plan clear in your mind?

- Do you have reminders and prompts to keep yourself on track?

- Have you thought about how you will monitor progress?

This is the business end of the programme, and it is the part of the journey where only you can find the way. Here are some other things that you need to be aware of:

High-risk situations

Identifying high-risk situations and circumstances that increase the risk of relapse is an essential skill when in change mode. External high-risk situations are people, places or food cues, and uncomfortable feelings or states such as fatigue, loneliness, boredom and anxiety. Therefore, being aware of high-risk people and places and having plans for when you encounter them is very important, as is improving your ability to identify internal feelings that have previously led to lapses.

Risky relapse situations are individual to each person, but common risks abound such as being alone (or out of sight of family and friends) in the presence of lots of food. For many people, frequent socialising makes moderation very difficult. Often, relapse is the result of an upsetting or emotional event, and this is obviously difficult to avoid, but an awareness that it is likely to be a trigger can act to be pre-emptive. As has been mentioned, excessive TV viewing is a passive activity that is highly associated with boredom, snacking and overconsumption, and a common catalyst for relapse.

I think now would be a good time to list all the people, places and events around which you think might lead you to temptation. This list does not mean that you must avoid these people and places, but it will give you time to prepare accordingly if they become unavoidable.

Another way of identifying high-risk situations is to keep a daily record of feelings such as cravings or emptiness, noting their intensity (1-10), when they occur, time, place, situation, and your mood or state at the time. In the early stages, I would encourage a constant vigilance of high-risk situations and don't fall for the misleading notion that you can just avoid risky situations – high-risk situations are part of life.

317

Experiment with being hungry and start to get accustomed to the slightly uncomfortable and unusual feelings that hunger brings. This will be an important part of learning to manage the inevitable internal signals of being in a negative energy phase. This is where fasting can help, as it can and will assist in teaching you how to deal with hunger so that you don't simply respond mindlessly when you get these nebulous feelings of want and need.

When in high-risk situations: feel the breath, find the calm, use the strength.

Coping with low-mood states

The relationship between low mood and overeating is well established[310] and it is considered a vicious cycle. The best way to break a vicious cycle is to take one of the wheels off! If low mood is lurking, then immediate action can and often will avert a full-on dark day. Awareness of emotional states and their impact on your ability to control food choices is an important tool in your arsenal. Therefore, if you do find yourself in or moving towards a low state, remember the section on CBT and REBT about 'thought chaperoning': Catch it – Check it – Change it. Practise this daily on small shadows, so that you don't get caught out when a very dark cloud looms.

Distraction techniques can help, and deep breathing and mindfulness is a very powerful tool to derail mood disturbances. Also, try to take some time out if you are feeling stressed and this is adding to your low mood. Taking a walk or doing something active, fun, or engaging are not always possible, but if you can, then they are very effective in defusing the sequence of processes that lead to low mood. Calling a trusted friend or mentor to share sad or angry feelings may be helpful. Challenging negative thoughts and the use of positive self-talk are also helpful during times of stress. Also, developing ways to resolve recurring conflicts can be important if these are a source of regular low mood.

Ineffective problem-solving skills or poor coping abilities can also facilitate maladaptive measures that are underpinning weight, such as using CRAP to cope. Therefore, working to hone problem-solving skills will greatly enhance relapse prevention. In the face of challenging situations or problems, think about breaking them down into their base components, gathering information, generating and evaluating options, and finally planning. Most people feel much more positive and optimistic when they have a plan, in contrast to just worrying and stressing about the problem. All these techniques will give you time to think through your options and provide an alternative to reaching for CRAP.

Building pleasant activities

In circumstances where there has been an over-dependence on CRAP food, or heightened sensory pleasure from eating, or regular episodes of excessive eating, then food and eating may have supplanted some normal life activities. In such cases, it would be risky to withdraw from dysfunctional eating behaviours without having other pleasurable, substitute activities in place to compensate, otherwise a significant void is likely to appear. In addition to having extra time on your hands, the void may be accompanied by feelings of emptiness, loneliness, anxiety or boredom – in other words, high-risk situations. Therefore, developing or rediscovering enjoyable activities, particularly those with a social aspect, will help to occupy time and bring pleasure and satisfaction, which will be an important rock to avoid relapse.

Summary: Well, that was a lot to take in!

I'm sat having a drink with my wife at our regular break-fast on Friday afternoon, and she asks me: "So, how are you going to summarise your book?" "Well," I say, "I can probably do that on the back of that napkin…"

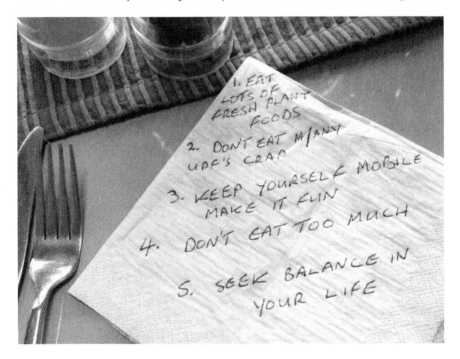

References

1. Lobstein, T., et al., *World Obesity Atlas,* World Obesity Federation, Editor. 2023.
2. Wang, Y., et al., *Will All Americans Become Overweight or Obese? Estimating the Progression and Cost of the US Obesity Epidemic.* Obesity, 2008. **16**(10): p. 2323-2330.
3. Li, M., et al., *Trends in body mass index, overweight and obesity among adults in the USA, the NHANES from 2003 to 2018: a repeat cross-sectional survey.* BMJ Open, 2022. **12**(12): p. e065425.
4. Europe, W.R.O.f., *WHO European Regional Obesity Report,* in *CC BY-NC-SA 3.0 IGO.* 2022: Copenhagen:.
5. Lusk, J.L. and B. Ellison, *Who is to blame for the rise in obesity?* Appetite, 2013. **68**: p. 14-20.
6. Vuorinen, A.L., et al., *Frequency of self-weighing and weight change: a cohort study on 10,000 smart scale users.* J Med Internet Res, 2021.
7. Purcell, K., et al., *The effect of rate of weight loss on long-term weight management: a randomised controlled trial.* The Lancet Diabetes & Endocrinology, 2014.
8. Wicherski, J., S. Schlesinger, and F. Fischer, *Association between Breakfast Skipping and Body Weight-A Systematic Review and Meta-Analysis of Observational Longitudinal Studies.* Nutrients, 2021. **13**(1).
9. Cummins, C.B., et al., *One Size Does Not Fit All: Sociodemographic Factors Affecting Weight Loss in Adolescents.* J Obes, 2020. **2020**: p. 3736504.
10. Dao, M.C., et al., *Association of counselor weight status and demographics with participant weight loss in a structured lifestyle intervention.* Obes Res Clin Pract, 2021. **15**(1): p. 69-72.
11. Finkelstein, E.A., et al., *Obesity and severe obesity forecasts through 2030.* Am J Prev Med, 2012. **42**(6): p. 563-70.
12. d'Errico, M., M. Pavlova, and F. Spandonaro, *The economic burden of obesity in Italy: a cost-of-illness study.* Eur J Health Econ, 2022. **23**(2): p. 177-192.
13. Okunogbe A, et al., *The Economic Impact of Overweight & Obesity in 2020 and 2060* in *World Obesity Federation,* W.O. Federation, Editor. 2022.
14. Borer, K.T., *Why We Eat Too Much, Have an Easier Time Gaining Than Losing Weight, and Expend Too Little Energy: Suggestions for Counteracting or Mitigating These Problems.* Nutrients, 2021. **13**(11).
15. Theis, D.R.Z. and M. White, *Is Obesity Policy in England Fit for Purpose? Analysis of Government Strategies and Policies, 1992-2020.* Milbank Q, 2021. **99**(1): p. 126-170.
16. Zoe Harcome, *The Obesity Epidemic. What caused it, how can we stop it?* 2010: Columbus Publishing Ltd. ISBN 978-1-907797-00-2.
17. Peng, W., et al., *Obesity intervention efforts in China and the 2022 World Obesity Day.* Global Health Journal, 2022. **6**(3): p. 118-121.
18. Pan, X.-F., L. Wang, and A. Pan, *Epidemiology and determinants of obesity in China.* The Lancet Diabetes & Endocrinology, 2021. **9**(6): p. 373-392.
19. Magkos, F., et al., *The Environmental Foodprint of Obesity Obesity.* Obesity, 2020. **28**: p. 73-79.
20. Harris, F., et al., *The Water Footprint of Diets: A Global Systematic Review and Meta-analysis.* Adv Nutr, 2020. **11**(2): p. 375-386.
21. Lares-Michel, M., et al., *Eat Well to Fight Obesity... and Save Water: The Water Footprint of Different Diets and Caloric Intake and Its Relationship With Adiposity.* Front Nutr, 2021. **8**: p. 694775.
22. Freigang, R., et al., *Misclassification of Self-Reported Body Mass Index Categories.* Dtsch Arztebl Int, 2020. **117**(15): p. 253-260.
23. Nevill, A.M., M.J. Duncan, and T. Myers, *NICE's recent guidelines on "the size of your waist" unfairly penalizes shorter people.* Obes Res Clin Pract, 2022. **16**(4): p. 277-280.
24. Leibel, R.L. and J. Hirsch, *Diminished energy requirements in reduced-obese patients.* Metabolism, 1984. **33**(2): p. 164-70.
25. Weinsier, R.L., et al., *Do adaptive changes in metabolic rate favor weight regain in weight-reduced individuals? An examination of the set-point theory.* Am J Clin Nutr, 2000. **72**(5): p. 1088-94.
26. Edwards, K.L., et al., *Impact of starting BMI and degree of weight loss on changes in appetite-regulating hormones during diet-induced weight loss.* Obesity (Silver Spring), 2022. **30**(4): p. 911-919.
27. Oustric, P., et al., *Changes in food reward during weight management interventions – a systematic review.* Obesity Reviews, 2018. **19**(12): p. 1642-1658.
28. Brownell, K.D., et al., *The effects of repeated cycles of weight loss and regain in rats.* Physiol Behav, 1986. **38**(4): p. 459-64.
30. Kanter, R. and B. Caballero, *Global gender disparities in obesity: a review.* Adv Nutr, 2012. **3**(4): p. 491-8.

31. Tsai, S.A., et al., *Gender Differences in Weight-Related Attitudes and Behaviors Among Overweight and Obese Adults in the United States.* American Journal of Men's Health, 2016. **10**(5): p. 389-398.

32. Kemnitz, J.W., *Body weight set point theory.* Bol Asoc Med P R, 1985. **77**(10): p. 438-40.

33. Levin, B.E. and A.A. Dunn-Meynell, *Defense of body weight against chronic caloric restriction in obesity-prone and -resistant rats.* American Journal of Physiology-Regulatory, Integrative and Comparative Physiology, 2000. **278**(1): p. R231-R237.

34. Fildes, A., et al., *Probability of an Obese Person Attaining Normal Body Weight: Cohort Study Using Electronic Health Records.* American Journal of Public Health, 2015. **105**(9): p. e54-e59.

35. Swinburn, B. and G. Egger, *The runaway weight gain train: too many accelerators, not enough brakes.* BMJ, 2004. **329**(7468): p. 736-9.

36. Mendoza-Herrera, K., et al., *The Leptin System and Diet: A Mini Review of the Current Evidence.* Front Endocrinol (Lausanne), 2021. **12**: p. 749050.

37. Zhao, S., et al., *Leptin: Less Is More.* Diabetes, 2020. **69**(5): p. 823-829.

38. Chateau-Degat, M.L., et al., *Cardiovascular burden and related risk factors among Nunavik (Quebec) Inuit: insights from baseline findings in the circumpolar Inuit health in transition cohort study.* Can J Cardiol, 2010. **26**(6): p. 190-6.

39. Key, T.J., et al., *Dietary habits and mortality in 11,000 vegetarians and health conscious people: results of a 17 year follow up.* Bmj, 1996. **313**(7060): p. 775-9.

40. Guenther, P.M., et al., *The Healthy Eating Index-2010 is a valid and reliable measure of diet quality according to the 2010 Dietary Guidelines for Americans.* The Journal of nutrition, 2014. **144**(3): p. 399-407.

41. Martínez-González, M., et al., *A 14-Item Mediterranean Diet Assessment Tool and Obesity Indexes among High-Risk Subjects: The PREDIMED Trial.* PloS one, 2012. **7**: p. e43134.

42. Clarys, P., et al., *Comparison of nutritional quality of the vegan, vegetarian, semi-vegetarian, pesco-vegetarian and omnivorous diet.* Nutrients, 2014. **6**(3): p. 1318-1332.

43. Fiolet, T., et al., *Consumption of ultra-processed foods and cancer risk: results from NutriNet-Santé prospective cohort.* Bmj, 2018. **360**: p. k322.

44. Mohamed Elfadil, O., et al., *Processed Foods - Getting Back to The Basics.* Curr Gastroenterol Rep, 2021. **23**(12): p. 20.

45. Rico-Campà, A., et al., *Association between consumption of ultra-processed foods and all cause mortality: SUN prospective cohort study.* BMJ, 2019. **365**: p. l1949.

46. Srour, B., et al., *Ultra-processed food intake and risk of cardiovascular disease: prospective cohort study (NutriNet-Santé).* BMJ, 2019. **365**: p. l1451.

47. Monteiro, C.A., *Nutrition and health. The issue is not food, nor nutrients, so much as processing.* Public Health Nutrition, 2009. **12**(5): p. 729-731.

48. Kuhnle, G.G., et al., *Association between sucrose intake and risk of overweight and obesity in a prospective sub-cohort of the European Prospective Investigation into Cancer in Norfolk (EPIC-Norfolk).* Public Health Nutr, 2015. **18**(15): p. 2815-24.

49. Lustig, R.H., *Fat Chance The bitter truth about sugar.* 2013, USA: Hudson Street Press.

50. Schlosser, E., *Fast Food Nation.* The true cost of Amarica's Diet. 1998, USA: Houghton Mifflin.

51. Basu, S., et al., *Relationship of soft drink consumption to global overweight, obesity, and diabetes: a cross-national analysis of 75 countries.* Am J Public Health, 2013. **103**(11): p. 2071-7.

52. *Sugar the Facts NHS England.* Available from: https://www.nhs.uk/live-well/eat-well/food-types/how-does-sugar-in-our-diet-affect-our-health/#:~:text=Adults%20should%20have%20no%20more,day%20(5%20sugar%20cubes).

53. Goiana-da-Silva, F., et al., *Projected impact of the Portuguese sugar-sweetened beverage tax on obesity incidence across different age groups: A modelling study.* PLoS Med, 2020. **17**(3): p. e1003036.

54. Fernández Sánchez-Escalonilla, S., C. Fernández-Escobar, and M. Royo-Bordonada, *Public Support for the Imposition of a Tax on Sugar-Sweetened Beverages and the Determinants of Such Support in Spain.* Int J Environ Res Public Health, 2022. **19**(7).

55. Allcott, H., B.B. Lockwood, and D. Taubinsky, *Should We Tax Sugar-Sweetened Beverages? An Overview of Theory and Evidence.* Journal of Economic Perspectives, 2019. **33**(3): p. 202-27.

56. Du, H. and E. Feskens, *Dietary determinants of obesity.* Acta Cardiol, 2010. **65**(4): p. 377-86.

57. Biltoft-Jensen, A., et al., *Defining Energy-Dense, Nutrient-Poor Food and Drinks and Estimating the Amount of Discretionary Energy.* Nutrients, 2022. **14**(7).

58. Gao, M., et al., *Associations between dietary patterns and the incidence of total and fatal cardiovascular disease and all-cause mortality in 116,806 individuals from the UK Biobank: a prospective cohort study.* BMC Medicine, 2021. **19**(1): p. 83.

59. Ng, A.P., M. Jessri, and M.R. L'Abbe, *Using partial least squares to identify a dietary pattern associated with obesity in a nationally-representative sample of Canadian adults: Results from the Canadian Community Health Survey-Nutrition 2015.* PLoS One, 2021. **16**(8): p. e0255415.

60. Ashkan Afshin, e.a., *Health effects of dietary risks in 195 countries, 1990–2017: a systematic analysis for the Global Burden of Disease Study 2017.* 2019. **393**(10184): p. P1958-1972.

61. Murray, C.J.L., et al., *Global burden of 87 risk factors in 204 countries and territories, 1990–2019: a systematic analysis for the Global Burden of Disease Study 2019.* The Lancet, 2020. **396**(10258): p. 1223-1249.

62. Pang, B., et al., *The effectiveness of graphic health warnings on tobacco products: a systematic review on perceived harm and quit intentions.* BMC Public Health, 2021. **21**(1): p. 884.

63. Taillie, L.S., et al., *Do sugar warning labels influence parents' selection of a labeled snack for their children? A randomized trial in a virtual convenience store.* Appetite, 2022. **175**: p. 106059.

64. Richard Johnson, M.D., *The Fat Switch.* 2012, Toledo, OH, USA: Mercola.

65. www.unep.org/thinkeatsave *(accessed June 2020).*

66. Robinson, E., P. Aveyard, and S.A. Jebb, *Is plate clearing a risk factor for obesity? A cross-sectional study of self-reported data in US adults.* Obesity (Silver Spring, Md.), 2015. **23**(2): p. 301-304.

67. Sheen, F., C.A. Hardman, and E. Robinson, *Food waste concerns, eating behaviour and body weight.* Appetite, 2020. **151**: p. 104692.

68. Clark, D. *Household expenditure breakdown in the UK 2020, by decile.* 2022 15/08/2023].

69. Alpaugh, M., et al., *Cooking as a Health Behavior: Examining the Role of Cooking Classes in a Weight Loss Intervention.* Nutrients, 2020. **12**(12).

70. Monbiot, G., *Regenesis.* 2022, UK: Penguin Random House.

71. Stamatakis, K.A., G.A. Kaplan, and R.E. Roberts, *Short sleep duration across income, education, and race/ethnic groups: population prevalence and growing disparities during 34 years of follow-up.* Ann Epidemiol, 2007. **17**(12): p. 948-55.

72. National Sleep Foundation, *Sleep in America* in *Sleep Foundation Washington,*. 2005.

73. Covassin, N., et al., *Effects of Experimental Sleep Restriction on Energy Intake, Energy Expenditure, and Visceral Obesity.* J Am Coll Cardiol, 2022. **79**(13): p. 1254-1265.

74. Du, C., R.M. Tucker, and C.L. Yang, *How Are You Sleeping? Why Nutrition Professionals Should Ask Their Patients About Sleep Habits.* J Am Nutr Assoc, 2022: p. 1-11.

75. Nedeltcheva, A.V., et al., *Insufficient Sleep Undermines Dietary Efforts to Reduce Adiposity.* Annals of Internal Medicine, 2010. **153**(7): p. 435-441.

76. Tasali, E., et al., *Effect of Sleep Extension on Objectively Assessed Energy Intake Among Adults With Overweight in Real-life Settings: A Randomized Clinical Trial.* JAMA Intern Med, 2022. **182**(4): p. 365-374.

77. Chevance, G., et al., *Day-to-day associations between sleep and physical activity: a set of person-specific analyses in adults with overweight and obesity.* J Behav Med, 2022. **45**(1): p. 14-27.

78. Buman, M.P. and A.C. King, *Exercise as a Treatment to Enhance Sleep.* American Journal of Lifestyle Medicine, 2010. **4**(6): p. 500-514.

79. Sampasa-Kanyinga, H., et al., *Bidirectional associations of sleep and discretionary screen time in adults: Longitudinal analysis of the UK biobank.* J Sleep Res, 2022: p. e13727.

80. Bacaro, V., et al., *Sleep duration and obesity in adulthood: An updated systematic review and meta-analysis.* Obes Res Clin Pract, 2020. **14**(4): p. 301-309.

81. Thomas, C., et al., *The health, cost and equity impacts of restrictions on the advertisement of high fat, salt and sugar products across the transport for London network: a health economic modelling study.* Int J Behav Nutr Phys Act, 2022. **19**(1): p. 93.

82. Lauber, K., et al., *Corporate political activity in the context of unhealthy food advertising restrictions across Transport for London: A qualitative case study.* PLoS Med, 2021. **18**(9): p. e1003695.

83. Brownell, K. and K.E. Warner, *The Perils of Ignoring History: Big Tobacco Played Dirty and Millions Died. How Similar Is Big Food?* The Milbank Quarterly, Vol. 87, No. 1, (pp. 259–294), 2009.

84. Norr, R., *Cancer by the Carton.* Reader's Digest, 1952.

85. Phaniendra, A., D.B. Jestadi, and L. Periyasamy, *Free radicals: properties, sources, targets, and their implication in various diseases.* Indian J Clin Biochem, 2015. **30**(1): p. 11-26.

86. Tobore, T.O., *Towards a comprehensive theory of obesity and a healthy diet: The causal role of oxidative stress in food addiction and obesity.* Behavioural Brain Research, 2020. **384**: p. 112560.

87. Pasarca, M., et al., *Adipogenic human adenovirus Ad-36 incduces commitment, differentiation, and lipid accumulation in human adipose derived stem cell. .* Stem cells, 2008. **26**: p. 969-978.

88. Mitra, A. and K. Clarke, *Viral obesity: fact or fiction?* Obes Rev, 2010. **11**: p. 289-296.

89. Jiang, S., et al., *Association between dietary mineral nutrient intake, body mass index, and waist circumference in U.S. adults using quantile regression analysis NHANES 2007-2014.* PeerJ, 2020. **8**: p. e9127.

90. Han, S.-J. and S.-H. Lee, *Nontraditional Risk Factors for Obesity in Modern Society.* Journal of Obesity & Metabolic Syndrome, 2021. **30**(2): p. 93.

91. Trasande, L., *Endocrine disrupting chemicals: new knowledge of health effects and policy implications.* Endocrine Abstracts, 2022. **86**.

92. World Health Organisation, *State of the science of endocrine disrupting chemicals.* 2012.

324

93. McAllister, E.J., et al., *Ten putative contributors to the obesity epidemic*. Crit Rev Food Sci Nutr, 2009. **49**(10): p. 868-913.

94. Burgoine, T., et al., *Changing foodscapes 1980-2000, using the ASH30 Study*. Appetite, 2009. **53**(2): p. 157-65.

95. Huang, Y., et al., *Differences in energy and nutrient content of menu items served by large chain restaurants in the USA and the UK in 2018*. Public Health Nutr, 2022: p. 1-9.

96. Muc, M., et al., *A bit or a lot on the side? Observational study of the energy content of starters, sides and desserts in major UK restaurant chains*. BMJ Open, 2019. **9**(10): p. e029679.

97. Stylianou, K.S., V.L. Fulgoni, and O. Jolliet, *Small targeted dietary changes can yield substantial gains for human health and the environment*. Nature Food, 2021. **2**(8): p. 616-627.

98. Anekwe, C.V., et al., *Socioeconomics of Obesity*. Curr Obes Rep, 2020. **9**(3): p. 272-279.

99. Han, S. and D. Hruschka, *Deprivation or discrimination? Comparing two explanations for the reverse income-obesity gradient in the US and South Korea*. J Biosoc Sci, 2022. **54**(1): p. 1-20.

100. Pinhas-Hamiel, O., et al., *Socioeconomic inequalities and severe obesity-Sex differences in a nationwide study of 1.12 million Israeli adolescents*. Pediatr Obes, 2020. **15**(12): p. e12681.

101. Badran, M. and I. Laher, *Obesity in arabic-speaking countries*. J Obes, 2011. **2011**: p. 686430.

102. Chithambo, T.P. and S.J. Huey, *Black/White Differences in Perceived Weight and Attractiveness among Overweight Women*. Journal of Obesity, 2013. **2013**: p. 320326.

103. Phelan, S., et al., *In their own words: Topic analysis of the motivations and strategies of over 6,000 long-term weight-loss maintainers*. Obesity (Silver Spring), 2022. **30**(3): p. 751-761.

104. Sebti, Y., et al., *The Circadian Clock and Obesity*. Handb Exp Pharmacol, 2022. **274**: p. 29-56.

105. Buettner, C., *Is Hyperinsulinemia Required to Develop Overeating-Induced Obesity?* Cell metabolism, 2012. **16**(6): p. 691-692.

106. Chaix, A., et al., *Time-restricted feeding is a preventative and therapeutic intervention against diverse nutritional challenges*. Cell Metab, 2014. **20**(6): p. 991-1005.

107. Przulj, D., et al., *Time restricted eating as a weight loss intervention in adults with obesity*. PLoS One, 2021. **16**(1): p. e0246186.

108. Stanek, A., et al., *The Role of Intermittent Energy Restriction Diet on Metabolic Profile and Weight Loss among Obese Adults*. Nutrients, 2022. **14**(7).

109. Davenport, C.B., *Body Build and its Inheritance*. Proceedings of the National Academy of Sciences of the United States of America, 1923. **9**(7): p. 226-230.

110. Maes, H.H., M.C. Neale, and L.J. Eaves, *Genetic and environmental factors in relative body weight and human adiposity*. Behav Genet, 1997. **27**: p. 325-351.

111. *Obesity rates by country*: https://worldpopulationreview.com/country-rankings/obesity-rates-by-country, in *World Population Review*. Accessed 24/04/2023,.

112. Thirlby, R.C. and J. Randall, *A genetic "obesity risk index" for patients with morbid obesity*. Obes Surg, 2002. **12**(1): p. 25-9.

113. Lillioja, S. and C. Bogardus, *Obesity and insulin resistance: lessons learned from the Pima Indians*. Diabetes Metab Rev, 1988. **4**: p. 517-540.

114. Neel, J.V., *Diabetes Millitus: a 'thrifty' genotype rendered detrimental by 'progress'?* Am J Hum Genet, 1962. **14**: p. 353-362.

115. Pierce, W.D., et al., *Evolution and obesity: resistance of obese-prone rats to a challenge of food restriction and wheel running*. International Journal of Obesity, 2010. **34**(3): p. 589-592.

116. Painter, R.C., T.J. Roseboom, and O.P. Bleker, *Prenatal exposure to the Dutch famine and disease in later life: An overview*. Reproductive Toxicology, 2005. **20**(3): p. 345-352.

117. Speliotes, E.K., et al., *Association analyses of 249,796 individuals reveal 18 new loci associated with body mass index*. Nat Genet, 2010. **42**(11): p. 937-948.

118. Locke, A.E., et al., *Genetic studies of body mass index yield new insights for obesity biology*. Nature, 2015. **518**(7538): p. 197-206.

119. Stunkard, A.J., et al., *An adoption study of human obesity*. The New England Journal of Medicine, 1986 **314**(4): p. 193-8.

120. Stunkard, A.J., et al., *The body-mass index of twins who have been reared apart*. New England Journal of Medicine, 1990. **322**: p. 1483-1487.

121. Bouchard, C., et al., *The response to exercise with constant energy intake in identical twins*. Obes Res, 1994. **2**: p. 400-410.

122. Hainer, V., et al., *Intrapair resemblance in very low calorie diet-induced weight loss in female obese identical twins*. Int J Obes Relat Metab Disord, 2000. **24**: p. 1051-1057.

123. Bouchard, C., et al., *The response to long-term overfeeding in identical twins*. New England Journal of Medicine, 1990. **322**(21): p. 1477-1482.

124. Walter, S., et al., *Association of a Genetic Risk Score With Body Mass Index Across Different Birth Cohorts*. Jama, 2016. **316**(1): p. 63-9.

125. Kopelman, P.G., *Obesity as a medical problem*. Nature. Vol. 2000. **404**(6778): p. 635-643.

126. Baratali, L., M. Mean, and P. Marques-Vidal, *Impact of dietary and obesity genetic risk scores on weight gain.* Am J Clin Nutr, 2021. **114**(2): p. 741-751.

127. Heianza, Y., et al., *Healthful plant-based dietary patterns, genetic risk of obesity, and cardiovascular risk in the UK biobank study.* Clin Nutr, 2021. **40**(7): p. 4694-4701.

128. Livingstone, K.M., et al., *Unhealthy Lifestyle, Genetics and Risk of Cardiovascular Disease and Mortality in 76,958 Individuals from the UK Biobank Cohort Study.* Nutrients, 2021. **13**(12).

129. Schlinkert, C., et al., *Snacks and The City: Unexpected Low Sales of an Easy-Access, Tasty, and Healthy Snack at an Urban Snacking Hotspot.* Int J Environ Res Public Health, 2020. **17**(20).

130. Samaras, K., et al., *Genetic and Environmental Influences on Total-Body and Central Abdominal Fat: The Effect of Physical Activity in Female Twins.* Annuals of Internal Medicine, 1999. **130**(11): p. 873-882.

131. Li, S., et al., *Physical Activity Attenuates the Genetic Predisposition to Obesity in 20,000 Men and Women from EPIC-Norfolk Prospective Population Study.* Journal.P Med, 2010.

132. Reddon, H., et al., *Physical activity and genetic predisposition to obesity in a multiethnic longitudinal study.* Scientific Reports, 2016. **6**(1): p. 18672.

133. Carnell, S. and J. Wardle, *Measuring behavioural susceptibility to obesity: validation of the child eating behaviour questionnaire.* Appetite, 2007. **48**(1): p. 104-13.

134. Haslam, D., *Obesity: a medical history.* Obesity Reviews, 2007. **8**(s1): p. 31-36.

135. Fontaine, K.R., et al., *Years of life lost due to obesity.* JAMA, 2003. **289**(2): p. 187-193.

136. Collaborators, G.B.D.R.F., *Global, regional, and national comparative risk assessment of 79 behavioural, environmental and occupational, and metabolic risks or clusters of risks, 1990-2015: a systematic analysis for the Global Burden of Disease Study 2015.* Lancet (London, England), 2016. **388**(10053): p. 1659-1724.

138. Petrus, P., et al., *Transforming Growth Factor-β3 Regulates Adipocyte Number in Subcutaneous White Adipose Tissue.* Cell Reports, 2018. **25**(3): p. 551-560.e5.

139. Gustafson, B. and U. Smith, *Regulation of white adipogenesis and its relation to ectopic fat accumulation and cardiovascular risk.* Atherosclerosis, 2015. **241**(1): p. 27-35.

140. Chait, A. and L.J. den Hartigh, *Adipose Tissue Distribution, Inflammation and Its Metabolic Consequences, Including Diabetes and Cardiovascular Disease.* Front Cardiovasc Med, 2020. **7**: p. 22.

141. Fuster, J.J., et al., *Obesity-Induced Changes in Adipose Tissue Microenvironment and Their Impact on Cardiovascular Disease.* Circulation research, 2016. **118**(11): p. 1786-1807.

142. Rupp H, *Insulin resistance, hyperinsulinemia, and cardiovascular disease. The need for novel dietary prevention strategies. .* Basis Res Cardiol 87: 99-105, 1992.

143. Pischon, T., et al., *General and abdominal obesity and and riks of death in Europe.* N Engl J Med, 2008. **359**: p. 2105-2120.

144. Dandona P, A.A., Mohanty P, *The anti-inflammatory and potential anti-atherogenic effect of insulin: a new paradigm. .* Diabetologia; 45:924 -930., 2002.

145. Dandona, P., et al., *Metabolic syndrome: a comprehensive perspective based on interactions between obesity, diabetes, and inflammation.* Circulation, 2005. **111**(11): p. 1448-54.

146. Reljic, D., et al., *Effects of very low volume high intensity versus moderate intensity interval training in obese metabolic syndrome patients: a randomized controlled study.* Sci Rep, 2021. **11**(1): p. 2836.

147. Watkins, P., et al., eds. *Diabetes and its Management* 6th Edition ed. 2003, Blackwell Publishing: Oxford.

148. Roper N, B.R., Kelly W, Unwin N, Connolly M, *Excess mortality in a population with diabetes and the impact of material deprivation.* British Medical Journal. Vol., 2001. **Volume 322.**

149. Sun, H., et al., *IDF Diabetes Atlas: Global, regional and country-level diabetes prevalence estimates for 2021 and projections for 2045.* Diabetes Research and Clinical Practice, 2022. **183**: p. 109119.

150. Unwin, D., et al., *What predicts drug-free type 2 diabetes remission? Insights from an 8-year general practice service evaluation of a lower carbohydrate diet with weight loss.* BMJ Nutrition, Prevention & Health, 2023. **6**(1): p. 46-55

151. Cerf, M.E., *Beta cell dysfunction and insulin resistance.* Frontiers in endocrinology, 2013. **4**: p. 37-37.

152. Abdullah, A., et al., *The magnitude of association between overweight and obesity and the risk of diabetes: a meta-analysis of prospective cohort studies.* Diabetes Res Clin Pract, 2010. **89**(3): p. 309-19.

153. Ganz, M.L., et al., *The association of body mass index with the risk of type 2 diabetes: a case-control study nested in an electronic health records system in the United States.* Diabetol Metab Syndr, 2014. **6**(1): p. 50.

154. Lingvay, I., et al., *Obesity management as a primary treatment goal for type 2 diabetes: time to reframe the conversation.* Lancet, 2022. **399**(10322): p. 394-405.

155. Klein, S., et al., *Why does obesity cause diabetes?* Cell Metab, 2022. **34**(1): p. 11-20.

155a Brown, A., et al., *Dietary strategies for remission of type 2 diabetes: A narrative review.* J Hum Nutr Diet, 2022. **35**(1): p. 165-178

156. Huang, Y., et al., Red and processed meat consumption and cancer outcomes: Umbrella review. Food Chemistry, 2021. 356: p. 129697

157. Shi, W., et al., Red meat consumption, cardiovascular diseases, and diabetes: a systematic review and meta-analysis. European Heart Journal, 2023. 44(28): p. 2626-2635

158. Mari-Sanchis, A., et al., Meat Consumption and Risk of Developing Type 2 Diabetes in the SUN Project: A Highly Educated Middle-Class Population. PLoS One, 2016. 11(7): p. e0157990

159. Zhang, R., et al., Processed and Unprocessed Red Meat Consumption and Risk for Type 2 Diabetes. International Journal of Environmental Research and Public Health, 2021. 18(20): p. 10788.

159a Baleato, C., et al., Plant-Based Dietary Patterns versus Meat Consumption and Prevalence of Impaired Glucose Intolerance and Diabetes Mellitus: A Cross-Sectional Study . Nutrients, 2022. 14: p. 4152

160. Lim, E., et al., *Reversal of type 2 diabetes: normalisation of beta cell function in association with decreased pancreas and liver triacylglycerol.* Diabetologia: p. 1-9.

161. Davenport, L., *Heart Benefits Follow T2D Remission With Rapid Weight Loss.* Medscape, 2021.

162. Jackson, S.E., C. Kirschbaum, and A. Steptoe, *Hair cortisol and adiposity in a population-based sample of 2,527 men and women aged 54 to 87 years.* Obesity, 2017. 25(3): p. 539-544.

163. American Psychological Association. *Stress in America 2022. Concerned for the future, beset by inflation.* 2022; Available from: https://www.apa.org/news/press/releases/stress/2022/concerned-future-inflation.

164. Dun, R. *What Are You So Scared of? Saber-Toothed Cats, Snakes, and Carnivorous Kangaroos - The evolutionary legacy of having been prey.* 2012; Available from: https://slate.com.

165. Rosmond, R., *Role of stress in the pathogenesis of the metabolic syndrome.* Psychoneuroendocrinology, 2005. 30(1): p. 1-10.

166. Kiecolt-Glaser, J.K., et al., *Daily Stressors, Past Depression, and Metabolic Responses to High-Fat Meals: A Novel Path to Obesity.* Biological Psychiatry, 2015. 77(7): p. 653-660.

167. Kuroki, M., *Obesity and bankruptcy: Evidence from US counties.* Econ Hum Biol, 2020. 38: p. 100873.

168. Kahan, S. and R.M. Puhl, *The damaging effects of weight bias internalization.* Obesity (Silver Spring), 2017. 25(2): p. 280-281.

169. Tomiyama, A.J., *Stress and Obesity.* Annual Review of Psychology, 2019. 70(1): p. 703-718.

170. Mahmood, S., Y. Li, and M. Hynes, *Adverse Childhood Experiences and Obesity: A One-to-One Correlation?* Clin Child Psychol Psychiatry, 2022: p. 13591045221119001.

171. Fogelman, N., et al., *A Longitudinal Study of Life Trauma, Chronic Stress and Body Mass Index on Weight Gain over a 2-Year Period.* Behav Med, 2020: p. 1-9.

172. Takemoto, E., et al., *Post-traumatic stress disorder and the association with overweight, obesity, and weight change among individuals exposed to the World Trade Center disaster, 2003-2016.* Psychol Med, 2021. 51(15): p. 2647-2656.

173. Stunkard, A.J., W.R. LaFleur, and T.A. Wadden, *Stigmatization of obesity in medieval times: Asia and Europe.* International Journal of Obesity, 1998. 22(12): p. 1141-1144.

174. Puhl, R.M. and C.A. Heuer, *The stigma of obesity: a review and update.* Obesity (Silver Spring), 2009. 17(5): p. 941-64.

175. Puhl, R. and Y. Suh, *Health Consequences of Weight Stigma: Implications for Obesity Prevention and Treatment.* Current Obesity Reports, 2015. 4(2): p. 182-190.

176. Flint, S.W. and S. Reale, *Weight stigma in frequent exercisers: Overt, demeaning and condescending.* Journal of Health Psychology, 2016.

177. Prunty, A., et al., *Enacted weight stigma and weight self stigma prevalence among 3821 adults.* Obesity Research & Clinical Practice, 2020. 14(5): p. 421-427.

178. Ogden, J. and C. Clementi, *The Experience of Being Obese and the Many Consequences of Stigma.* J Obes, 2010(Online Aug 2010).

179. Wott, C.B. and R.A. Carels, *Overt Weight Stigma, Psychological Distress and Weight Loss Treatment Outcomes.* Journal of Health Psychology, 2010. 15(4): p. 608-614.

180. Sutin, A.R., et al., *Perceived weight discrimination, changes in health, and daily stressors.* Obesity, 2016: p. n/a-n/a.

181. Cohen, R. and S. Shikora, *Fighting Weight Bias and Obesity Stigma: a Call for Action.* Obesity Surgery, 2020. 30(5): p. 1623-1624.

182. Puhl, R.M. and K.D. Brownell, *Confronting and coping with weight stigma: An investigation of overweight and obese adults.* Obesity, 2006. 14: p. 1802-1815.

183. Kyle, R.G., R.A. Neall, and I.M. Atherton, *Prevalence of overweight and obesity among nurses in Scotland: A cross-sectional study using the Scottish Health Survey.* Int J Nurs Stud, 2016. 53: p. 126-33.

184. Thirsk, L.M., et al., *Cognitive and implicit biases in nurses' judgment and decision-making: A scoping review.* Int J Nurs Stud, 2022. 133: p. 104284.

185. Puhl, R.M. and C.A. Heuer, *The Stigma of Obesity: A Review and Update.* Obesity, 2009. 17(5): p. 941-964.

186. Puhl, R. and K.D. Brownell, *Bias, Discrimination, and Obesity.* Obes Res, 2001. 9(12): p. 788-805.

187. Carels, R.A., et al., *Changes in Weight Bias and Perceived Employability Following Weight Loss and Gain.* Obesity Surgery, 2015. 25(3): p. 568-570.

188. Latif, E., *Obesity and happiness: does gender matter?* Economics and Business Letters, 2014. 3(1): p. 59-67.

189. Hughes, C.A., et al., *Changing the narrative around obesity in the UK: a survey of people with obesity and healthcare professionals from the ACTION-IO study.* BMJ Open, 2021. 11(6): p. e045616.

191. Warr, W., et al., *A systematic review and thematic synthesis of qualitative studies exploring GPs' and nurses' perspectives on discussing weight with patients with overweight and obesity in primary care.* Obes Rev, 2021. **22**(4): p. e13151.

192. Janssen, F., et al., *Future life expectancy in Europe taking into account the impact of smoking, obesity, and alcohol.* Elife, 2021. **10**.

193. Kaeberlein, M., *How healthy is the healthspan concept?* GeroScience, 2018. **40**(4): p. 361-364.

194. Subramanian, D.V., *Developing the African Turquoise killifish (N. furzeri) as a model for Alzheimer's Disease* 2022.

195. Halagappa, V.K.M., et al., *Intermittent fasting and caloric restriction ameliorate age-related behavioral deficits in the triple-transgenic mouse model of Alzheimer's disease.* Neurobiology of Disease, 2007. **26**(1): p. 212-220.

196. Weindruch, R., *The retardation of aging by caloric restriction: studies in rodents and primates.* Toxicol Pathol, 1996. **24**(6): p. 742-5.

197. *Caloric Restriction in Humans: Impact on Physiological, Psychological, and Behavioral Outcomes.* Antioxidants & Redox Signaling, 2011. **14**(2): p. 275-287.

198. Fontana, L. and L. Partridge, *Promoting health and longevity through diet: from model organisms to humans.* Cell, 2015. **161**(1): p. 106-118.

199. McCay, C.M. and M.F. Crowell, *Prolonging the Life Span.* The Scientific Monthly, 1934. **39**: p. 405-414.

200. Mattison, J.A., et al., *Impact of caloric restriction on health and survival in rhesus monkeys from the NIA study.* Nature, 2012. **advance online publication**.

201. Colman, R.J., et al., *Caloric Restriction Delays Disease Onset and Mortality in Rhesus Monkeys.* Science, 2009. **325**(5937): p. 201-204.

202. Larson-Meyer, D.E., et al., *Effect of calorie restriction with or without exercise on insulin sensitivity -cell function, fat cell size, and ectopic lipid in overweight subjects.* Diabetes Care, 2006. **29**: p. 1337-1344.

203. Johnson, J.B., et al., *Alternate day calorie restriction improves clinical findings and reduces markers of oxidative stress and inflammation in overweight adults with moderate asthma.* Free Radic Biol Med, 2007. **42**: p. 665-674.

204. Fontana, L., *Calorie restriction and cardiometabolic health.* European Journal of Cardiovascular Prevention & Rehabilitation, 2008. **15**(1): p. 3-9 10.1097/HJR.0b013e3282f17bd4.

205. Redman, L.M. and E. Ravussin, *Caloric Restriction in Humans: Impact on Physiological, Psychological, and Behavioral Outcomes.* Antioxidants & Redox Signaling, 2011. **14**(2): p. 275-287.

206. Dorling, J.L., C.K. Martin, and L.M. Redman, *Calorie restriction for enhanced longevity: The role of novel dietary strategies in the present obesogenic environment.* Ageing Res Rev, 2020: p. 101038.

207. Antoni, R., et al., *Intermittent v. continuous energy restriction: differential effects on postprandial glucose and lipid metabolism following matched weight loss in overweight/obese participants.* British Journal of Nutrition, 2018. **119**(5): p. 507-516.

208. Mattson, M.P., et al., *Meal frequency and timing in health and disease.* Proc Natl Acad Sci U S A, 2014. **111**(47): p. 16647-53.

209. Haywood, D., et al., *A Conceptual Model of Long-Term Weight Loss Maintenance: The Importance of Cognitive, Empirical and Computational Approaches.* Int J Environ Res Public Health, 2021. **18**(2).

210. Levy, B.R., et al., *Longevity increased by positive self-perceptions of aging.* J Pers Soc Psychol, 2002. **83**(2): p. 261-70.

211. Dzau, V.J., et al., *Enabling Healthful Aging for All - The National Academy of Medicine Grand Challenge in Healthy Longevity.* N Engl J Med, 2019. **381**(18): p. 1699-1701.

212. Tam, B.T., J.A. Morais, and S. Santosa, *Obesity and ageing: Two sides of the same coin.* Obesity Reviews, 2020. **21**(4): p. e12991.

213. Stenholm, S., et al., *Midlife Obesity and Risk of Frailty in Old Age During a 22-Year Follow-up in Men and Women: The Mini-Finland Follow-up Survey.* The Journals of Gerontology: Series A, 2013. **69**(1): p. 73-78.

214. Li, Y., et al., *Impact of Healthy Lifestyle Factors on Life Expectancies in the US Population.* Circulation, 2018. **138**(4): p. 345-355.

215. Bull, M.J. and N.T. Plummer, *Part 1: The Human Gut Microbiome in Health and Disease.* Integr Med (Encinitas), 2014. **13**(6): p. 17-22.

216. Heikkilä, M.P. and P.E. Saris, *Inhibition of Staphylococcus aureus by the commensal bacteria of human milk.* J Appl Microbiol, 2003. **95**(3): p. 471-8.

217. Iovine, N.M. and M.J. Blaser, *Antibiotics in animal feed and spread of resistant Campylobacter from poultry to humans.* Emerg Infect Dis, 2004. **10**(6): p. 1158-9.

218. Weiss, G.A. and T. Hennet, *Mechanisms and consequences of intestinal dysbiosis.* Cellular and Molecular Life Sciences, 2017. **74**(16): p. 2959-2977.

219. Valdes, A.M., et al., *Role of the gut microbiota in nutrition and health.* BMJ, 2018. **361**: p. k2179.

220. Tang, W.H., et al., *Intestinal microbial metabolism of phosphatidylcholine and cardiovascular risk.* N Engl J Med, 2013. **368**(17): p. 1575-84.

221. Blaser, M.J., *Antibiotic use and its consequences for the normal microbiome.* Science, 2016. **352**(6285): p. 544-545.

222. Obregon-Tito, A.J., et al., *Subsistence strategies in traditional societies distinguish gut microbiomes.* Nat Commun, 2015. **6**: p. 6505.

223. Sonnenburg, E.D., et al., *Diet-induced extinctions in the gut microbiota compound over generations.* Nature, 2016. **529**(7585): p. 212-5.

224. Korpela, K., et al., *Intestinal microbiome is related to lifetime antibiotic use in Finnish pre-school children.* Nat Commun, 2016. **7**: p. 10410.

225. Strachan, D.P., *Hay fever, hygiene, and household size.* Bmj, 1989. **299**(6710): p. 1259-60.

226. Stiemsma, L.T., et al., *The hygiene hypothesis: current perspectives and future therapies.* Immunotargets Ther, 2015. **4**: p. 143-57.

227. *Global Probiotics Market: Trends, consumer behaviour and growth opportunities.* Available from: https://www.lumina-intelligence.com/blog/probiotics/global-probiotics-market-trends-consumer-behaviour-and-growth-opportunities/#: ~ :text = Overall%20the%20global%20probiotic%20supplements,2024%20 (Global%20Market%20Insights).

228. Kristensen, N.B., et al., *Alterations in fecal microbiota composition by probiotic supplementation in healthy adults: a systematic review of randomized controlled trials.* Genome Medicine, 2016. **8**(1): p. 52.

229. Cabral, L.Q.T., et al., *Probiotics have minimal effects on appetite-related hormones in overweight or obese individuals: A systematic review of randomized controlled trials.* Clin Nutr, 2021. **40**(4): p. 1776-1787.

230. Lang, J.M., J.A. Eisen, and A.M. Zivkovic, *The microbes we eat: abundance and taxonomy of microbes consumed in a day's worth of meals for three diet types.* PeerJ, 2014. **2**: p. e659.

231. Bindels, L.B., et al., *Towards a more comprehensive concept for prebiotics.* Nat Rev Gastroenterol Hepatol, 2015. **12**(5): p. 303-10.

232. Ray, K., *Gut microbiota: Filling up on fibre for a healthy gut.* Nat Rev Gastroenterol Hepatol, 2018. **15**(2): p. 67.

233. Levy, M., et al., *Dysbiosis and the immune system.* Nat Rev Immunol, 2017. **17**(4): p. 219-232.

234. Silva, Y.P., A. Bernardi, and R.L. Frozza, *The Role of Short-Chain Fatty Acids From Gut Microbiota in Gut-Brain Communication.* Endocrinology, 2020. **Neuroendocrine Science**.

235. Alcock, J., C.C. Maley, and C.A. Aktipis, *Is eating behavior manipulated by the gastrointestinal microbiota? Evolutionary pressures and potential mechanisms.* Bioessays, 2014. **36**(10): p. 940-9.

236. Santacruz, A., et al., *Interplay between weight loss and gut microbiota composition in overweight adolescents.* Obesity 17: 1906–1915. 2009.

237. Lebwohl, B., et al., *Long term gluten consumption in adults without celiac disease and risk of coronary heart disease: prospective cohort study.* BMJ, 2017. **357**: p. j1892.

238. Threapleton, D.E., et al., *Dietary fibre intake and risk of cardiovascular disease: systematic review and meta-analysis.* Bmj, 2013. **347**: p. f6879.

239. Luke, A. and R.S. Cooper, *Physical activity does not influence obesity risk: time to clarify the public health message.* International Journal of Epidemiology, 2014. **42**(6): p. 1831-1836.

240. Prentice, A.M. and S.A. Jebb, *Obesity in Britain: gluttony or sloth?* British Medical Journal, 1995. **311**(7002): p. 437-439.

241. Government, U. *Physical activity: applying All Our Health.* 2022; Available from: https://www.gov.uk/government/publications/physical-activity-applying-all-our-health/physical-activity-applying-all-our-health.

242. Heady, J.A., et al., *Coronary Heart Disease in London Busmen: A Progress Report with Particular Reference to Physique* British Journal of Preventive and Social Medicine, 1961. **15**(4): p. 143-153.

243. Julian, V., et al., *Effects of Movement Behaviors on Overall Health and Appetite Control: Current Evidence and Perspectives in Children and Adolescents.* Curr Obes Rep, 2022. **11**(1): p. 10-22.

244. Ahmadi, M.N., J.M.R. Gill, and E. Stamatakis, *Association of Changes in Physical Activity and Adiposity With Mortality and Incidence of Cardiovascular Disease: Longitudinal Findings From the UK Biobank.* Mayo Clin Proc, 2022. **97**(5): p. 847-861.

245. Roake, J., et al., *Sitting Time, Type, and Context Among Long-Term Weight-Loss Maintainers.* Obesity (Silver Spring), 2021. **29**(6): p. 1067-1073.

246. Hamer, O., et al., *Fear-related barriers to physical activity among adults with overweight and obesity: A narrative synthesis scoping review.* Obes Rev, 2021. **22**(11): p. e13307.

247. Thedinga, H.K., R. Zehl, and A. Thiel, *Weight stigma experiences and self-exclusion from sport and exercise settings among people with obesity.* BMC Public Health, 2021. **21**(1): p. 565.

248. Colberg, S.R., et al., *Exercise and type 2 diabetes: the American College of Sports Medicine and the American Diabetes Association: joint position statement.* Diabetes Care, 2010. **33**(12): p. e147-67.

249. Unick, J.L., et al., *Randomized Trial Examining the Effect of a 12-wk Exercise Program on Hedonic Eating.* Med Sci Sports Exerc, 2021. **53**(8): p. 1638-1647.

250. Kempen, K.P., W.H. Saris, and K.R. Westerterp, *Energy balance during an 8-wk energy-restricted diet with and without exercise in obese women.* The American Journal of Clinical Nutrition, 1995. **62**(4): p. 722-729.

251. Pontzer, H., et al., *Constrained Total Energy Expenditure and Metabolic Adaptation to Physical Activity in Adult Humans.* Curr Biol, 2016. **26**(3): p. 410-7.

252. Melanson, E.L., *The effect of exercise on non-exercise physical activity and sedentary behavior in adults.* Obes Rev, 2017. **18 Suppl 1**(Suppl 1): p. 40-49.

253. Chakravarthy, M.V. and F.W. Booth, *Eating, exercise, and thrifty genotypes*, Division of Endocrinology. Metabolism and Lipid Research. Department of Internal Medicine, Editor. 2004, Washington University School of Medicine, St. Louis 63110: Missouri 65211

254. Grummon, A.H., et al., *Changes in Calorie Content of Menu Items at Large Chain Restaurants After Implementation of Calorie Labels.* JAMA Netw Open, 2021. **4**(12): p. e2141353.

255. Fico, B.G., M. Alkatan, and H. Tanaka, *No Changes in Appetite-Related Hormones Following Swimming and Cycling Exercise Interventions in Adults with Obesity.* Int J Exerc Sci, 2020. **13**(2): p. 1819-1825.

256. Schumacher, L.M., et al., *Sustaining Regular Exercise During Weight Loss Maintenance: The Role of Consistent Exercise Timing.* J Phys Act Health, 2021. **18**(10): p. 1253-1260.

257. Oppert, J.M., et al., *Exercise training in the management of overweight and obesity in adults: Synthesis of the evidence and recommendations from the European Association for the Study of Obesity Physical Activity Working Group.* Obes Rev, 2021: p. e13273.

258. Gómez-Bruton, A., et al., *How important is current physical fitness for future quality of life? Results from an 8-year longitudinal study on older adults.* Exp Gerontol, 2021. **149**: p. 111301.

259. O'Donoghue, G., et al., *What exercise prescription is optimal to improve body composition and cardiorespiratory fitness in adults living with obesity? A network meta-analysis.* Obes Rev, 2021. **22**(2): p. e13137.

260. Lee. NM, et al., *Public Views on Food Addiction and Obesity: Implications for Policy and Treatment.* PLoS ONE, 2013. **8**(e74386).

261. Hebebrand, J., et al., *"Eating addiction", rather than "food addiction", better captures addictive-like eating behavior.* Neuroscience & Biobehavioral Reviews, 2014. **47**: p. 295-306.

262. Som, M., et al., *Food addiction among morbidly obese patients: prevalence and links with obesity complications.* J Addict Dis, 2022. **40**(1): p. 103-110.

263. Pedram, P., et al., *Food Addiction: Its Prevalence and Significant Association with Obesity in the General Population.* PLoS ONE, 2013. **8**(9): p. e74832.

264. Carter, A., C.A. Hardman, and T. Burrows, *Food Addiction and Eating Addiction: Scientific Advances and Their Clinical, Social and Policy Implications.* Nutrients, 2020. **12**(5): p. 1485.

265. Rogers P J, S.H.J., *Food craving and food "addiction": A critical review of the evidence from a biopsychosocial perspective.* Pharmacology Biochemistry And Behavior, 2000. **66**(1): p. 3-14.

266. Gearhardt, A.N. and A.G. DiFeliceantonio, *Highly processed foods can be considered addictive substances based on established scientific criteria.* Addiction, 2022.

267. Schulte, E.M. and A.N. Gearhardt, *Attributes of the food addiction phenotype within overweight and obesity.* Eat Weight Disord, 2021. **26**(6): p. 2043-2049.

268. Brunton, P.A., et al., *An intraoral device for weight loss: initial clinical findings.* British Dental Journal, 2021.

269. Cloninger, C.R., *Neurogenetic adaptive mechanisms in alcoholism.* Science, 1987. **236**: p. 410-416.

270. Gearhardt, A.N., et al., *The addiction potential of hyperpalatable foods.* Curr Drug Abuse Rev, 2011. **4**(3): p. 140-5.

271. Stice, E., et al., *Weight Gain Is Associated with Reduced Striatal Response to Palatable Food.* J. Neurosci., 2010. **30**(39): p. 13105-13109.

272. Volkow, N.D., R.A. Wise, and R. Baler, *The dopamine motive system: implications for drug and food addiction.* Nat Rev Neurosci, 2017. **18**(12): p. 741-752.

273. Johnson, P.M. and P.J. Kenny, *Dopamine D2 receptors in addiction-like reward dysfunction and compulsive eating in obese rats.* Nat Neurosci, 2010. **13**: p. 635-641.

274. Ong, Z.Y. and B.S. Muhlhausler, *Maternal "junk-food" feeding of rat dams alters food choices and development of the mesolimbic reward pathway in the offspring.* FASEB journal : official publication of the Federation of American Societies for Experimental Biology, 2011. **25**(7): p. 2167-2179.

275. Vucetic, Z., et al., *Maternal high-fat diet alters methylation and gene expression of dopamine and opioid-related genes.* Endocrinology, 2010. **151**(10): p. 4756-64.

276. Lenoir, M., et al., *Intense sweetness surpasses cocaine reward.* PLoS One, 2007. **2**(8): p. e698.

277. Onaolapo, A.Y., O.J. Onaolapo, and O.A. Olowe, *Chapter 9 - An overview of addiction to sugar*, in *Dietary Sugar, Salt and Fat in Human Health*, H.G. Preuss and D. Bagchi, Editors. 2020, Academic Press. p. 195-216.

278. Katherine, K. and M.M. Ann, *Eating right to live sober.* 1985: Madrona Pub.

279. Jegatheesan, P. and J.P. De Bandt, *Fructose and NAFLD: The Multifaceted Aspects of Fructose Metabolism.* Nutrients, 2017. **9**(3): p. 230.

280. Lustig, R.H., et al., *Isocaloric fructose restriction and metabolic improvement in children with obesity and metabolic syndrome.* Obesity, 2016. **24**(2): p. 453-460.

281. Mela, D.J., *Why do we lilke what we like?* Journal of the Science of Food and Agriculture, 2000. **81**(1): p. 10-16.

282. di Tomaso, E., M. Beltramo, and D. Piomelli, *Brain cannabinoids in chocolate.* Nature, 1996. **382**: p. 677-678.

283. Rogers, P., et al., *Relationships between food craving and anticipatory salivation, eating patterns, mood and body weight in women and men.* Appetite, 1994. **23**: p. 319-325.

284. *The serenity prayer - Living Sober.* Available from: https://www.aa.org/sites/default/files/2021-10/b-7_livingsober_18-32.pdf.

285. Tarman, V. and P. Werdell, *Food Junkies. The truth about food addiction.* 2014, Ontario, Canada: Dundurn.

286. Unwin, J., et al., *Low carbohydrate and psychoeducational programs show promise for the treatment of ultra-processed food addiction.* Front. Psychiatry, 2022. **13:1005523**.

287. Ravussin, E., et al., *Determinants of 24-hour energy expenditure in man. Methods and results using a respiratory chamber.* Journal of Clinical Investigation, 1986. **78**(6): p. 1568-1578.

288. Ravussin, E. and B. Swinburn, eds. *Energy metabolism.* Obesity; theory and therapy, ed. A. Stunkard and T.A. Wadden. 1993, Raven Press Ltd.: New York. 97-123.

289. Beaton, G.H., *Approaches to analysis of dietary data: relationship between planned analyses and choice of methodology.* Am J Clin Nutr, 1994. **59**(1 Suppl): p. 253s-261s.

290. Tudor, K., et al., *Brief interventions for obesity when patients are asked to pay for weight loss treatment: an observational study in primary care with an embedded randomised trial.* British Journal of General Practice, 2020: p. bjgp20X708792.

291. Rounds, T., M. Crane, and J. Harvey, *The Impact of Incentives on Weight Control in Men: A Randomized Controlled Trial.* Am J Mens Health, 2020. **14**(1): p. 1557988319895147.

292. Relton, C., M. Strong, and J. Li, *The 'Pounds for Pounds' weight loss financial incentive scheme: an evaluation of a pilot in NHS Eastern and Coastal Kent.* Journal of Public Health, 2011. **33**(4): p. 536-542.

293. Livingston, G., *Never Binge Again.* unknown: Psy Tech Inc. and Never Ever Again, Inc.

294. Jang, H.J., et al., *The Relationship between Psychological Factors and Weight Gain.* Korean J Fam Med, 2020.

295. Betancourt-Núñez, A., et al., *Emotional Eating and Dietary Patterns: Reflecting Food Choices in People with and without Abdominal Obesity.* Nutrients, 2022. **14**(7).

296. Beshara, M., A.D. Hutchinson, and C. Wilson, *Does mindfulness matter? Everyday mindfulness, mindful eating and self-reported serving size of energy dense foods among a sample of South Australian adults.* Appetite, 2013. **67**: p. 25-9.

297. Touray, M.M.L., et al., *Overweight/Obesity and Time Preference: Evidence from a Survey among Adults in the UK.* Obes Facts, 2022. **15**(3): p. 428-441.

298. Jim Collins, *Good To Great.* 2001, London: Collins Business (Random House).

299. Freud, S., *The Ego and the Id.* The Standard Edition of the Complete Psychological Works of Sigmund Freud, Volume XIX, ed. I.J.S.e.a. (Trans.). 1923, London: Hogarth Press.

300. Rogers, C.R., *On Becoming a Person: A Therapist's View of Psychotherapy.* 1961, Boston: Houghton Mifflin.

301. Mark Manson. *3 Reasons Why You Make Terrible Decisions (And How to Stop).* Available from: https://markmanson.net/decision-making.

302. Levy, A., et al., *A quantitative review of overjustification effects in persons with intellectual and developmental disabilities.* J Appl Behav Anal, 2017. **50**(2): p. 206-221.

303. Rumjaun, A. and F. Narod, *Social Learning Theory—Albert Bandura,* in *Science Education in Theory and Practice: An Introductory Guide to Learning Theory,* B. Akpan and T.J. Kennedy, Editors. 2020, Springer International Publishing: Cham. p. 85-99.

304. Watson, J., *Behaviorism.* (2009) [1958], Chicago: Universtiy of Chicago Press.

305. Skinner, B.F., *Operant behavior.* American Psychologist, 1963. **18**(8): p. 503-515.

306. Prochaska, J. and W. Velicer, *The transtheoretical model of health behavior change.* Am J Health Promot, 1997. **12**: p. 38 - 48.

307. Albert Ellis, *Rational Emotive Behavior Therapy: It Works for Me - It Can Work for You.* 2004, New York: Prometheus Books.

308. Turner, M.J., *Rational Emotive Behavior Therapy (REBT), Irrational and Rational Beliefs, and the Mental Health of Athletes.* Front Psychol, 2016. **7**: p. 1423.

309. Miller, W.R., *Motivational Interviewing with problem drinkers.* Behavioural Psychotherapy, 1983. **11**: p. 147-172.

310. de Wit, L., et al., *Body Mass Index and risk for onset of mood and anxiety disorders in the general population: Results from the Netherlands Mental Health Survey and Incidence Study-2 (NEMESIS-2).* BMC Psychiatry, 2022. **22**(1): p. 522.

About the author

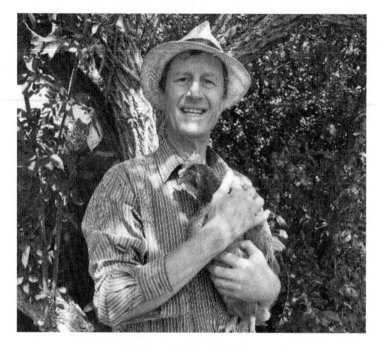

At home on the allotment

A weight management practitioner of 25 years Alan has practiced and researched weight management extensively and continues to support many adults and children to lose weight using novel behavioural and practical methodologies that he has developed.

Alan has taught for training centres and Universities across the UK and presented at seminars both home and overseas. In 2000 he founded the Weight Management Centre in London, which assisted over 20,000 adults and children to successfully lose weight.

Alan holds a master's degree in Obesity & Weight Management from the Department of Clinical Sciences at the University of Chester and has authored several educational works on the subject, including the first UK accredited level 4 Obesity and Diabetes Management Qualification. Alan is a fellow of the Chartered Institute for Sport and Physical Activity (CIMSPA) having 40 years of membership.

Printed in Great Britain
by Amazon

30321023R00190